Participation and Well Being Among Children and Youth With Childhood Onset Disabilities

Participation and Well Being Among Children and Youth With Childhood Onset Disabilities

Editors

Dana Anaby
Mats Granlund

MDPI • Basel • Beijing • Wuhan • Barcelona • Belgrade • Manchester • Tokyo • Cluj • Tianjin

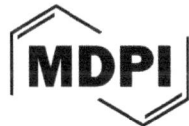

Editors
Dana Anaby
School of Physical and
Occupational Therapy
McGill University
Montreal
Canada

Mats Granlund
Jönköping University
Jönköping University
Jönköping
Sweden

Editorial Office
MDPI
St. Alban-Anlage 66
4052 Basel, Switzerland

This is a reprint of articles from the Special Issue published online in the open access journal *International Journal of Environmental Research and Public Health* (ISSN 1660-4601) (available at: www.mdpi.com/journal/ijerph/special_issues/Children_Disabilities).

For citation purposes, cite each article independently as indicated on the article page online and as indicated below:

LastName, A.A.; LastName, B.B.; LastName, C.C. Article Title. *Journal Name* **Year**, *Volume Number*, Page Range.

ISBN 978-3-0365-1444-4 (Hbk)
ISBN 978-3-0365-1443-7 (PDF)

© 2021 by the authors. Articles in this book are Open Access and distributed under the Creative Commons Attribution (CC BY) license, which allows users to download, copy and build upon published articles, as long as the author and publisher are properly credited, which ensures maximum dissemination and a wider impact of our publications.

The book as a whole is distributed by MDPI under the terms and conditions of the Creative Commons license CC BY-NC-ND.

Contents

About the Editors vii

Preface to "Participation and Well Being Among Children and Youth With Childhood Onset Disabilities" ix

Melanie Burrough, Clare Beanlands and Paul Sugarhood
Experiences of Using Pathways and Resources for Engagement and Participation (PREP) Intervention for Children with Acquired Brain Injury: A Knowledge Translation Study
Reprinted from: *International Journal of Environmental Research and Public Health* **2020**, *17*, 8736, doi:10.3390/ijerph17238736 1

Colin Hoehne, Brittany Baranski, Louiza Benmohammed, Liam Bienstock, Nathan Menezes, Noah Margolese and Dana Anaby
Changes in Overall Participation Profile of Youth with Physical Disabilities Following the PREP Intervention
Reprinted from: *International Journal of Environmental Research and Public Health* **2020**, *17*, 3990, doi:10.3390/ijerph17113990 19

Chi-Wen Chien, Yuen Yi Cynthia Lai, Chung-Ying Lin and Fiona Graham
Occupational Performance Coaching with Parents to Promote Community Participation and Quality of Life of Young Children with Developmental Disabilities: A Feasibility Evaluation in Hong Kong
Reprinted from: *International Journal of Environmental Research and Public Health* **2020**, *17*, 7993, doi:10.3390/ijerph17217993 37

Roopa Srinivasan, Vrushali Kulkarni, Sana Smriti, Rachel Teplicky and Dana Anaby
Cross-Cultural Adaptation and Evaluation of the Participation and Environment Measure for Children and Youth to the Indian Context—A Mixed-Methods Study
Reprinted from: *International Journal of Environmental Research and Public Health* **2021**, *18*, 1514, doi:10.3390/ijerph18041514 63

Shakila Dada, Kirsty Bastable, Liezl Schlebusch and Santoshi Halder
The Participation of Children with Intellectual Disabilities: Including the Voices of Children and Their Caregivers in India and South Africa
Reprinted from: *International Journal of Environmental Research and Public Health* **2020**, *17*, 6706, doi:10.3390/ijerph17186706 79

Alecia Samuels, Shakila Dada, Karin Van Niekerk, Patrik Arvidsson and Karina Huus
Children in South Africa with and without Intellectual Disabilities' Rating of Their Frequency of Participation in Everyday Activities
Reprinted from: *International Journal of Environmental Research and Public Health* **2020**, *17*, 6702, doi:10.3390/ijerph17186702 93

Shakila Dada, Kirsty Bastable and Santoshi Halder
The Role of Social Support in Participation Perspectives of Caregivers of Children with Intellectual Disabilities in India and South Africa
Reprinted from: *International Journal of Environmental Research and Public Health* **2020**, *17*, 6644, doi:10.3390/ijerph17186644 105

Florian Allonsius, Arend de Kloet, Gary Bedell, Frederike van Markus-Doornbosch, Stefanie Rosema, Jorit Meesters, Thea Vliet Vlieland and Menno van der Holst
Participation Restrictions among Children and Young Adults with Acquired Brain Injury in a Pediatric Outpatient Rehabilitation Cohort: The Patients' and Parents' Perspective
Reprinted from: *International Journal of Environmental Research and Public Health* **2021**, *18*, 1625, doi:10.3390/ijerph18041625 123

Tair Shabat, Haya Fogel-Grinvald, Dana Anaby and Anat Golos
Participation Profile of Children and Youth, Aged 6–14, with and without ADHD, and the Impact of Environmental Factors
Reprinted from: *International Journal of Environmental Research and Public Health* **2021**, *18*, 537, doi:10.3390/ijerph18020537 141

Ghaidaa Khalifa, Peter Rosenbaum, Kathy Georgiades, Eric Duku and Briano Di Rezze
Exploring the Participation Patterns and Impact of Environment in Preschool Children with ASD
Reprinted from: *International Journal of Environmental Research and Public Health* **2020**, *17*, 5677, doi:10.3390/ijerph17165677 157

Mats Granlund, Christine Imms, Gillian King, Anna Karin Andersson, Lilly Augustine, Rob Brooks, Henrik Danielsson, Jennifer Gothilander, Magnus Ivarsson, Lars-Olov Lundqvist, Frida Lygnegård and Lena Almqvist
Definitions and Operationalization of Mental Health Problems, Wellbeing and Participation Constructs in Children with NDD: Distinctions and Clarifications
Reprinted from: *International Journal of Environmental Research and Public Health* **2021**, *18*, 1656, doi:10.3390/ijerph18041656 173

Ai-Wen Hwang, Chia-Hsieh Chang, Mats Granlund, Christine Imms, Chia-Ling Chen and Lin-Ju Kang
Longitudinal Trends of Participation in Relation to Mental Health in Children with and without Physical Difficulties
Reprinted from: *International Journal of Environmental Research and Public Health* **2020**, *17*, 8551, doi:10.3390/ijerph17228551 193

Yael Fogel, Naomi Josman and Sara Rosenblum
Exploring the Impacts of Environmental Factors on Adolescents' Daily Participation: A Structural Equation Modelling Approach
Reprinted from: *International Journal of Environmental Research and Public Health* **2020**, *18*, 142, doi:10.3390/ijerph18010142 209

Ai-Wen Hwang, Chia-Feng Yen, Hua-Fang Liao, Wen-Chou Chi, Tsan-Hon Liou, Ben-Sheng Chang, Ting-Fang Wu, Lin-Ju Kang, Shu-Jen Lu, Rune J. Simeonsson, Tze-Hsuan Wang and Gary Bedell
Structural Validity of an ICF-Based Measure of Activity and Participation for Children in Taiwan's Disability Eligibility Determination System
Reprinted from: *International Journal of Environmental Research and Public Health* **2020**, *17*, 6134, doi:10.3390/ijerph17176134 221

About the Editors

Dana Anaby

Dana Anaby is an associate professor at the School of Physical and Occupational Therapy at McGill University, Canada. She holds a PhD in rehabilitation sciences from the University of British Columbia and had post-doctoral training at CanChild Centre for Childhood Disability Research. Dr. Anaby's research encompasses the areas of participation and well being among children and youth with physical disabilities, with a special focus on leisure participation and the impact of the environment. Her studies involve testing intervention plans to enhance community engagement such as the PREP (Pathways and Resources for Engagement and Participation) as well as developing participation- and environmental-focused assessments. She also leads knowledge translation initiatives promoting participation-based practices. Dana holds the FRQ-S Research Scholars Salary Award. She oversees a series of studies funded by the Canadian Institutes of Health Research, testing the multiple benefits of the PREP.

Mats Granlund

Mats Granlund is a senior professor at the School of Health and Welfare at Jönköping University, Jönköping, Sweden. He is a full professor of disability research and psychology and is the leader of the CHILD research group. His research focuses on positive everyday functioning in children, adolescents, and adults with disabilities or in need of special support for other reasons. Together with a management team, Mats is responsible for around 20 research projects that deal with various factors in the individual, in the interaction between the individual and the environment, and in the environment that affects the positive everyday functioning of people in need of special support. His research includes collaboration with leading scholars at several universities in Europe, North America, Australia, and Africa. He also collaborates with the WHO, 15 European partners, and the Swedish National Board of Health and Welfare on the health classification system-ICF.

Preface to "Participation and Well Being Among Children and Youth With Childhood Onset Disabilities"

Dear Colleagues,

Welcome to this Special Issue on "Participation and Well Being Among Children and Youth With Childhood Onset Disabilities". Participation, defined as involvement in life situations, is considered beneficial to children's development, health, and well being. Prior research has shown that the participation of children and youth with various types of disabilities is often restricted around the world. Factors affecting the participation patterns of those with childhood-onset disabilities are also well-documented and include personal, familial, and environmental factors. This Special Issue advances the current body of knowledge through high-quality multi-disciplinary research that enhances our understanding of 1) the impact of participation on subjective well being, 2) effective interventions to improve children's participation and emotional well being, and 3) knowledge translation (KT) strategies and implementation processes aimed at bringing changes in clinical practice towards a greater focus on participation for this population.

This Special Issue includes a collection of 14 peer-reviewed articles that bring new knowledge/evidence on the participation of children and youth with various type of disabilities such as physical disabilities, intellectual disabilities, acquired brain injuries, autism spectrum disorders, attention deficit hyperactivty disorders, and executive function deficits. This special collection is based on research conducted from different parts of the world including high-resource countries (Canada, The Netherlands, Israel, Taiwan, and Hong-Kong) and low-resource regions (South Africa and India). It focuses on methods for measuring participation in different cultural contexts, provides knowledge about benefits of new interventions to improve participation, and illustrates KT strategies facilitating the uptake of new evidence regarding participation in clinical day-to-day practice.

While new cutting-edge evidence generated globally is compiled here, concerted efforts are still needed to advance our understanding of the direct impact of participation in meaningful activities on one's well being. Specifically, intervention studies aimed at improving participation and, therefore, subjective well being, are needed, especially those that focus on mental or psychosocial elements of well being (e.g., mood/emotional status, self-esteem, friendships, and life satisfaction) rather than solely aspects of physical well being (e.g., fitness, energy, pain, and physical functioning). It is clear that our field is moving away from typical impairment-based interventions and therapist-prescribed exercise programs towards real-life client-engaging interventions that are meaningful for the child/youth and can build capacity and foster health and happiness. Thus, we hope to see future lines of inquiry to advance best practices for improving health and well being of children and youth with disabilities through participation-based approaches.

Dana Anaby, Mats Granlund
Editors

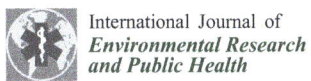

Article

Experiences of Using Pathways and Resources for Participation and Engagement (PREP) Intervention for Children with Acquired Brain Injury: A Knowledge Translation Study

Melanie Burrough [1,*], Clare Beanlands [2] and Paul Sugarhood [2]

1. The Children's Trust, Neurorehabilitation, Tadworth Court, Surrey KT20 5RU, UK
2. Occupational Therapy Division, Department of Allied Health, Social Care and Advanced Practice, School of Health and Social Care, London South Bank University, London SE1 0AA, UK; clare.beanlands@lsbu.ac.uk (C.B.); p.sugarhood@lsbu.ac.uk (P.S.)
* Correspondence: mburrough@thechildrenstrust.org.uk; Tel.: +441-737-365-072

Received: 18 October 2020; Accepted: 20 November 2020; Published: 24 November 2020

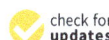

Abstract: *Background:* Children with acquired brain injury experience participation restrictions. Pathways and Resources for Participation and Engagement (PREP) is an innovative, participation focused intervention. Studies have examined PREP in Canadian research contexts, however little is known about implementation in real-life clinical settings. This study aimed to understand experiences of clinicians implementing PREP in a UK clinical context, with a focus on implementation processes and key factors for successful implementation. *Methods:* A qualitative single-site 8-week knowledge translation intervention study, guided by an action research framework, explored clinicians' experiences of implementation. Six occupational therapists (OTs) working in a neurorehabilitation setting participated. The therapists provided two intervention sessions per week, over four weeks for one child on their caseload. Planning, implementation and evaluation were explored through two focus groups. Thematic analysis was used to analyse data. *Results:* Two themes, "key ingredients before you start" and "PREP guides the journey", were identified before introducing PREP to practice. Four additional themes were related to PREP implementation: "shifting to a participation perspective", "participation moves beyond the OT", "environmental challengers and remedies" and "whole family readiness". A participation ripple effect was observed by building capacity across the multi-disciplinary team and families. The involvement of peers, social opportunities and acknowledging family readiness were key factors for successful implementation. *Conclusions:* The findings illustrate practical guidance to facilitate the uptake of participation-based evidence in clinical practice. Further research is required to understand aspects of knowledge translation when implementing participation interventions in other UK clinical settings.

Keywords: participation; participation interventions; knowledge translation; environment; acquired brain injury; occupational therapy

1. Introduction

Over 1.2 million people suffer brain injuries in the UK annually, with up to 50% of incidences observed in children and young people (CYP) [1]. The most common causes of acquired brain injury (ABI) result from acute trauma, brain tumours, infections, anoxia and childhood stroke [2]. It is estimated that at least 350 children per year in the UK suffer a severe ABI requiring in-patient neurorehabilitation to support recovery [2].

Participation, defined as involvement in a life situation [3] is considered fundamental for children's development of physical and mental health, happiness and life satisfaction. Eighty per cent of CYP in one study experienced reduced social participation after neurorehabilitation, with all families identifying difficulties with attitudes and social support [4]. Participation following ABI is less frequent when compared with typically developing peers [5], with restrictions in structured community activities, social events, play and household chores [6]. CYP with ABI are more likely to experience participation restrictions due to ongoing physical, communication, emotional and behavioural needs [5], increasing the risk of social isolation and poor health.

Interventions in neurorehabilitation to remedy long-term effects of ABI have traditionally aimed to remediate body functions, attempting to change impairments such as motor, cognitive and sensory deficits [7]. Emerging research however suggests that clinicians working in children's rehabilitation should primarily offer interventions to improve children's participation across a range of home, school and community occupations [8]. Attendance in diverse meaningful activities and involvement [9] are key attributes to participation interventions.

One participation intervention, known as Pathways and Resources for Engagement and Participation [10] (PREP), has shown that children's participation can be influenced by modification of the environment only [11]. PREP is an innovative participation intervention protocol which encompasses five steps: (1) make goals, (2) make a plan, (3) make it happen, (4) measure process and outcomes and (5) move forward ([10], p.6).

PREP differs from traditional remedial approaches as it aims to identify strengths and barriers within a child's natural environment, as opposed to changing underlying impairments such as motor coordination or cognition. PREP offers a practical framework to set participation goals in chosen occupations [10]. A coaching approach is adopted when working with the child and family to agree on an intervention plan with solution-focused strategies to reduce environmental barriers.

Key research offers early evidence for PREP with youth aged 12–18 years old. Two interrupted-time series studies found that following 12 weeks of intervention, goals set in leisure domains using the Canadian Occupational Performance Measure (COPM) [12] demonstrated statistically significant improvements for youth [7,13]. Barriers to goal satisfaction were noted in poor societal attitudes, community opportunities and physical accessibility [13]. A recent formative study also highlighted that not only does PREP support changes in participation, but changes were also observed in motor function, cognition and activity performance [14].

Another study examined clinician perspectives when using PREP over a 12-week intervention period, for CYP aged 12 to 17 years old with physical disabilities [8]. Clinicians experienced a new understanding of participation interventions [8]. Notably, therapists *"did not perceive it as "true" therapy if "hands-on" treatment was not provided"* ([8], p. 13,396) questioning the readiness and knowledge translation required when introducing a participation intervention in practice.

There are no available studies exploring participation interventions in children's neurorehabilitation, therefore highlighting a gap in practice. PREP offers emerging evidence when working with youth with physical disabilities; however, it has not yet been studied in a real-life clinical context for CYP with ABI. This study therefore aimed to understand experiences of OTs implementing PREP in a UK neurorehabilitation setting for children aged 0–18 years old. Although debate exists around the complex concept of knowledge translation [15], this study assumed a knowledge translation definition of forming partnerships between researcher and participants, with a flow of information exchange [16] to influence evidence-based clinical practice.

Study objectives were to:

- Establish planning required before introducing PREP to routine clinical practice;
- Implement PREP in a neurorehabilitation setting and evaluate clinician experiences;
- Identify key factors that influence PREP implementation.

2. Materials and Methods

2.1. Study Design

This study was a qualitative single-site 8-week knowledge translation intervention study, guided by an action research (AR) framework. The study took place in a 25 bed neurorehabilitation setting for CYP aged 0–18 years old with ABI. CYP received a goal-led 24 h rehabilitation programme, supported by an integrated team of professionals, including neurorehabilitation consultants, occupational therapists, physiotherapists, speech and language therapists, psychologists, music therapists, nurses and carers.

A criterion sample of qualified OTs working within the neurorehabilitation setting and treating CYP with ABI were asked to participate. The size of the sample was limited by the total number of OTs working within the setting. All six OTs working within the setting participated. Participants were invited to participate via a letter sent by an independent non-clinical professional. A participation information sheet detailed the research question, aims and methods. Informed consent was obtained by providing OTs with a two-week period before being offered the opportunity to provide written consent to participate. Participants were invited to take part in two focus groups, a follow-up meeting and an intervention phase, over a total period of seven weeks. All six had the right to withdraw from the study at any time.

The first focus group was conducted initially to explore and prepare for the introduction of PREP to practice. Action planning took place two weeks later, during a follow-up meeting. Initial themes were shared with participants from focus group 1 and group participants designed and agreed upon an implementation action plan (Tables A1 and A2). The participants selected one child on their caseload to offer two 45 min PREP intervention sessions per week, over a four-week period. PREP intervention was offered as part of routine neurorehabilitation treatment, therefore informed consent from the CYP and families was not required. The CYP selected had already received a multi-disciplinary initial assessment, were undertaking active rehabilitation treatment and were not preparing for immediate discharge home.

Participation goals were set by using either goal attainment scaling (GAS) [17] or the COPM [12] before introducing PREP intervention. Three OTs set a participation goal directly with a CYP on their caseload. Three OTs set participation goals with parents, caregivers and family members as they were unable to directly set goals due to their level of cognitive impairment following an ABI or developmental ability. A second focus group was conducted following the four-week PREP intervention period and evaluated the OT's experiences.

2.2. Procedures

AR frameworks assume collaborative approaches and the formation of mutual enquiry [18]. At the time of study, the first author held 12 years of post-qualification experience and was the professional lead, band 8 OT within the service. As the first author also held a caseload and team manager responsibilities, the relationship between the first author and participants needed to be carefully considered. A mutual partnership between the study participants and the first author was sought, aiming to empower participants and reduce perceptions of seniority. With this in mind a professionalising action research framework was selected to guide the process. Professionalising action research 'seeks improvement in professional practice ... on behalf of service users' ([19], p. 155), whilst promoting partnership between the first author and participants.

In accordance with professionalising action research, a work-based action research cycle was selected [20], providing a cyclical and reflective framework for PREP implementation (Figure 1). This cycle was chosen as it was developed for use in work-based professional settings. The AR cycle consisted of one preliminary step and four main phases.

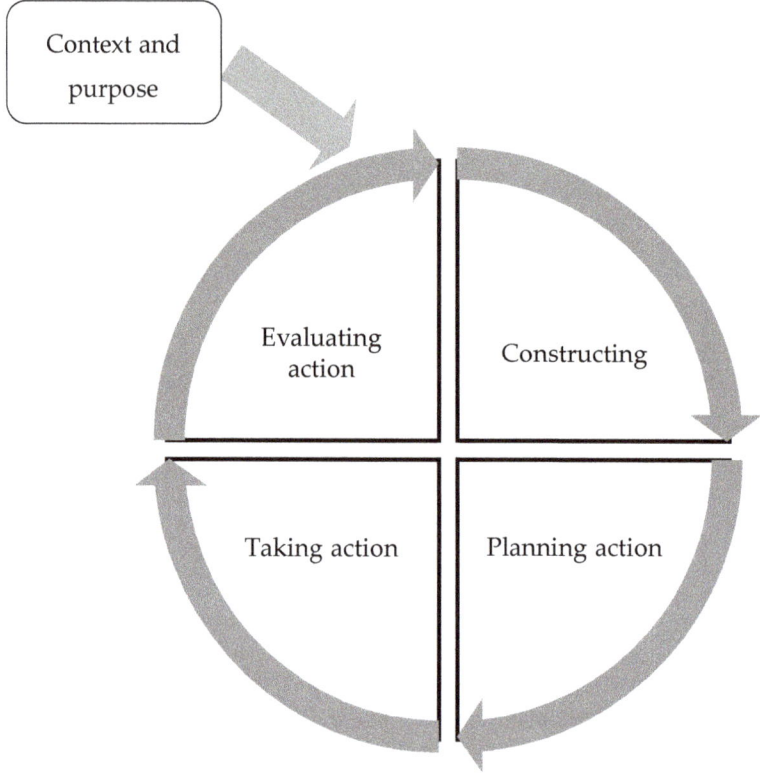

Figure 1. Action Research Cycle adapted from ([20], p. 9).

2.2.1. Constructing

One cycle of AR was completed over seven weeks, consisting of four phases. The constructing phase involved participants defining and critiquing participation interventions. PREP was selected as participants felt it provided structured intervention, well-suited to rehabilitation and members had not previously used this intervention.

2.2.2. Planning Action

The planning action phase lasted two weeks, and involved the first focus group to establish the planning required before introducing PREP to the routine clinical practice. After this two-week period, a subsequent follow-up meeting was held to clarify the focus group findings, share themes and agree on an implementation plan.

2.2.3. Taking Action

The taking action phase of the cycle was based on the implementation plan from the first focus group and was completed over four weeks. Two PREP intervention sessions were offered each week for one CYP on each participant's caseload. PREP was introduced to the multi-disciplinary team via e-mail and during team meetings to familiarise professionals in the wider team with this new intervention approach. During PREP implementation, participants requested peer support, therefore peer group support sessions were organised and facilitated by a clinical researcher, independent of the study. Budget funds were made available for PREP activities.

2.2.4. Evaluating Action

Finally, the evaluation phase was completed over two weeks. Actions were evaluated through a second focus group involving the first author and all participants. Reflections examined all stages of the action research cycle, implementation of the action plan and participant experiences.

In children's occupational therapy there are current challenges—in the generation of evidence-based research and the integration of this into clinical practice [21]. The AR framework therefore provided an opportunity for OTs to translate knowledge into practice and enhance the potential for sustainable change.

2.3. Data Collection

Focus groups were deemed suitable for AR to provide joint discussion around shared implementation experiences, whilst triggering critical reflections. The first author assumed the role of focus group moderator and guidelines were agreed to ensure all members adhered to confidentiality. The first author advised that seniority was not considered advantageous and aimed to draw out all of the OTs during discussions. The first focus group, lasting 1.5 h, included five semi-structured questions to explore the introduction of PREP to practice (Table A3). The focus group questions were adapted from an existing research study exploring clinician perspectives of using PREP within a research setting [8], in order to reduce moderator leading questions and allow for probing.

The second focus group used nine semi-structured questions (Table A4) to evaluate participant experiences of implementing PREP in practice. The second focus group lasted 2 h, and questions were again adapted from existing research [8] with a focus on implementing PREP in a neurorehabilitation setting, evaluating the OT's experiences and identifying factors that influenced PREP implementation.

The findings were digitally recorded and then transcribed verbatim by the first author. Confidential data such as child or organisational names were replaced with pseudonyms. All digital recordings were transferred and stored on an encrypted PC to comply with data protection principles.

2.4. Data Analysis

The content of each transcript were read and re-read by the first author to increase familiarisation, note initial ideas and search for patterns. Braun and Clarke's six step thematic analysis [22] was applied to analyse focus group transcripts. To gain an in-depth understanding of the data, transcripts and initial codes were derived by the first author, highlighting data relevant to the research question across the whole data set and collating particular quotes that were relevant to each code. Complete coding was undertaken to ensure relevant words and phrases were coded. At this point, transcripts and initial codes were shared with the second and third authors to check independently of the first author. All authors then searched the codes for potential themes, drawing data together which was relevant to each suggested theme.

The next stage involved drawing together a thematic map for themes. The initial themes derived from focus group 1 were shared with the participants during the follow-up meeting, providing an opportunity to member check themes and further refine themes. Further defining and naming of themes from both transcripts took place with the second and third authors, with discussions around definitions for each overarching theme. During the six-step analysis, themes and subthemes were reflected upon, checked with the original transcripts and analysed with direct quotes to ensure that thematic mapping derived meaning from the entire data set.

Data were collected from the criterion sample at set points during the AR cycle. This did not allow for continued recruitment or data collection until the concept of saturation could be achieved. However, the in-depth focus group discussions using open questions created sufficient data to gain a plausible understanding of the issues. The iterative nature of data collection and analysis allowed for detailed exploration of themes as they emerged and developed over the course of the study.

2.5. Study Rigour

As the aims of this study were to implement PREP in this particular neurorehabilitation setting, the findings cannot readily be generalised to different population groups. No exclusion criteria were set and all OTs regardless of gender, ethnicity, age and experience were eligible. The study sample was limited by the number of occupational therapists working within the setting.

The study established trustworthiness through principles of credibility and transparency by member checking, following the first focus group. The project was time limited, therefore themes from focus group 2 could not be shared with participants in the same way as focus group 1. Triangulation was considered in gaining a variety of participant views, although increasing findings through representation of different data collection methods and study co-design was not possible due to time constraints.

The first author was aware of the close connection to participants during routine clinical practice, throughout each stage of the AR process and during data analysis. In routine clinical practice the first author also provided support and supervision to the team of OTs, which may have influenced study findings. As part of the implementation action plan participants identified the importance of peer support during the taking action phase. A clinical researcher, independent from the study, facilitated peer support groups during the action phase, which provided a space for reflective thinking, without the influence of the first author. The first author and clinical researcher met to reflect on the peer group sessions before the second focus group, giving the first author an external perspective of the taking action phase.

A reflective diary was completed by the first author throughout the study to increase reflexivity [23]. Reflective diary themes considered the potential influence of the first author and the participant relationship on study findings. Themes highlighted the need to draw out all participant views during focus group discussions. The first author reflected on the routine responsibility of professional lead OT, whilst balancing the role of focus group moderator. Diary experiences and reflections were shared and discussed with the other authors to increase transparency. This supported the first author with allowing for enough time and space to draw out all participant views and experiences.

2.6. Ethical Considerations

Ethical approval was granted from the School of Health and Social Care Ethics Committee at London South Bank University on 10th May 2017, study number 17/A/32. Permission from the organisation's research board was given. All participants gave their informed consent for inclusion before they participated in the study. This study was classified as a service evaluation; therefore, Health Research Authority approval was not required.

3. Results

3.1. Sample Characteristics

Six OTs participated in the study, with varied levels of experience and seniority. Table 1 outlines participant characteristics.

3.2. Emerging Themes

Six themes were identified from the data. Two overarching themes related to establishing the planning required before introducing PREP to routine clinical practice and four themes related to implementing PREP and evaluating OT experiences of implementation. Each theme will be reported on in turn. All names have been replaced with pseudonyms.

Table 1. Sample Participant Characteristics.

Participant Characteristics	Number
Gender	
Male	0
Female	6
Experience in Clinical Practice	
0 years up to 2 years	0
3 years up to 5 years	1
6 years up to 8 years	1
9 years up to 11 years	1
12 years up to 20 years	2
21 years or more	1
Level of Seniority (according to agenda for change banding scale)	
5	0
6	2
7	3
8	1
Occupation	
Full time occupational therapist	3
Part time occupational therapist	3

Two themes, before introducing PREP to practice, included: "key ingredients before you start" and "PREP guides the journey" (Figure 2). Four additional themes were related to PREP implementation: "shifting to a participation perspective", "participation moves beyond the OT", "environmental challengers and remedies" and "whole family readiness" (Figure 3).

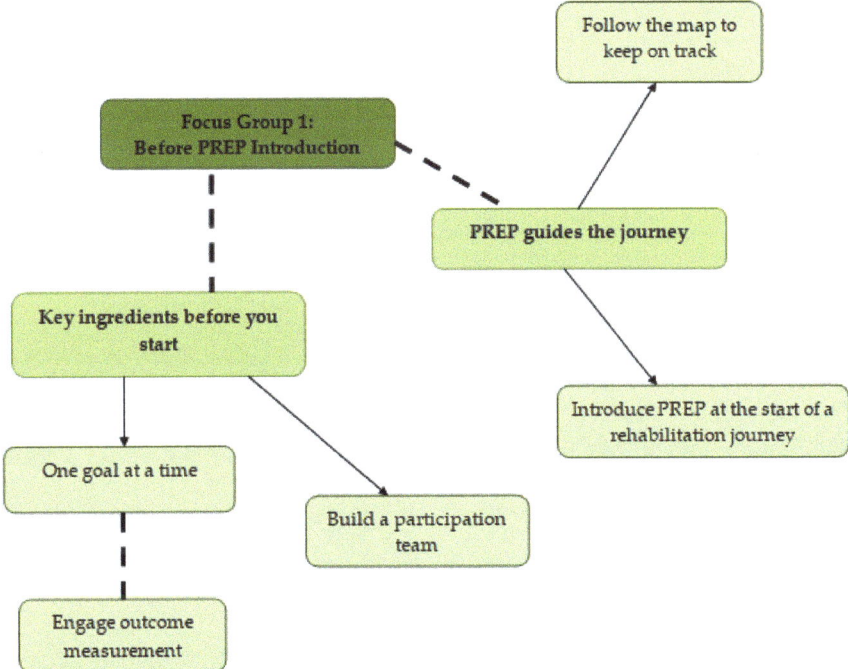

Figure 2. Structure of themes generated by the data in focus group 1: before PREP introduction.

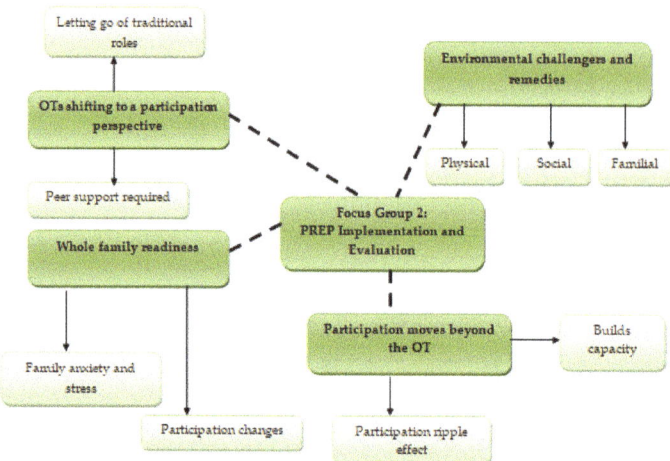

Figure 3. Structure of themes generated by the data in focus group 2: PREP implementation.

3.3. Key Ingredients before You Start

An overarching theme emerged from the planning stage of the action research cycle when preparing to implement PREP for the first time: *key ingredients before you start*. Key ingredients in preparation for PREP use were suggested to set and work on one participation goal at a time, engage outcome measurement and build a participation team.

One key ingredient was recognised as working on one participation goal at a time. This took a different direction than usual routine practice, which involved working on multiple activity focused goals. Sarah highlighted:

"You get to the end of a placement where you feel like you have moved ever so slowly or not at all in these large number of (goal) areas."

Sarah went on to say that:

"One participation goal might be greater than helping the family move forward with five or six."

Using PREP intervention to work on one participation goal at a time appeared to offer opportunity for focused, high intensity therapy to increase children's participation. Katy suggested:

"It drives that intensity doesn't it? in terms of intervention, which we know people need, but if you're covering a number of goals, how do you get that intensity of intervention, you know giving lots of repetition, lots of practice."

Katy's view of using PREP to work on one goal at a time supported the need for children to receive intensive, repeated input when receiving participation focused intervention.

Similarly Hannah gave examples of working on participation goals such as visiting the local park with family. Hannah commented that PREP intervention is:

"Very clear focused, repetitive and you make progress."

Working on one participation goal was recognised as needing early prioritisation, to guide therapist and family focus during the rehabilitation journey. Another key ingredient to prepare for PREP introduction was considered to be engaging in the use of outcome measurements such as the COPM. The engagement of outcome measurements supported OTs with underpinning changes in participation goals. Sarah reflected when preparing outcome measurement for PREP intervention it enables OTs to:

"Stay focused, do the COPM, that's your core thing."

Sarah also described that the suggestion of completing COPM more frequently

"Felt like a big shift."

However, there were different feelings about how frequently outcome measurement was required when preparing to introduce PREP to the CYP and families. When considering outcome measurement using the COPM, Beth described frequency of measurement as:

"Not as regularly as twice a week, parents would find that too much"

In contrast Emma felt that when introducing PREP intervention, outcome measurement should:

"Be more than once a week."

There appeared to be consensus when engaging in outcome measurement before PREP introduction; however, OTs felt that they required different time frequencies in outcome measurement according to the individual CYP and family needs.

Prior to PREP implementation, the OTs recognised the need for the key ingredient of building a participation team. It was suggested that an integrated approach, drawing on members of the multi-disciplinary team, the child, family and supports in the community (for example sports coaches) was needed. Alice commented that there should be:

"Shared responsibility for a participation team" and this needed to be developed during implementation *"because I feel like the understanding and that shared responsibility of the participation team isn't there yet."*

Communication and collaboration appeared to form initial building blocks for a participation team.

3.4. PREP Guides the Journey

The PREP manual was seen as a map and practical guide to keep the OTs on track. Sarah outlined the PREP process as:

"You set goals, you make a plan, you make it happen and then you check it."

Before implementation, the PREP process was considered as a tool for keeping OTs focused by working through goal setting and treatment planning logically. Katy highlighted:

"If you do work through the resources you've got in this you'll be looking at it thinking oh I actually haven't done what I'm meant to be doing this week, I've got to keep on this, this is my plan, I'm using this tool, you've got something really specifically to focus you."

Beth commented that PREP will *"structure the plan of intervention"* and reported *"if someone else needs to follow the process that you have done, it starts to kind of break down the different components."*

It appears that PREP offers a concise map to form a measurable treatment plan, with the opportunity to involve different members of the multi-disciplinary team to follow the process if needed.

Finally, in order for PREP to guide the journey, it was felt that PREP should be introduced at the start of a rehabilitation journey to clarify family expectations. Beth highlighted that early expectations of neurorehabilitation programmes can include a focus on *"walking and talking."* At the start of rehabilitation Hannah commented:

"They're not used to thinking about participation yet, helping them to understand that. If you're going to the park, they're not just going to the park for fun, it's showing them why we're doing that and the skills we're using and how that's rehab."

Introducing PREP early on appeared to introduce participation goals and intervention early on in the rehabilitation journey. Alice however recognised that participation may have changed and questioned whether the child would be: *"prepared to take on or participate in something in not its true or original form."*

Four themes were identified when implementing PREP and evaluating OT experiences of implementation: *shifting to a participation perspective; participation moved beyond the OT; environmental challengers and remedies; and whole family readiness* (Figure 3).

3.5. Shifting to a Participation Perspective

Adopting PREP intervention meant letting go of traditional, remedial therapy approaches focused on component skills or impairments in mobility or cognition and shifting to a participation perspective. For some therapists PREP offered an intervention approach to focus on participation. Sarah illustrated:

"PREP kind of underpins why we're in this job because you want people despite health problems to enjoy life and participate in what life has to offer ... "

Emma recognised that PREP offered a new, flexible approach to work on participation even when a young person may not have achieved skill mastery:

"Playing play station 4 ... he's indicated that he would really like just to try and see what he can do, I probably wouldn't have thought about doing that because I know it's going to be really really difficult."

For others however shifting to a participation perspective felt anxiety provoking, particularly when attempting coaching to empower families to solve problems. Beth reflected on her own *"hesitations"* and Alice highlighted:

"Not having experience of coaching techniques, of managing difficult situations or having those tricky conversations with parents, because I don't have that knowledge and experience I think is probably why I didn't do some much of that ... "

Therapists identified that peer support, facilitated by an experienced therapist would address feelings of apprehension and changes to intervention practices.

3.6. Participation Moved Beyond the OT

PREP built capacity with families and the multi-disciplinary team by using the pathway to form solutions independently of the therapist. Not only did the therapists feel that young people demonstrated more insight into participation challenges than they anticipated, some therapists felt that CYP and families began to generalise problem-solving techniques to other participation opportunities. One young person initially achieved his participation goal of going to a local fast food outlet with his family. Soon after this the young person and his family identified other community experiences that they wanted to achieve whilst undergoing neurorehabilitation. Alice reflected:

"I was very taken aback by how he had come up with all of these strategies, it was so important that they'd come from him. He's gone to the bakery, to the harvester (restaurant), to the seaside at weekends. His Mum and sister have done it, they'll say 'well where shall we go next and then he comes up with the next idea and then what do we need to do? oh well I need to be able to walk outside, I need to be able to stand up to put the pennies in the slot machine you know he's coming up with those things."

Beth discussed a participation goal around a Father and young person making a train journey from the rehabilitation centre to home:

"I went and spoke to Dad about if I was doing that trip what I would do and I would look for. Dad took that on board and I spoke to him yesterday and he said 'yea it was fine' he already knew that (name) would know the way home and was physically able to do it but his concerns were still (name's) behaviour and communication difficulties."

Beth went on to describe how she developed a strategy with this young person:

"Maybe you could learn how you say I have difficulty with talking and he said words are hard so he's made his own little script for that."

Once therapists shared knowledge of local community activities and leisure opportunities, CYP and families appeared to increase their active involvement in participation experiences. After one CYP achieved his original participation goal, he started to apply his skills to familiarise himself with car journeys to participate in community outings, Alice described:

"They built up their car parking, car driving practice, they built up every night by themselves, they visited local areas"

Therapists perceived attitudinal changes of professionals during increased young person and family involvement, leading to greater ownership and shared management of participation challenges.

Through the development of a shared participation vision and action plan, PREP was perceived by one therapist as causing *"ripple effects" (Sarah)*. To illustrate, Emma highlighted:

"I had some positive engagement with care staff who identified there were some things they could do with the young people outside of sessions that they wouldn't have done otherwise."

In some cases, members of the multi-disciplinary team began contributing to PREP planning and used strategies without OT involvement. Ripple effects were seen not only for CYP and families but also reaching wider members of the multi-disciplinary team.

3.7. Environmental Challengers and Remedies

A number of environmental factors were recognised as challengers and barriers to successful participation. Hannah recognised that PREP *"helped get that real participation goal, think about the barriers and facilitators and steps towards it."* Most barriers were perceived to be physical environmental restrictions including 'noisy environments,' 'wheelchair accessibility' and 'the temporary nature of the rehabilitation centre'. Other barriers however reflected social factors such as 'his friends aren't here,' whilst other CYP were worried about societal reactions to communication difficulties following a brain injury.

Some environmental factors were observed to remedy participation challenges. Social and familial relationships appeared to hold great importance in remedying participation challenges. For one young person, social engagement appeared to hold greater importance than the activity itself, as Alice suggested:

"Riding your bike is not the meaningful part, it was more about doing it, that feeling of belonging, being with the people that they wanted it to be with, that sense of socialisation in the way that he wanted it to be."

Being with family and peers was perceived as crucial for this young person to feel valued and involved:

"It was that he wanted, to go with his Mum and his sister, he wanted to be able to have that whole experience, it wasn't about could he order, could he eat it safely, could he sit in the car, he wanted to tell Mum off every time that she sung in the car on the way there." (Alice)

Although some CYP were unable to engage with peers in their typical home, school and community environments, they often wanted to participate with new peers during rehabilitation. Sarah illustrated that one young person reported *"no, no we really want to do it together."*

3.8. Whole Family Readiness

The concept of family readiness influenced therapist abilities to implement PREP. Notably, family anxiety and stress were acknowledged as key influencers to engagement in participation, goal setting and finding solutions. For instance, Emma highlighted:

"The families have got so much going on, the family I worked with they've got lots of other anxieties and worries, for them to try and focus and think about something else was quite hard."

Factors such as re-housing, changes in schooling and the young person's mood were identified as areas of consideration before introducing PREP. Changes to participation patterns and loss were also acknowledged. Some young people wanted to participate *"when they were better,"* whilst others were aware of *"who they were and now that's different"* (Emma). Alice reflected on perceiving children's participation in a new way after brain injury:

"Whether the child is going to be able to participate in the way they did before and if they can't are they happy to accept the change in how they participate? That wasn't what he'd done before so in his eyes well that wasn't achieving it."

Contrastingly, resilience and strong family networks appeared to reduce family anxiety and stress to increase readiness for PREP intervention. One family had another child with a disability and Sarah found that they drew on past experiences to overcome participation challenges:

"The family had their own experiences prior to injury with another sibling in the family who has special needs, and so adjustment to their young boys' brain injury was very different to other families. Their acceptance of needing to do things differently, to be innovative about the way you do things, their personal circumstances have really meant that they don't have that as a barrier, adjusting to disability."

4. Discussion

This study aimed to understand how OTs implemented PREP, a participation intervention, in a UK clinical context. The study explored planning required before introducing PREP to routine clinical practice and evaluated the OT's experiences of implementation when working with CYP aged 0 to 18 years old with ABI in a neurorehabilitation setting. Study findings highlight important messages for practice, when introducing a participation intervention for the first time.

Several key ingredients were acknowledged in order to introduce PREP to practice, notably setting and working on one participation goal at a time, engaging outcome measurement and mobilising a participation team. Enabling the child and family to form a team to work on one participation goal appeared to increase the intensity and focus of the intervention. Notably active ingredients such as caregiver support and a supportive environment for the child have previously been recognized to improve CYP participation outcomes [24], echoing the value in identifying a supportive participation team to work on the goal with the child.

Implementation of PREP initiated new directions in practice. Although participation outcomes were enhanced, participants often felt anxious when adopting new ways of working, sometimes feeling that they may overlook rehabilitation goals in activity or body functions and structure domains [3]. Reluctance to shift to a participation perspective is consistent with previous research, challenging the nature of the environment and therapeutic need to work on personal factors [8]. Two practical steps were recognised to support early adoption of PREP. Firstly, peer support offered space for reflection, problem solving and sharing PREP strategies. Additionally, training on coaching techniques was suggested to enhance knowledge in order to explore participation challenges.

PREP enabled extension of knowledge and built capacity with others. Knowledge sharing allowed CYP and families to generalise problem-solving techniques to new participation challenges. One young person successfully achieved his participation goal of going to a local fast food outlet, through developing participation strategies with his therapist. Following this success he then participated in other community experiences such as visiting the local bakery, restaurant and seaside without input from his therapist. Capacity building was also seen within the multi-disciplinary team. Another participant commented that care staff continued with participation strategies outside of intervention sessions. PREP was described as causing "ripple effects" suggesting that immediate successes grew outwardly with the support of the identified participation team. The participation team and knowledge sharing appear to be fundamental for successful implementation.

PREP was observed to prepare CYP for transition between neurorehabilitation and discharge to their local home, school and community. Previous research has shown that parents require support to build confidence in managing a range of complex difficulties following neurorehabilitation [25]. This study's findings suggest that PREP offers promising findings to equip families to support self-management of participation challenges following discharge. This approach is congruent with person-centered care principles of empowering families to self-manage health needs following illness [26]. Focusing on participation goals for discharge could therefore offer long-term quality of life and health benefits to families. Participation interventions appear to address the need for personalised care, which may result in a lesser need for intensive professional input in the community.

The environment was recognised as a salient factor during PREP intervention. Although environmental restrictions were experienced, environmental remedies were recognised as facilitators. Physical and social barriers included feelings of anxiety when leaving the neurorehabilitation centre, combined with unfamiliar and noisy environments. Existing peer relationships were not always present post ABI due to geographical distances, limiting support when working on participation goals. Once environmental challengers were identified, strengths could be drawn on to overcome these barriers. In this study feelings of belonging and engagement often overcame participation barriers. Some CYP requested to work on participation goals with peers also receiving neurorehabilitation. One CYP reported that, when bike riding, being with friends and socialising was more important than the activity itself. Another CYP visited a local restaurant and reflected that spending time with family and singing during a car journey made all the difference to his happiness and enjoyment. Identifying and drawing on strengths within the social and familial environment appeared to remedy initial participation challenges.

It is noteworthy that even though social skills may be disrupted or impaired post ABI, social experiences for young people receiving neurorehabilitation were most significant in remedying participation difficulties. Understanding social norms and boundaries can be challenging following ABI [27] however social opportunities and peer support were key participation influencers. Findings show that peer support can remedy participation challenges due to benefits of enjoyment, socialisation and the sense of belonging. In neurorehabilitation specifically, therapists may consider implementing participation interventions involving existing peer groups or creating opportunities for new friendships with peers who have experienced ABI.

Finally, family readiness was integral before PREP introduction. Family factors including anxiety, stress, mood and life changes such as re-housing and schooling were identified. Some families identified life adjustments, reflecting that aspects of participation may be lost or changed. Literature highlights that many caregivers experience grief, loss and family strain following ABI, often requiring a period of adjustment to their child's disability [28]. Conversely, one family drew on past experiences of supporting a sibling with a disability to help them overcome new challenges, increasing readiness for PREP intervention and reducing family anxiety. Consequently, when introducing PREP therapists recognised the need to actively listen to the family and CYP during their rehabilitation journey, whilst acknowledging difficulties along the way.

4.1. Key Implications for Practice

Key guidance and recommendations were identified for sharing application of knowledge when introducing PREP to clinical practice:

- Key ingredients including 'working on one participation goal at a time, engaging outcome measurement and building a participation team' can prepare therapists to introduce a participation intervention in a neurorehabilitation practice setting.
- Peer support and formal training around parent coaching should be offered to support clinicians with adopting PREP intervention.
- Sharing knowledge of problem-solving and participation strategies will enhance capacity building of others, such as the multi-disciplinary team, parents, caregivers and the child or young person to increase opportunities for participation success.
- Participation interventions are perceived as valuable by OTs to prepare CYP for participation in their local home, school and community following discharge from neurorehabilitation.
- Opportunities for socialisation with existing peer groups or peers who have experienced ABI should be created to support benefits of enjoyment and belonging when implementing participation interventions.
- Family readiness is a key factor to consider when implementing participation interventions.
- Therapists should actively listen to and acknowledge family difficulties during the rehabilitation journey to help the family plan for achievable and client-centred participation interventions.

4.2. Limitations and Future Direction

This study contributes to a knowledge gap by offering guiding principles of how OTs can facilitate the uptake of PREP in a children's neurorehabilitation setting in the UK. Many earlier studies considered PREP use with youth. Key implications for practice from this study were considered for CYP ranging from 0–18 years old, however further studies may offer more specific guidance to differentiate recommendations for PREP use between younger children and youth.

Although key ingredients have been proposed for the introduction of PREP to clinical practice, they may not be transferable for use in other areas of paediatric occupational therapy practice. It would be valuable for future studies to examine perceptions of the proposed key ingredients to investigate transferability. Further action research cycles could offer the opportunity to evaluate key ingredients to introduce PREP to practice in different paediatric practice settings in the UK.

As this study did not examine the perspectives of CYP and families, future qualitative research would add further triangulation of views and experiences. Furthermore, a longitudinal study would be of interest to follow-up CYP participation experiences following discharge. It would be useful to understand whether families benefited from PREP intervention following discharge, and whether or not participation strategies were effective in home, school or community environments.

Finally clinicians would benefit from further practice guidelines to support implementation of participation interventions. This study somewhat offers a starting point for clinicians working with CYP who have experienced ABI to offer participation interventions in their clinical practice.

5. Conclusions

This study examined how occupational therapists can introduce and implement participation interventions in a children's neurorehabilitation setting. The study specifically examined PREP, a participation intervention aiming to improve children's participation through the identification of environmental barriers and facilitators [10]. This knowledge translation study considered knowledge and application to clinical practice to further contribute to the evidence base for participation focused interventions.

Findings offer practical principles to apply knowledge when supporting early adoption of participation interventions in practice, whilst building capacity to support generalisation of PREP strategies beyond therapist led intervention. The involvement of peers, social opportunities and acknowledging family readiness were key factors for successful implementation. Therapy-led peer support and training in coaching were identified to remedy challenges when adopting a new participation perspective and directions in practice.

Author Contributions: Conceptualization, M.B; methodology, M.B.; formal analysis, M.B.; writing—original draft preparation, M.B; writing—review and editing, M.B., C.B. and P.S.; supervision, C.B. and P.S. All authors have read and agreed to the published version of the manuscript.

Funding: This research received no external funding.

Conflicts of Interest: The authors declare no conflict of interest.

Appendix A

Table A1. Follow-up meeting and implementation action plan (Shared candidate themes so far).

Cases Identified for PREP Implementation (Anonymised)	Therapist Allocation (Anonymised)
Child 1 (Male, aged 14)	Beth
Child 2 (Male, aged 17)	Hannah
Child 3 (Male, aged 11)	Sarah
Child 4 (Male, aged 16)	Emma
Child 5 (Male, aged 16)	Katy
Child 6 (Male, aged 10)	Alice

Table A2. Implementation Action Plan.

Action Description	Action Steps	Who?	Resources Required?
Number of goals set	One participation goal will be set for each child, unless they already have one participation goal already set through GAS due to timing of placement	All	COPM, GAS
Frequency of COPM rating	Discretion of the treating OT, aim for minimum of once per week	All	COPM
Goal rating to monitor progress	The COPM scales (performance and satisfaction) will be used to rate progress. This will be done with parents and children/ young person where possible.	All	COPM GAS
Frequency of PREP intervention	Two sessions per week. Sessions are typically for 30 min	OTs to book sessions onto MDT timetable for the child weekly	Planning time to organise intervention sessions
Group support	Organise a check in meeting after lunch time with clinical researcher external to group, to share goals and support implementation	Professional from research	Room booking for one hour per week Research time
Inform the MDT	E-mail to therapists, nursing, care and psychosocial teams Place on agenda for rehab staff meeting	Moderator Moderator	
Inform the MDT	Poster in communal staff areas for awareness of PREP. Post blog on the intranet	P1 P1	Time to make poster
Address problems during action cycle	To be done in check in session Option to email moderator during action cycle with any questions	All	
Budget for community activities	Make available funds if needed, OT's to keep track of any spend		Funds in OT budget

Appendix B

Table A3. Semi-structured questions for focus group 1.

Questions
1. What are your impressions of the PREP so far?
2. What do we think about the structure of the PREP intervention?
3. What do we need to consider before introducing the PREP intervention in our setting?
4. What may the challenges be in implementing the PREP in practice?
5. Agree on how we might define our implementation plan and time frame for implementation (How we will introduce PREP to practice)
Focus group questions adapted [8].

Appendix C

Table A4. Semi-structured questions for focus group 2.

Questions
1. Could we begin by discussing the introduction of the PREP intervention? The PREP is focused on setting goals, identifying barriers and facilitators to participation. Can we discuss this?
2. The PREP is focused on developing strategies to overcome environmental barriers. What are our thoughts on this?
3. When we implemented the PREP intervention, what was easy? What was more difficult?
4. Could we discuss your experiences of using parent coaching as part of the PREP intervention?
5. The PREP intervention focuses on changing the child's natural environment. Could we discuss our experiences of using this context-focused intervention?
6. What was the response of the children and family to the intervention? What was the response of the MDT?
7. Overall, what do we feel went well and what do we feel did not go so well?
8. What changes in practice do we feel have been made after implementing the PREP intervention? Are there any issues for using the PREP in the future?
9. Is there anything that you would like to add to what you have already said about experiences of implementing the PREP intervention?
Focus group questions adapted [8].

Appendix D

Abbreviation List

1. Acquired brain injury (ABI)
2. Action research (AR)
3. Canadian Occupational Performance Measure (COPM)
4. Children and young people (CYP)
5. Goal attainment scaling (GAS)
6. Occupational Therapist (OT)
7. Pathways and Resources for Participation and Engagement (PREP)

References

1. National Institute for Health and Care Excellence. Head Injury: Triage, Assessment, Investigation and Early Management of Head Injury in Children, Young People and Adults. Available online: https://www.nice.org.uk/guidance/cg176/resources/costing-report-pdf-191714653 (accessed on 7 April 2020).
2. Hayes, L.; Shaw, S.; Pearce, M.; Forsyth, R. Requirements for and current provision of rehabilitation services for children after severe acquired brain injury in the UK: A population based study. *Arch. Dis. Child.* **2017**, *102*, 813–820. [CrossRef] [PubMed]
3. World Health Organization. International Classification of Functioning, Disability and Health (icf). Available online: https://www.who.int/classifications/icf/en/ (accessed on 10 May 2020).
4. Wells, R.; Minnes, P.; Phillips, M. Predicting social and functional outcomes for individuals sustaining paediatric traumatic brain injury. *Dev. Neurorehabil.* **2009**, *12*, 12–23. [CrossRef] [PubMed]
5. Galvin, J.; Froude, E.; McAleer, J. Children's participation in home, school and community life after acquired brain injury. *Aust. Occup. Ther. J.* **2010**, *57*, 118–126. [CrossRef] [PubMed]
6. Foo, W.; Galvin, J.; Olsen., J. Participation of children with ABI and the relationship with discharge functional status. *Dev. Neurorehabil.* **2012**, *15*, 1–12. [CrossRef] [PubMed]
7. Law, M.; Anaby, D.; Imms, C.; Teplicky, R.; Turner, L. Improving the participation of youth with physical disabilities in community activities: An interrupted time series design. *Aust. Occup. Ther. J.* **2015**, *62*, 105–115. [CrossRef]
8. Anaby, D.; Law, M.; Teplicky, R.; Turner, L. Focussing on the environment to improve youth participation: Experiences and perspectives of occupational therapists. *Int. J. Environ. Res. Public Health* **2015**, *12*, 13387–13398. [CrossRef]
9. Imms, C.; Granlund, M.; Wilson, P.; Steenbergen, B.; Rosenbaum, P.; Gordon, A. Participation, both a means and an end: A conceptual analysis of processes and outcomes in childhood disability. *Dev. Med. Child Neurol.* **2017**, *59*, 16–25. [CrossRef]
10. Law, M.; Anaby, D.; Teplicky, R.; Turner, L. *Pathways and Resources for Engagement and Participation, a Practice Model for Occupational Therapists*; Reference Manual: CanChild, ON, Canada, 2016; pp. 1–47.
11. Anaby, D.; Law, M.; Feldman, D.; Majnemer, A.; Avery, L. The effectiveness of the Pathways and Resources for Engagement and Participation (PREP) intervention: Improving participation of adolescents with physical disabilities. *Dev. Med. Child Neurol.* **2018**, *60*, 513–519. [CrossRef]
12. Law, M.; Baptiste, S.; Carswell, A.; McColl, M.; Polatajko, H.; Pollock, N. *Canadian Occupational Performance Outcome Measure*, 5th ed.; CAOT Publications ACE: Toronto, ON, Canada, 2014.
13. Anaby, D.; Law, M.; Majnemer, A.; Feldman, D. Opening doors to participation of youth with physical disabilities: An intervention study. *Can. J. Occup. Ther.* **2016**, *83*, 83–90. [CrossRef]
14. Anaby, D.; Avery, L.; Willem Gorter, J.; Levin, M.; Teplicky, R.; Turner, L.; Cormier, I.; Hanes, J. Improving body functions through participation in community activities among young people with physical disabilities. *Dev. Med. Child Neurol.* **2019**, *62*, 640–646. [CrossRef]
15. Greenhalgh, T.; Wieringa, S. Is it time to drop the 'knowledge translation' metaphor? A critical literature review. *J. R. Soc. Med.* **2011**, *104*, 501–509. [CrossRef] [PubMed]
16. Woolf, S. The meaning of translational research and why it matters. *Am. Med. Assoc.* **2008**, *299*, 211–213. [CrossRef] [PubMed]
17. Kiresuk, T.; Sherman, R. Goal attainment scaling: A general method for evaluating comprehensive community mental health programs. *Community Mental Health J.* **1968**, *4*, 443–453. [CrossRef] [PubMed]
18. Biljon, H.; Casteleijn, D.; Du Toit, S.; Rabothata, S. An action research approach to profile an occupational therapy vocational rehabilitation service in public healthcare. *S. Afr. J. Occup. Ther.* **2015**, *45*, 40–47. [CrossRef]
19. Hart, E.; Bond, M. Making sense of action research through the use of a typology. *J. Adv. Nurs.* **1995**, *23*, 152–159. [CrossRef]
20. Coghlan, D.; Brannick, T. *Doing Action Research in Your Own Organization*, 4th ed.; Sage Publications Inc.: London, UK, 2014; pp. 1–18.
21. Dunford, C.; Bannigan, K. Children and young people's occupation health and well-being: A research manifesto for developing the evidence base. *World Fed. Occup. Ther. Bull.* **2011**, *64*, 46–52. [CrossRef]
22. Braun, V.; Clarke, V. Using thematic analysis in psychology. *Qual. Res. Psychol.* **2006**, *3*, 77–101. [CrossRef]

23. Koch, T.; Kralik, D. *Participatory Action Research in Healthcare*; Blackwell Publishing: Oxford, UK, 2006; pp. 1–194.
24. Armitage, S.; Swallow, V.; Kolehmainen, N. Ingredients and change processes in occupational therapy for children: A grounded theory study. *Scand. J. Occup. Ther.* **2017**, *24*, 208–213. [CrossRef]
25. Woods, D.; Catroppa, C.; Godfrey, C.; Anderson, V. Long-term maintenance of treatment effects following intervention for families with children who have acquired brain injury. *Soc. Care Neurodisabil.* **2015**, *5*, 70–82. [CrossRef]
26. NHS England. New Care Models: Empowering Patients and Communities. A Call to Action for a Directory of Support. Available online: https://www.england.nhs.uk/wp-content/uploads/2015/12/vanguards-support-directory.pdf (accessed on 7 April 2020).
27. Tonks, J.; Williams, W.; Frampton, I.; Yates, P.; Wall, S.; Slater, A. Reading emotions after childhood brain injury: Case series evidence of dissociation between cognitive abilities and emotional expression processing skills. *Brain Injury* **2008**, *22*, 325–332. [CrossRef]
28. Lahey, S.; Beaulieu, C.; Sandbach, K.; Colaiezzi, A.; Balkan, S. The role of the psychologist with disorders of consciousness in inpatient pediatric neurorehabilitation: A case series. *Rehabil. Psychol.* **2017**, *62*, 238–248. [CrossRef] [PubMed]

Publisher's Note: MDPI stays neutral with regard to jurisdictional claims in published maps and institutional affiliations.

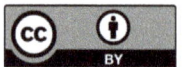

© 2020 by the authors. Licensee MDPI, Basel, Switzerland. This article is an open access article distributed under the terms and conditions of the Creative Commons Attribution (CC BY) license (http://creativecommons.org/licenses/by/4.0/).

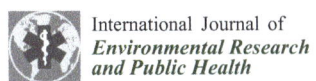

Article

Changes in Overall Participation Profile of Youth with Physical Disabilities Following the PREP Intervention

Colin Hoehne [1], Brittany Baranski [2], Louiza Benmohammed [3], Liam Bienstock [2], Nathan Menezes [2], Noah Margolese [2] and Dana Anaby [2,4,*]

[1] Health Sciences Centre, Winnipeg, MB R3A 1R9, Canada
[2] School of Physical & Occupational Therapy, McGill University, Montreal, QC H3G 1Y5, Canada
[3] CIUSSS du Nord-de-l'Île-de-Montréal, Montreal, QC H4K 1B3, Canada
[4] Centre de Recherche Interdisciplinaire en Réadaptation de Montréal Métropolitain (CRIR), Montreal, QC H3S1M9, Canada
* Correspondence: dana.anaby@mcgill.ca

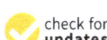

Received: 8 May 2020; Accepted: 30 May 2020; Published: 4 June 2020

Abstract: The Pathways and Resources for Engagement and Participation (PREP), an environmental-based intervention, is effective in improving the participation of youth with disabilities in specific targeted activities; however, its potential impact on overall participation beyond these activities is unknown. This study examined the differences in participation levels and environmental barriers and supports following the 12-week PREP intervention. Existing data on participation patterns and environmental barriers and supports, measured by the Participation and Environment Measure for Children and Youth, pre-and post-PREP intervention, were statistically analyzed across 20 youth aged 12 to 18 (mean = 14.4, standard deviation (SD) = 1.82) with physical disabilities in three settings: home, school and community. Effect sizes were calculated using Cohen's d. Following PREP, youth participated significantly less often at home (d = 2.21; 95% Confidence Interval (CI) [1.79, 2.96]), more often (d = 0.57; 95% CI [−0.79, −0.14]) and in more diverse activities (d = 0.51; 95% CI [−1.99, −0.51]) in the community. At school, significantly greater participation was observed in special school roles (t = −2.46. p = 0.024). Involvement and desire for change remained relatively stable across all settings. A substantial increase in community environmental supports was observed (d = 0.67), with significantly more parents reporting availability of, and access to information as a support (χ^2 = 4.28, p = 0.038). Findings lend further support to the effectiveness of environmental-based interventions, involving real-life experiences.

Keywords: social participation; adolescence; intervention

1. Introduction

Participation, defined as involvement in life situations [1], involves being with others [2], and is critical to the development of physical, emotional and social well-being in youth with and without disabilities [3,4]. Through participation, youth can develop a sense of self, feelings of success and connectedness to their community [5]. Participation of youth is of particular importance not only because their participation levels decrease as they enter adolescence [6] but also because they face a challenging transitional phase to adulthood [7]. Indeed, youth living with disabilities report lower participation levels than those without disabilities at home, school and in the community [8,9]. Specifically, they experience lower participation frequency, lower involvement levels and poorer satisfaction with their participation profile [10].

Some of the key factors that determine the participation profile of youth with disabilities lie within their environment [11]. Recent scoping reviews reveal a range of common environmental barriers and supports which can affect participation [12–14]. Examples of barriers include physical inaccessibility, unsupportive attitudes of others and lack of knowledge about ways to adapt activities and equipment. Examples of supports include social support from family and friends and availability of information. Therefore, minimizing environmental barriers and building upon supports are promising intervention strategies for improving participation, especially for youth with disabilities, who might not yet have the necessary skills to manage environmental barriers to participation themselves [15]. Consequently, interventions that aim to improve participation via environmental modifications have emerged in the last decade. Examples include context-focused therapy for young children with cerebral palsy [16] and Teens Making Environment and Activity Modifications (TEAM) for youth with developmental disabilities [15]. The Pathways and Resources for Engagement and Participation (PREP) is another example of an environment-based participation-targeting intervention, which is designed for individuals across different ages and abilities [17] and employs a strength-based approach. This 12-week intervention provides youth and caregivers with one-on-one coaching to foster problem solving and self-advocacy skills in order to remove environmental barriers to, and build supports for participation [18].

In our recent study [19], PREP has been shown to improve the performance of youth with physical disabilities (n = 28) in three targeted, self-chosen, leisure community-based activities; yet, it has not been established whether this intervention could impact areas beyond its three targeted activities, resulting in overall changes in participation profile. Our prior research with a sub-sample of this cohort provides preliminary evidence of such an effect. Parents, through individual interviews (n = 12) [20], reported positive improvements in their child's physical, emotional and social states following PREP. Another investigation of youth receiving PREP (n = 13) [21] indicated a shift in the types of activities performed, such as increased participation in social- and school-related activities, as measured using the Aday app, which is a 24 h activity log.

To complement these findings, the goal of this study is to systematically examine the effect of PREP on overall participation patterns using a standardized assessment. This was done by investigating a novel, distinct aspect of our existing dataset (n = 28) [19]. Specifically, our primary objectives were to examine the effect of PREP on (1) youths' overall participation patterns in terms of frequency, involvement and desire for change in the home, school and community settings, and (2) the number of environmental barriers and supports to participation reported in these settings. A secondary objective was also set, exploring the association between baseline youth characteristics known to influence participation (in terms of physical functioning, motivation and family functioning) and rates of change of participation.

2. Materials and Methods

2.1. Design

A subsequent analysis of existing data generated by an Interrupted Time Series study previously conducted by Anaby et al. [19] was employed to detect overall changes in participation patterns following the 12-week PREP intervention. Specifically, participation patterns were examined at the first week of baseline (which lasted 4 weeks) as well as 4 weeks after the completion of the PREP intervention (12 weeks), resulting in a 20-week delay between pre- and post-points of time. The original dataset included 28 youths with mobility restrictions (i.e., due to cerebral palsy, spina bifida, musculoskeletal disorders), who were recruited from five major rehabilitation centers and two high schools in Greater Montreal, from both Anglophone and Francophone families. Youth who also had cognitive and/or communication impairments were included. Youth within the first-year post-severe brain injury, or within 4 months post orthopedic surgery, were excluded from the selection process, as their participation and functional levels may not have been stable.

Of the 28 participants from the original study, a total of eight participants were excluded from the current study. Six participants were excluded because additional questionnaires (Dimensions of Mastery Questionnaire—DMQ, Activities Scale for Kids—ASK, Family Environment Scale—FES) were not administered to them at baseline. Two additional participants were excluded from the analysis as either pre- or post-intervention Participation and Environment Measure for Children and Youth (PEM-CY) data was incomplete. Thus, our current study included data from 20 participants. The included (n = 20) and excluded (n = 8) groups had an equal female-to-male ratio. The mean ages were similar (n = 20, mean = 14.4), (n = 8, mean = 15.13), and both groups had the same median age (median = 14.5). Mann–Whitney U tests indicated no significant differences between the groups in terms of number of health conditions (U = 74.5; p = 0.80258) and functional issues (U = 54.5; p = 0.20408). For further details on the original study design, see Anaby et al. [19].

2.2. Intervention

The PREP is a 5-step intervention, i.e., (1) Make goals, (2) Map out a plan, (3) Make it happen, (4) Measure process and outcomes and (5) Move forward, aimed at improving participation in self-chosen activities by changing aspects of the environment and by engaging and coaching youth/parents. An occupational therapist met with each youth/family individually at their home/community where they jointly set three community-based participation goals that the youth aspired to engage in yet found difficult. Examples of desired activities included joining a sledge hockey team, taking cooking classes, going to the movies with friends and enjoying music in a social group, among others. A collaborative plan was then devised to identify and implement solution-based strategies for removing environmental barriers and leveraging existing supports. The therapist and family also built a "participation team" comprised of a range of stakeholders (i.e., family members, teachers, community instructors, volunteers, etc.) to assist in the execution of the plan. Further information about the intervention can be found in the PREP manual [17] and the online learning module [22].

To ensure treatment fidelity and adherence to PREP principles, all therapists (n = 6) completed a 6 h PREP training program. Ongoing expert consultation was also provided throughout the study. Additionally, intervention forms, completed by therapists, documenting strategies used in their interventions were reviewed. As expected, all intervention strategies illustrated modifications of the environment and none focused on changing the youth's impairment. Effective environmental strategies included improving physical accessibility, adapting activity equipment, finding available programs, providing information about transportation, informing community agencies about how they could adapt their programs and provide accessible services and improving attitudes of others through education [19].

2.3. Procedure and Data Collection

Informed consent and assent were obtained from parents and youth, approved by the Research Ethics Board of the Centre for Interdisciplinary Research in Rehabilitation of Greater Montreal. At baseline, during the first meeting with the therapist, several assessment measures were completed, including the Participation and Environment Measure—Children and Youth (PEM-CY) to measure participation patterns, Family Environment Scale (FES) to assess family functioning (contextual factors), Activities Scale for Kids (ASK) to measure physical functioning (activity limitation) and the Dimensions of Mastery Questionnaire (DMQ) to measure level of motivation (personal factors). The PEM-CY was also completed at follow-up (week 20).

2.4. Measures

The PEM-CY is a parent-report measure that assesses participation frequency, involvement and desire for change across 25 sets of activities occurring in three different settings: home (10 activities), school (5 activities) and community (10 activities). Frequency is rated on an 8-point Likert scale (0 = never, 7 = daily) and level of involvement is ranked on a 5-point Likert scale (1 = minimally involved, 5 = very involved). Desire for change includes a 6-point nominal scale describing the type of change desired; however, for the purpose of this study it was treated dichotomously to indicate if a change in each activity was desired (yes/no). The PEM-CY also measures environmental factors, including barriers and supports to participation, within each of the three settings (12 items for home, 17 items for school and 16 items for community). The PEM-CY demonstrated moderate to good reliability (test re-test reliability, 0.58–0.95, internal consistency 0.59–0.91) as well as ability to distinguish between children with and without disabilities, supporting aspects of construct validity [23]. Factorial structure of participation frequency and involvement across all three settings was confirmed [11]. This measure has been used with children with Spina Bifida [24].

The FES is a valid and reliable self-report questionnaire used to assess the social environment of families [25]. It is composed of 90 self-report items that can be separated into 10 subscales. This study focused on two of the subscales of family functioning, Active–Recreation Orientation (i.e., family's participation in social and recreational activities) and Intellectual–Cultural Orientation (i.e., family's interest in political, intellectual and cultural activities), as there is evidence that these two subscales influence participation outcomes among children with physical disabilities [26]. For each subscale, a summary score was generated by converting true/false answers into a standardized score ranging from 0 to 100, where a score of 60 or more indicates that the subscale area is present to a high degree in the family. This measure has also been used with children with musculoskeletal disorders such as rheumatoid arthritis [27].

The DMQ is a parent-report tool used to measure a child's self-perceived motivation. This measure contains 45 items, which assess the level of persistence to solve problems, mastery of tasks and the feelings associated with attempts of mastery. Parents indicate the degree that each item applies to their child using a five-point Likert scale. A general summary score ranging from 1 to 5 was generated, with scores of 5 indicating higher mastery motivation. This measure has been used with children with cerebral palsy [28], has adequate reliability and validity [29], and has been shown to be associated with children's participation [30].

Aspects of activity limitation which are associated with participation [31] were measured using the ASK. The ASK is a valid and reliable self-report tool designed to measure physical functional issues for children and youth, experiencing activity limitations due to musculoskeletal disorders [32]. It includes 30 functional activities separated into 7 sub-domains (e.g., personal care and transfers) that rate independent performance of each activity using a 5-point scale. A summary score ranging from 0 to 100 is generated, where 0 indicates the greatest disability. A global rating of physical disability is also generated: mild (75 to 100), moderate (35 to 74) and severe (<35).

2.5. Data Analysis

2.5.1. Primary Objective 1—Differences in Participation Levels in Each Setting following the PREP Intervention

Setting-level and item-level mean scores of diversity (number of activities actually done), frequency (ranged from 0 to 7), involvement (ranged from 1 to 5), and number of activities in which parents wanted to see change were calculated pre- and post-PREP intervention.

Setting-level changes, i.e., changes in mean participation levels across an entire setting (home, school, community), pre- and post-intervention were analyzed using a paired t-test; this is based on the central limit theorem assumption that with a sample of 20 youth, the sampling distribution of the mean approximates a normal distribution. In cases where the number of responders was less than 20, a non-parametric test was used (Wilcoxon). Values of $p < 0.05$ were considered significant and 95% Confidence Intervals (CI) were calculated. Cohen's d was used to estimate effect sizes, where $d = 0.2$ is considered a small effect, $d = 0.5$ is medium and $d = 0.8$ is large. SPSS Software Version 25 was used for all statistical calculations. Data was also analyzed descriptively to identify direction and amount of change.

Item-level mean scores were calculated for participation frequency and number of youths engaged in each of the activities, pre- and post-intervention. All item-level comparisons were graphed using radar plots to visually analyze the data. Items of activities were analyzed for significance when the amount of change was more likely to represent a change in one category/point within the frequency scale (e.g., from "once in a week" = 1 to "few times a week" = 2'). These values corresponded to a mean difference in frequency of greater than 0.5 points. Wilcoxon or paired t-tests were used depending on the number of responses per item. To reduce the number of item-level statistical comparisons, diversity scores (representing number of youths engaged in each activity) were only tested for statistical significance (using the Chi-square test) when a pre–post change was observed in at least 20% of the sample, an arbitrary set. Notably, item-level analyses were only performed for those setting-level mean scores which were statistically significant.

2.5.2. Primary Objective 2—Differences in Environmental Barriers and Supports in Each Setting following the PREP Intervention

Setting-level and Item-level scores for environmental barriers and supports were calculated pre- and post-intervention. Scores represent the number of parents (in percentages) who viewed the given environmental item as a barrier/support.

Setting-level mean scores, i.e., changes in the percentage of environmental barriers/supports reported in each setting (home, school, community) were analyzed using the same methods as objective 1: A paired t-test or a Wilcoxon test, as well as descriptively.

Item-level mean scores were calculated for each of the environmental barriers/supports, pre- and post-intervention. Items in which a change of at least 20% of the sample was observed were statistically analyzed using Chi-square tests. All Item-level comparisons were displayed using radar plots, in terms of percentage of parents who considered the given environmental item to be a barrier/support. These radar plots were used to analyze data visually.

2.5.3. Secondary Objective—Association between Youth's Characteristics at Baseline and Rates of Change of Participation

To examine the secondary objective, exploratory analysis was done to investigate factors associated with change in participation scores that were found significant in objective 1. Exploratory variables considered were: youth functional levels (number of functional issues reported, ASK total score of physical functioning) motivation (i.e., DMQ gross motor persistence, mastery pleasure, negative reaction, object-oriented persistence, social persistence with children, social persistence with adults) and aspects of family functioning (FES active–recreation orientation scale standard score, FES intellectual-cultural orientation scale standard score). To identify patterns/association between change in participation and the explanatory variables, change scores (post-score − pre-score) were calculated and plotted against the baseline scores on the explanatory variables. A loess smoothed line (with span of 0.75) was added to each scatterplot to help identify any patterns visually.

3. Results

3.1. Participants

Twenty youth (10 female) aged 12–18 years (mean = 14.4; standard deviation (SD) = 1.82) were included in this analysis. Up to seven health conditions were reported per youth (mean = 2.4, SD = 1.7; Interquartile range (IQR) 1 to 3), with the most common being orthopedic/movement impairments (70%), followed by speech/language impairments (50%), intellectual delay (25%) and vision impairment (25%). Number of functional issues ranged from 1 to 11 (mean = 5.1, SD = 3.01; IQR 3 to 7) including difficulty using hands to do activities (85%), moving around (72%), communicating with others (58%) and managing emotions (58%). The majority of the youth (68.8%) had a severe physical disability, as measured by the ASK. As shown in Table 1, levels of family functioning in terms of active–recreation and intellectual–cultural orientation were below 60, indicating a relativity low presence of these attributes. In terms of motivation, similar levels of mastery pleasure and gross motor persistence were observed, when compared to typically developing teens of a similar age [29].

The remaining domains of motivation approached normative levels, apart from negative reactions to failure. Further sociodemographic factors are also described in Table 1.

Table 1. Sample Characteristics (n = 20).

Variable	n	%
Class type		
Regular classroom	3	15
Both regular and special classroom	3	15
Special education class	13	65
Other (International program)	1	5
Community type		
Major urban	7	35
Suburban	7	35
Small town	2	10
Missing	4	20
Language		
English	2	10
French	7	35
Other (Spanish and Arabic)	2	10
Bilingual (English or French with Bulgarian, Arabic, Portuguese, Hebrew, or Creole)	9	45
Age of family member		
30–39	3	15
40–49	13	65
50–59	4	20
Education level of family member		
High school or less	3	15
Some college/university or technical training 1-year min	4	20
Graduate college/university	11	55
High school or less	2	10
	Mean	SD
Family Environment Scale (FES)		
Active-Recreation Orientation (n = 20)	48.85	11.86
Intellectual-Cultural Orientation (n = 20)	52.50	8.44
Dimensions of Mastery Questionnaire (DMQ)		
Persistence at object or cognitive tasks (n = 18)	3.57	0.82
Gross motor persistence (n = 19)	2.99	0.76
Social mastery motivation with adults (n = 20)	3.47	0.80
Social mastery motivation with peers/children (n = 18)	3.24	0.93
Mastery pleasure (n = 18)	3.90	0.73
Negative reactions in mastery situations (n = 19)	3.03	0.92
Activities Scale for Kids (ASK)		
ASK total score (n = 19)	mild	15.9%
	moderate	15.9%
	severe	68.8%

3.2. Differences in Participation and Environmental Scores in Each Setting

Following the PREP intervention, on average, youth participated significantly more often ($d = 0.57$, 95% CI [−0.79, −0.14]) and in greater ranges of activities ($d = 0.51$, 95% CI [−1.99, −0.51]) in the community setting with moderate effect sizes, and significantly less often in the home setting ($d = 2.1$, 95% CI [1.79, 2.96]), with a large effect size (Table 2). Youth also participated more often in school, yet a non-significant effect was observed. Levels of involvement and percentages of parents who desired change in activities remained relatively similar pre- and post-intervention across all settings.

Table 2. Setting-level Participation and Environment Measure for Children and Youth mean scores in the home, school, and community (n = 20).

	PEM-CY Scale (Range/Unit)	Pre Scores Mean (SD)	Post Scores Mean (SD)	95% CI	t	ES
Home	Frequency (0–7)	5.43 (1.11)	3.05 (1.02)	1.79, 2.96	8.456 ***	2.144
	Diversity (0–10)	9.20 (1.24)	9.00 (1.45)	−0.13, 0.52	1.285	0.16
	Level of involvement (1–5)	4.06 (0.48)	3.97 (0.82)	−0.22, 0.39	0.586	0.17
	Number of activities desired for change (0–10)	5.00 (2.38)	5.30 (2.54)	−1.39, 0.785	−0.578	0.12
	Number of environmental barriers (in %)	10.42 (14.02)	9.58 (11.24)	−4.05, 5.72	0.357	0.06
	Number of environmental supports (in %)	28.33 (20.84)	33.33 (17.10)	−15.77, 5.77	−0.972	0.24
School	Frequency (0–7)	2.84 (1.13)	3.05 (1.02)	−0.79, 0.36	−0.782	0.189
	Diversity (0–5)	3.05 (0.94)	3.10 (1.25)	−0.44, 0.34	−0.271	0.052
	Level of involvement (1–5)	3.70 (1.08)	3.55 (1.17)	−0.40, 0.70	0.571	0.14
	Number of activities desired for change (0–5)	2.95 (1.57)	2.70 (1.59)	−0.49, 0.99	0.705	0.16
	Number of environmental barriers (in %)	10.59 (9.27)	9.12 (8.20)	−3.07, 6.01	0.677	0.16
	Number of environmental supports (in %)	35.88 (18.39)	38.53 (19.88)	−13.12, 7.83	−0.529	0.14
Community	Frequency of participation (0–7)	1.68 (0.91)	2.15 (0.78)	−0.79, −0.14	−3.017 **	0.57
	Diversity (score 0–10)	4.50 (2.44)	5.75 (1.83)	−1.99, −0.51	−3.526 **	0.51
	Level of involvement (1–5)	3.73 (1.15)	3.97 (0.82)	−0.82, 0.33	−0.894	0.17
	Number of activities desired for change (0–10)	6.8 (2.28)	6.05 (2.96)	−0.74, 2.24	1.06	0.33
	Number of environmental barriers (in %)	17.50 (16.30)	15.00 (10.42)	−4.30, 9.30	0.769	0.15
	Number of environmental supports (in %)	23.75 (13.23)	32.19 (19.37)	−17.20, 0.33	−2.015 [a]	0.67

** $p < 0.01$; *** $p < 0.001$; [a] = 0.058; ES = Effect Size represented by Cohen's d.

The results that follow are organized according to scale, restricted to those scales where a statistically significant change was observed.

3.3. Differences in Frequency Scores

Following the PREP intervention a significant, moderate effect on participation was observed in the community setting (ES = 0.57, 95% CI [−0.79, −0.14]), where participation frequency increased, and a significant, large effect on participation was observed in the home setting (ES = 2.14, 95% CI [1.79, 2.96]), where participation frequency decreased. Additionally, a small, non-significant effect was observed in the school setting, indicating an increase in frequency levels (Table 2).

Changes in frequency at the Item-level (within each activity) indicated that across the three settings, nine activity sets out of 25 were found to have a pre-post difference equal to 0.5 or greater, five of which illustrated a statistically significant change (Figure 1). Children participated significantly less at home, specifically in *computer and video games* (Z = −2.33, p = 0.02), and *homework* (Z = −2.043, p = 0.041). They significantly took on more *special roles at school* (t = −2.46, p = 0.024) such as lunchroom supervisor or student mentor roles, among others. In the community setting, youth significantly participated more often in two activity sets: *organized physical activities* (t = −3.11, p = 0.006) and *classes and lessons* (t = −2.614, p = 0.018), and a positive non-significant change was observed in *organizations, groups, clubs, and volunteer or leadership activities* and *neighborhood outings*.

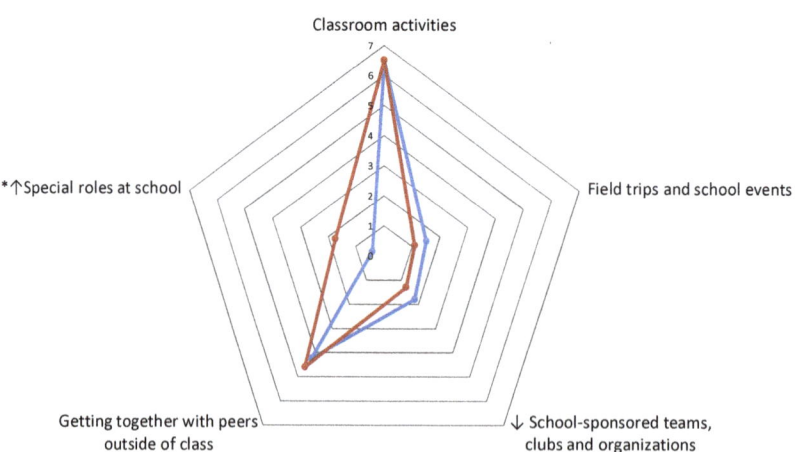

Figure 1. Cont.

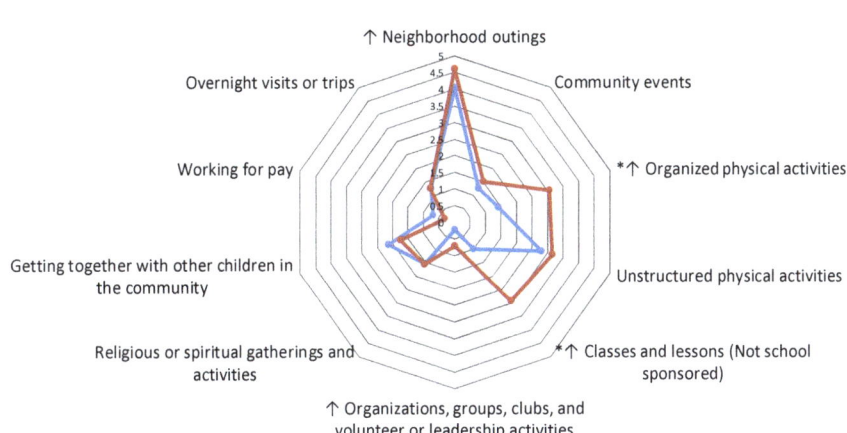

(c)

Figure 1. Frequency of participation in the home (a), school (b), and community settings (c) (n = 20). 0 = Never, 1 = Once in the last four months, 2 = Few times in the last four months, 3 = Once a month, 4 = Few times a month, 5 = Once a week, 6 = Few times a week, 7 = Daily. ↑/↓ = Mean increase/decrease of at least 0.5. * $p < 0.05$.

3.4. Differences in Diversity Scores

As previously mentioned, a significant moderate effect on participation diversity was observed in the community section (d = 0.51, 95% CI [−1.99, −0.51]), where youth took part in a greater number of activities following the intervention. The diversity scores of home and school activities remained similar post-intervention (Table 2).

Looking at the item-level scores, across the three settings, there were seven activity types out of 25 in which a change of 20% of the sample occurred, two of which were statistically significant based on Chi-square tests. Specifically, in the community, there were more youth participating in *organized physical activities* (χ^2 = 4.31, p = 0.037) and *classes/lessons* (χ^2 = 7.44, p = 0.006). Specific trends (non-significant) were also observed in all three settings. In the home, fewer youth participated in *indoor play and games*. In the school, fewer youth attended *field trips and school events*, and more youth took on *special roles at school*. In the community, there were more youth participating in *community events* and *unstructured physical activities* (Figure 2).

3.5. Differences in Environmental Barriers

While the mean number of setting-level barriers did not change significantly after PREP in any of the settings (Table 2), Item-level examination revealed a change in a range of barriers across all settings. In the community, parents reported a reduction in most barriers (11/16), with 20% fewer parents viewing *physical demands of activities*, and 25% fewer parents viewing *safety of the community* as barriers. Interestingly, a few specific environmental barriers in the home and school slightly increased following PREP, particularly those related to the cognitive and social demands of the activity (Figure 3).

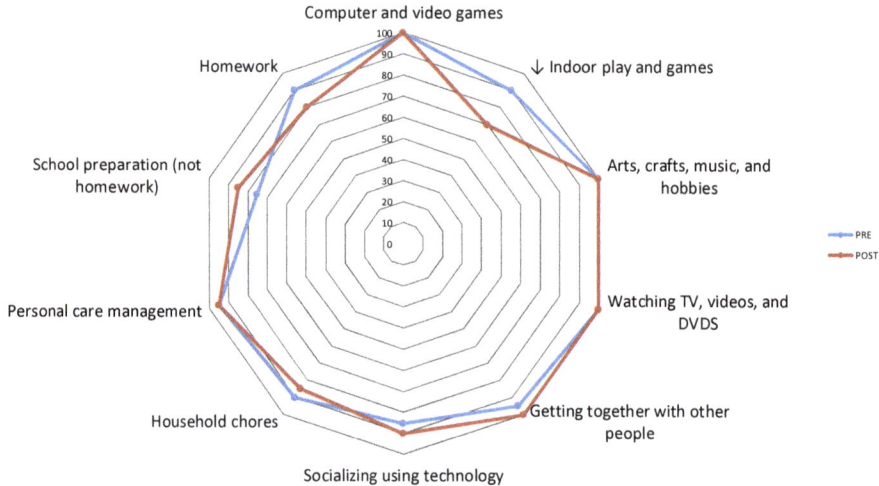

(a)

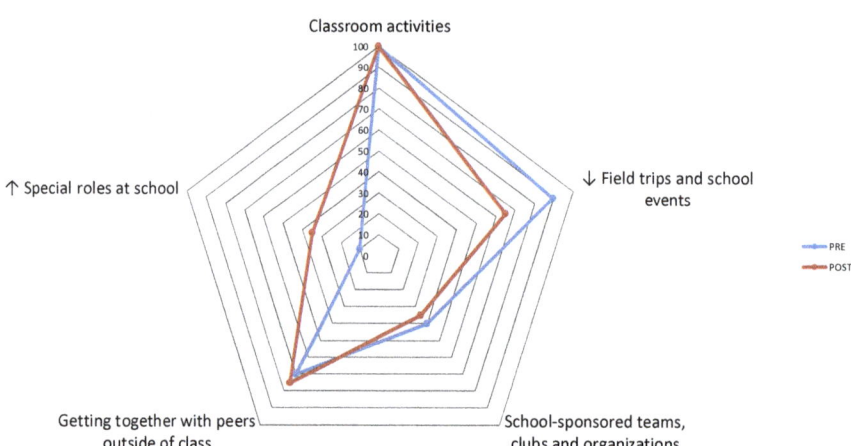

(b)

Figure 2. *Cont.*

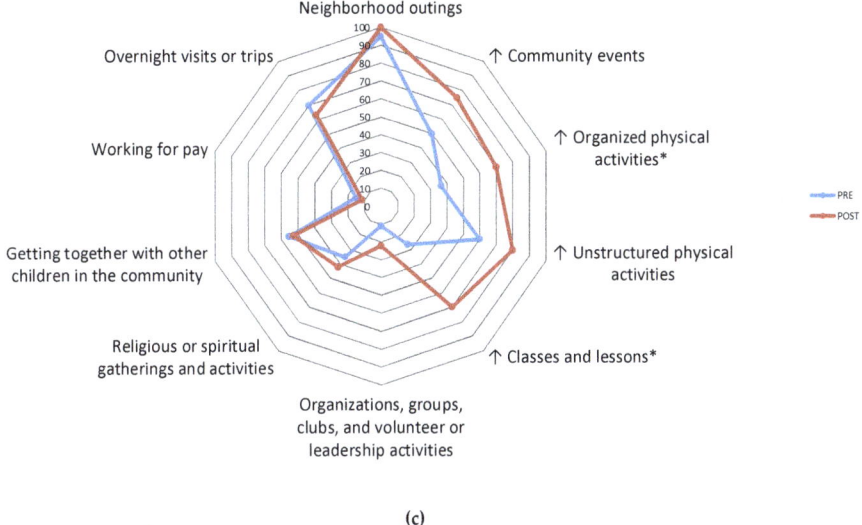

Figure 2. Percentage of youth (n = 18 to 20) participating in each activity in the home (**a**), school (**b**), and community (**c**) settings. ↑/↓ = Increase/decrease in at least 20% of sample. * $p < 0.05$.

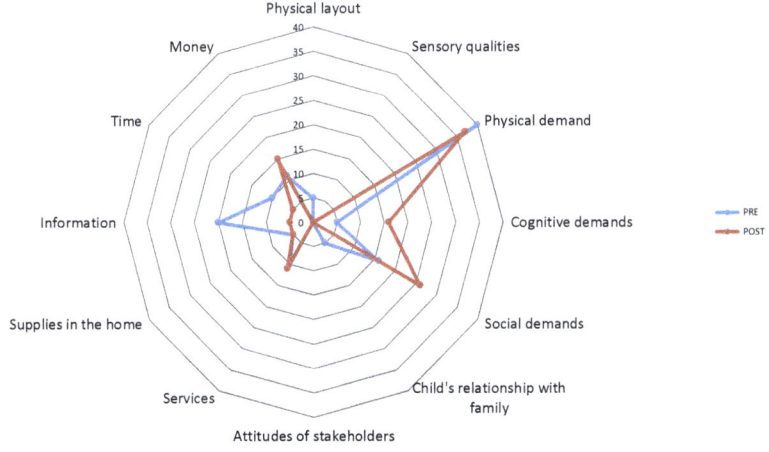

Figure 3. *Cont.*

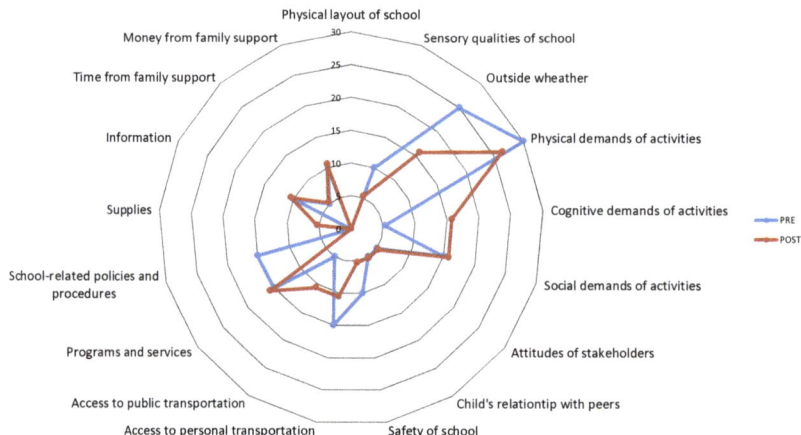

(b)

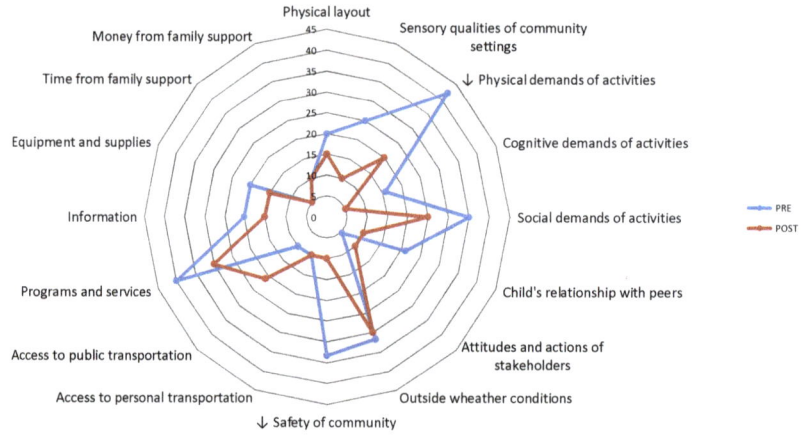

(c)

Figure 3. Percentage of parents (out of 20) who reported an environmental component as being a barrier in the home (**a**), school (**b**), and community (**c**) settings. ↓ = Decrease in at least 20% of sample. * $p < 0.05$.

3.6. Differences in Environmental Supports

As shown in Table 2, there was a non-significant increase in the mean number of supports in the home after PREP, with a small effect size ($d = 0.24$, 95% CI [−15.77, 5.77]). Mean number of supports remained fairly similar in the school and increased in the community with median effect size ($d = 0.67$,

95% CI [−17.20, 0.33]) approaching statistical significance ($p = 0.058$). Item-level comparisons indicated that parents reported an initial trend of increase in 8/12 supports in the home, 10/17 in the school and 12/16 in the community. Across all three settings, 20% of parents or more added a support in four environmental supports, one of which was statistically significant, i.e., availability of information (15% of parents pre versus 45% post, $\chi^2 = 4.28$, $p = 0.038$; Figure 4). Overall, more parents viewed *supplies* in the home (e.g., sports equipment, craft supplies), *physical layout* of the school, availability of community *programs* and community *information* as supports after PREP.

3.7. Secondary Objective—Association between Child's Characteristics at Baseline and Changes in Participation

Secondary objective analysis was performed on the three scores found to have statistically significant pre–post differences in objective 1 (i.e., home participation frequency, community participation frequency, and diversity). Visual examination of scatterplots indicated that none of the youth's characteristics at baseline were associated with rate of change in participation scores, with the exception of level of physical disability, measured by the ASK, where initial trends of association were observed. Specifically, youth with more severe disabilities tend to change slightly more in their participation frequency in the home setting, whereas in the community, changes to their participation appear less evident. Family functioning and youth motivation at baseline did not seem to influence change in participation patterns following PREP.

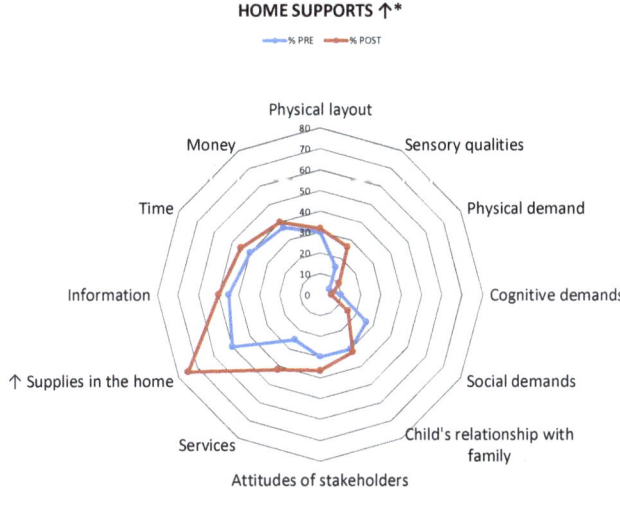

(a)

Figure 4. *Cont.*

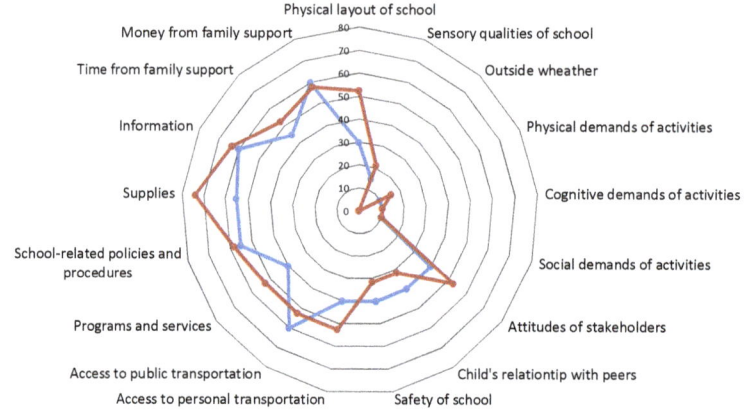

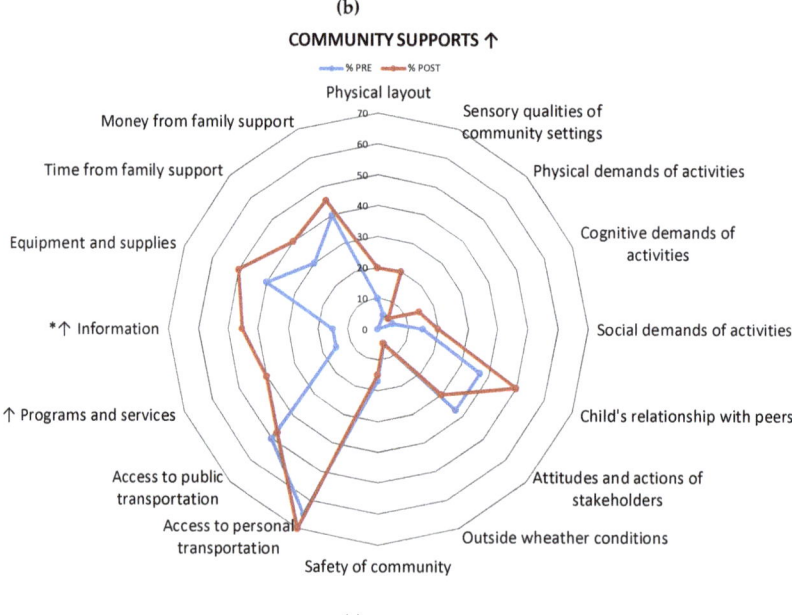

Figure 4. Percentage of parents (out of 20) who consider an environmental component as being a source of support in the home (**a**), school (**b**), and community (**c**) settings. ↑ = Increase in at least 20% of sample. * $p < 0.05$.

4. Discussion

4.1. Changes in Activities and Settings

After PREP, youth participation frequency significantly increased in the community setting, while it decreased in the home setting. This shift in participation patterns, supported by moderate to large effect sizes, is encouraging and positive as previous research shows that youth with physical disabilities tend to spend more time alone and at home [8]. Moreover, a change towards more community 'out-of-home' activities done with others is considered beneficial. In general, the majority of observed changes occurred in the community, which further supports the impact demonstrated by PREP in previous studies [19–21], and reflects the area in which the targeted activities took place (i.e., the community). The positive changes in specific activities within other settings such as the school (i.e., taking on special roles in school), found in this study, may indicate that youth and parents were applying skills they had gained during PREP in order to explore new opportunities in additional environments. This finding coincides with a qualitative study [20], in which parents whose child received the intervention, indicated that youth "had gained tools" to apply to other settings. Specifically, they expressed interest and showed initiative in taking on new roles and activities in school, for instance, an environment that was not directly targeted by PREP [20].

Youth also demonstrated changes in the types of activities that they were participating in. Participation frequency in sedentary leisure activities at home, such as *computer and video games* decreased, while frequency in active forms of leisure or social leisure in the community, such as *organized physical activities* and *classes and lessons* increased. These changes confirm a trend regarding decreased frequency of participation in digital media activities following PREP, which was initially observed in a previous study of a sub-sample of this cohort [21]. Overall, this initial shift in the types of activities undertaken supports patterns of participation and active lifestyle behaviors that are health-promoting.

Following PREP, involvement levels remained stable. This may be due, in part, to the length of study. It is possible that a 12-week period of time was not sufficient for the youth to experience the level of comfort and sense of social inclusion and belonging that comes with familiarity (of the new activity) often necessary to become fully involved [33]. As such, implementing additional prolonged follow-ups may allow changes to be observed in involvement scores, illustrating the subjective experience that is derived from the activity. Given that the PEM-CY was not completed by the youth themselves, it is possible that subtle changes in level of involvement, a highly subjective construct, would have been difficult to detect by a proxy. Regarding desire for change, it is difficult to determine whether changes occurred or not without qualitative data to complement interpretation. For example, an increase in the number of activities in which change is desired could indicate a newfound motivation, as PREP may have provided parents and youth with new insight into their participation capacity. Alternatively, an increase in activities parents wish to see change in, may indicate that parents and youth are less satisfied with the current level of participation. In-depth interviews, where participants could reflect on their PEM-CY results and the cause of changes observed, could complement interpretation.

4.2. Skill Implementation

Families likely implemented skills and knowledge obtained through PREP to modify their environments, as shown by the descriptive changes in certain barriers and supports across all settings. For example, the decrease observed in *physical demands* of activities as a barrier in the community setting likely results from coaching families (and other stakeholders) on ways of grading and adapting specific activities to youth's abilities, making activities more accessible and manageable. In addition, accessibility to resources, such as *supplies* in the home and *information* in the community (about activities, services and programs), were perceived as supports by more parents following PREP. This may reflect families gaining new knowledge about the resources available to them and new connections to other families with children with disabilities, allowing for the exchange of information, as well as developing more advanced advocacy skills. This is a valuable finding as parents who are equipped with knowledge and skills to improve their child's participation, often become "knowledge brokers", who confidently explore opportunities for their families [14].

As expected, environmental barriers encountered in the community displayed a pattern that suggests a post-intervention decrease. However, a few specific barriers were encountered more often in the home and school after PREP, especially those barriers related to the demands of the activity. These specific barriers may have been reported due to novel challenges encountered while starting new activities, such as *cognitive demands*. Additionally, at baseline, parents may not have considered that certain factors could act as barriers. Such an effect has also been reported by Kramer et al. [34], where parents identified significantly more barriers after applying a structured problem-identification strategy. It is plausible that the more one participates, the more barriers one encounters. Further studies are needed to examine this assumption.

4.3. The Impact of Child and Family Characteristics on Rates of Change

None of the children's characteristics measured at baseline were associated with rates of changes in PEM-CY scores that were found significant. This may suggest that the PREP intervention was beneficial to various youth and families regardless of their level of motivation and family functioning. Presumably, this speaks to the nature of the intervention where youth participate in an activity of choice (which can increase motivation) and where family barriers are addressed (as environmental barriers to remove). Physical functioning at baseline showed an initial trend of association with changes in participation outcomes which concur with previous research, where the effects of PREP were influenced by the number of functional issues at baseline [19]. This may be explained by the fact that PREP considers aspects of motivation and family environment but does not directly target functional issues. However, given the sample size, there was not enough power to detect clear patterns of association between child/family factors and changes in participation.

4.4. Limitations, Strengths and Future Directions

While this study included a relatively small sample size, we had sufficient power to detect changes in participation (primary objective), which has contributed an additional piece of evidence towards PREP's effectiveness as well as preliminary evidence towards its ability to foster positive change in participation beyond its three specific targeted activities. In addition, this was the first study to evaluate pre-post data using the PEM-CY, providing support for the potential ability of this tool to detect change following an intervention. However, as the PEM-CY is a parent-report measure, it may not have captured the youths' subjective experience, particularly in the desire for change and involvement scales, as those aspects of participation did not display significant differences post-intervention. Furthermore, the lack of qualitative information may have limited the interpretability of changes in these areas of participation. Overall, the results from this study are promising and warrant larger and prolonged trials in order to better capture all potential changes resulting from the PREP approach. In addition, combining results with qualitative interviews would better support interpretation of the PEM-CY, particularly with regards to parent's desire for change. Finally, further studies could also contribute evidence towards the PEM-CYs responsiveness to change.

5. Conclusions

This study contributes to a growing body of evidence that environmental-based interventions, such as PREP, are effective at enhancing participation. By equipping families with solution-based strategies, PREP may empower them to explore new opportunities beyond their initial target goals and potentially carry-over skills into other areas of participation. Further, larger and prolonged studies can be used to capture change in the subjective aspects of participation (i.e., involvement and desire for change). Consequently, this can support the multiple benefits that can be generated by one single intervention, improving the provision of rehabilitation services in pediatrics.

Author Contributions: Conceptualization, D.A.; methodology, D.A.; validation, D.A., C.H. and N.M. (Noah Margolese); formal analysis, C.H., L.B. (Louiza Benmohammed), L.B. (Liam Bienstock), N.M. (Nathan Menezes), N.M. (Noah Margolese), B.B. and D.A.; investigation, D.A.; resources, D.A.; data curation, D.A.; writing—original draft preparation, C.H., B.B., L.B. (Louiza Benmohammed), L.B. (Liam Bienstock), N.M. (Nathan Menezes); writing—review and editing, C.H., B.B., L.B. (Louiza Benmohammed), L.B. (Liam Bienstock), N.M. (Nathan Menezes), N.M. (Noah Margolese) and D.A.; visualization, C.H., B.B., L.B. (Louiza Benmohammed), L.B. (Liam Bienstock), N.M. (Nathan Menezes), N.M. (Noah Margolese) and D.A.; supervision, D.A.; project administration, D.A.; funding acquisition, D.A. All authors have read and agreed to the published version of the manuscript.

Funding: This research was funded by Canadian Institutes of Health Research, grant number 130571.

Acknowledgments: This study was funded by CIHR. It was conducted in partnership with Lethbridge-Layton-Mackay Rehabilitation Centre (Mackay site) and the Centre for Interdisciplinary Research in Rehabilitation of Greater Montreal (CRIR).

Conflicts of Interest: The authors declare no conflict of interest.

References

1. WHO. *International Classification of Functioning, Disability and Health*; WHO: Geneva, Switzerland, 2001.
2. Heah, T.; Case, T.; McGuire, B.; Law, M. Successful participation: The lived experience among children with disabilities. *Can. J. Occup. Ther.* **2007**, *74*, 38–47. [CrossRef] [PubMed]
3. Larson, R.W. Toward a psychology of positive youth development. *Am. Psychol.* **2000**, *55*, 170–183. [CrossRef] [PubMed]
4. Law, M. Participation in the occupations of everyday life. *Am. J. Occup. Ther.* **2002**, *56*, 640–649. [CrossRef] [PubMed]
5. Imms, C.; Mathews, S.; Richmond, K.N.; Law, M.; Ullenhag, A. Optimising leisure participation: A pilot intervention study for adolescents with physical impairments. *Disabil. Rehabil.* **2016**, *38*, 963–971. [CrossRef] [PubMed]
6. Jarus, T.; Anaby, D.; Bart, O.; Engel-Yeger, B.; Law, M. Childhood participation in after-school activities: What is to be expected? *Br. J. Occup. Ther.* **2010**, *73*, 344–350. [CrossRef]
7. Gorter, J.W.; Stewart, D.; Woodbury-Smith, M. Youth in transition: Care, health and development. *Child Care Health Dev.* **2011**, *37*, 757–763. [CrossRef]
8. Engel-Yeger, B.; Jarus, T.; Anaby, D.; Law, M. Differences in patterns of participation between youths with cerebral palsy and typically developing peers. *Am. J. Occup. Ther.* **2009**, *63*, 96–104. [CrossRef]
9. Michelsen, S.I.; Flachs, E.M.; Damsgaard, M.T.; Parkes, J.; Parkinson, K.; Rapp, M.; Arnaud, C.; Nystrand, M.; Colver, A.; Fauconnier, J.; et al. European study of frequency of participation of adolescents with and without cerebral palsy. *Eur. J. Paediatr. Neurol. EJPN Off. J. Eur. Paediatr. Neurol. Soc.* **2014**, *18*, 282–294. [CrossRef]
10. Bedell, G.; Coster, W.; Law, M.; Liljenquist, K.; Kao, Y.C.; Teplicky, R.; Anaby, D.; Khetani, M.A. Community participation, supports, and barriers of school-age children with and without disabilities. *Arch. Phys. Med. Rehabil.* **2013**, *94*, 315–323. [CrossRef]
11. Anaby, D.; Law, M.; Coster, W.; Bedell, G.; Khetani, M.; Avery, L.; Teplicky, R. The mediating role of the environment in explaining participation of children and youth with and without disabilities across home, school, and community. *Arch. Phys. Med. Rehabil.* **2014**, *95*, 908–917. [CrossRef]
12. Krieger, B.A.-O.; Piškur, B.; Schulze, C.; Jakobs, U.; Beurskens, A.; Moser, A. Supporting and hindering environments for participation of adolescents diagnosed with autism spectrum disorder: A scoping review. *PLoS ONE* **2018**, *13*, 1–30. [CrossRef] [PubMed]
13. Anaby, D.; Hand, C.; Bradley, L.; Direzze, B.; Forhan, M.; Digiacomo, A.; Law, M. The effect of the environment on participation of children and youth with disabilities: A scoping review. *Disabil. Rehabil.* **2013**, *35*, 1589–1598. [CrossRef]
14. Willis, C.; Girdler, S.; Thompson, M.; Rosenberg, M.; Reid, S.; Elliott, C. Elements contributing to meaningful participation for children and youth with disabilities: A scoping review. *Disabil. Rehabil.* **2017**, *39*, 1771–1784. [CrossRef] [PubMed]
15. Kramer, J.M.; Roemer, K.; Liljenquist, K.; Shin, J.; Hart, S. Formative evaluation of project TEAM (teens making environment and activity modifications). *Intell. Dev. Disabil.* **2014**, *52*, 258–272. [CrossRef]

16. Law, M.; Darrah, J.; Pollock, N.; Wilson, B.; Russell, D.J.; Walter, S.D.; Rosenbaum, P.; Galuppi, B. Focus on function: A cluster, randomized controlled trial comparing child- versus context-focused intervention for young children with cerebral palsy. *Dev. Med. Child Neurol.* **2011**, *53*, 621–629. [CrossRef] [PubMed]
17. Law, M.; Anaby, D.; Teplicky, R.; Turner, L. Pathways and Resources for Engagement and Participation (PREP): A Practice Model for Occupational Therapists. Available online: https://www.canchild.ca/en/shop/25-prep (accessed on 26 September 2016).
18. Law, M.; Anaby, D.; Imms, C.; Teplicky, R.; Turner, L. Improving the participation of youth with physical disabilities in community activities: An interrupted time series design. *Aust. Occup. Ther. J.* **2015**, *62*, 105–115. [CrossRef] [PubMed]
19. Anaby, D.; Law, M.; Feldman, D.; Majnemer, A.; Avery, L. The effectiveness of the Pathways and Resources for Engagement and Participation (PREP) intervention: Improving participation of adolescents with physical disabilities. *Dev. Med. Child Neurol.* **2018**, *60*, 513–519. [CrossRef]
20. Anaby, D.; Mercerat, C.; Tremblay, S. Enhancing youth participation using the PREP intervention: Parents' perspectives. *Int. J. Environ. Res. Public Health* **2017**, *14*. [CrossRef]
21. Anaby, D.; Vrotsou, K.; Kroksmark, U.; Ellegard, K. Changes in participation patterns of youth with physical disabilities following the Pathways and Resources for Engagement and Participation intervention: A time-geography approach. *Scand. J. Occup. Ther.* **2019**, 1–9. [CrossRef]
22. Anaby, D.; Law, M.; Teplicky, R.; Turner, L. PREP—Pathways and Resources for Engagement and Participation. Available online: https://www.prepintervention.ca/ (accessed on 12 June 2019).
23. Coster, W.; Bedell, G.; Law, M.; Khetani, M.A.; Teplicky, R.; Liljenquist, K.; Gleason, K.; Kao, Y.-C. Psychometric evaluation of the participation and environment measure for children and youth. *Dev. Med. Child Neurol.* **2011**, *53*, 1030–1037. [CrossRef]
24. Bakaniene, I.; Prasauskiene, A. Patterns and predictors of participation in children and adolescents with spina bifida. *Disabil. Rehabil.* **2019**, 1–9. [CrossRef] [PubMed]
25. Moos, R.H.; Moos, B.S. *Family Environment Scale Manual*, 4th ed.; Mind Garden, Inc.: Menlo Park, CA, USA, 2009.
26. King, G.; Law, M.; Hanna, S.; King, S.; Hurley, P.; Rosenbaum, P.; Kertoy, M.; Petrenchik, T. Predictors of the leisure and recreation participation of children with physical disabilities: A structural equation modeling analysis. *Child. Health Care* **2006**, *35*, 209–234. [CrossRef]
27. Gerhardt, C.A.; Vannatta, K.; McKellop, J.M.; Zeller, M.; Taylor, J.; Passo, M.; Noll, R.B. Comparing parental distress, family functioning, and the role of social support for caregivers with and without a child with juvenile rheumatoid arthritis. *J. Pediatr. Psychol.* **2003**, *28*, 5–15. [CrossRef]
28. Majnemer, A.; Shevell, M.; Law, M.; Poulin, C.; Rosenbaum, P. Level of motivation in mastering challenging tasks in children with cerebral palsy. *Dev. Med. Child Neurol.* **2010**, *52*, 1120–1126. [CrossRef] [PubMed]
29. Morgan, G.A.; Leech, N.L.; Barrett, K.C.; Busch-Rossnagel, N.A.; Harmon, R.J. *The Dimensions of Mastery Questionnaire*; Colorado State University: Fort Collins, CO, USA, 2000.
30. Majnemer, A.; Shevell, M.; Law, M.; Birnbaum, R.; Chilingaryan, G.; Rosenbaum, P.; Poulin, C. Participation and enjoyment of leisure activities in school-aged children with cerebral palsy. *Dev. Med. Child Neurol.* **2008**, *50*, 751–758. [CrossRef] [PubMed]
31. Beckung, E.; Hagberg, G. Neuroimpairments, activity limitations, and participation restrictions in children with cerebral palsy. *Dev. Med. Child Neurol.* **2002**, *44*, 309–316. [CrossRef] [PubMed]
32. Young, N.L.; Williams, J.I.; Yoshida, K.K.; Wright, J.G. Measurement properties of the activities scale for kids. *J. Clin. Epidemiol.* **2000**, *53*, 125–137. [CrossRef]
33. Palisano, R.J.; Begnoche, D.M.; Chiarello, L.A.; Bartlett, D.J.; McCoy, S.W.; Chang, H.-J. Amount and Focus of physical therapy and occupational therapy for young children with cerebral palsy. *Phys. Occup. Ther. Pediatr.* **2012**, *32*, 368–382. [CrossRef]
34. Kramer, J.M.; Helfrich, C.; Levin, M.; Hwang, I.T.; Samuel, P.S.; Carrellas, A.; Schwartz, A.E.; Goeva, A.; Kolaczyk, E.D. Initial evaluation of the effects of an environmental-focused problem-solving intervention for transition-age young people with developmental disabilities: Project TEAM. *Dev. Med. Child Neurol.* **2018**, *60*, 801–809. [CrossRef]

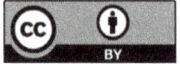

© 2020 by the authors. Licensee MDPI, Basel, Switzerland. This article is an open access article distributed under the terms and conditions of the Creative Commons Attribution (CC BY) license (http://creativecommons.org/licenses/by/4.0/).

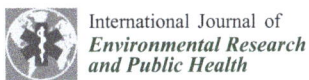

Article

Occupational Performance Coaching with Parents to Promote Community Participation and Quality of Life of Young Children with Developmental Disabilities: A Feasibility Evaluation in Hong Kong

Chi-Wen Chien [1,*], Yuen Yi Cynthia Lai [1], Chung-Ying Lin [1] and Fiona Graham [2]

[1] Department of Rehabilitation Sciences, The Hong Kong Polytechnic University, Hung Hom, Kowloon, Hong Kong (SAR), China; cynthia.yy.lai@polyu.edu.hk (Y.Y.C.L.); cylin36933@gmail.com (C.-Y.L.);
[2] Rehabilitation Teaching and Research Unit, University of Otago, Wellington South 6242, New Zealand; fi.graham@otago.ac.nz
* Correspondence: will.chien@polyu.edu.hk; Tel.: +852-2766-6703; Fax: +852-2330-8656

Received: 18 September 2020; Accepted: 28 October 2020; Published: 30 October 2020

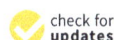

Abstract: Participation in community activities contributes to child development and health-related quality of life (HRQOL), but restricted participation has been reported in children with disabilities. Occupational performance coaching (OPC) is an intervention that targets participatory goals in child performance through coaching parents, with evidence of effectiveness for pediatric populations. Little is known about the feasibility of OPC in Hong Kong, or its effect on children's community participation and HRQOL. A mixed-methods case study design was applied to explore Hong Kong parents' experience of OPC in relation to goal achievement, community participation, and HRQOL change in children. Four parents of young children with developmental disabilities (aged five to six years) received OPC for three to eight sessions within one to three months. Quantitative pre- and post-intervention data were analyzed descriptively. Semi-structured interviews with parents were conducted at post-intervention, and analyzed using content analysis. Results showed a trend of improvement in goal performance, child involvement in community activities, and specific aspects of HRQOL among most participants. Parents perceived undertaking OPC positively, described gaining insights and skills, and felt supported. The findings suggest that OPC warrants further investigation for use in Hong Kong, to promote children's community participation and quality of life.

Keywords: occupational performance coaching; community participation; health-related quality of life; Hong Kong; preschool-aged children; developmental disability

1. Introduction

The opportunity to participate and be involved in community activities is necessary for the optimal physical, emotional, and psychological development of children [1–3]. Community participation allows children to make friends, learn skills, and develop independence and a sense of belonging. Yet, children with developmental disabilities (DD) as young as five, participate less frequently, and are less involved in community activities, compared to children with typical development [4–6]. While DD includes a heterogeneous group of impairments [7,8], lower community participation may, in itself, impede the development of children with DD [9,10], adversely affecting their health and quality of life [11,12]. Research that focuses on improving community participation for young children with DD is urgently needed [13,14].

A recent systematic review of community participation interventions in children and adolescents with DD [15], found 13 interventions that improved friendships, recreational participation, and quality of life. Few interventions were identified that were designed for and applied to children younger than six years. Current models providing early intervention services focus predominantly on body impairment, or incapacity to execute daily [16]. However, evidence indicates that these types of interventions do not necessarily contribute to improve children's participation in real-life, practical situations [17,18]. Instead, as changes in participation are considered multifactorial [2,19,20], approaches should be individually-tailored, family-centered, and ecologically-oriented.

Coaching has recently been highlighted as an evidence-based intervention that engages parents of young children in early intervention and pediatric rehabilitation [16,21,22]. Coaching is defined as partnering with clients in a thought-provoking and creative process that maximizes their personal and professional potential [23]. In pediatric rehabilitation, this takes place in family settings, by collaboratively working with parents on individualized participatory goals, identifying parents-directed solutions, and building their capacity to implement practical strategies [24].

Occupational performance coaching (OPC) [25] is one of several coaching interventions that are applicable to children with DD. OPC facilitates children's occupational performance and participation through coaching parents to implement change in the context of children's life situations. Key techniques in OPC include mindful listening, empathy, focusing on parents' priorities, collaborative performance analysis, and sharing knowledge. These techniques are used to heighten parents' engagement in the action-reflection process [25–27]. OPC is non-directive in that parents are not advised, instructed, or trained in any action or method. Instead, using goal-specific, open-ended questions, therapists guide parents to identify highly individualized and practical strategies to improve children's participation. As such, OPC takes an enablement-focused, family-centered, and ecologically-oriented approach to address participation difficulties faced by children with DD and their families [25].

Emerging evidence that supports the effectiveness of OPC includes case studies [28–30], time-series [31], and randomized controlled trial designs [32]. The effects of OPC on parents' wellbeing, including self-competence, have also been demonstrated [28,31,32]. However, the extent to which OPC leads to changes in community participation is unclear, given individualized measures of personally-identified participation goals were used in all of previous studies, with no subgroup analysis of community participation effects. Furthermore, few studies investigated whether OPC could improve children's quality of life or parents' emotional states. To date, existing evidence for OPC has been established in Germany [30], Australia [28], Canada [29], and Iran [32], but more research is needed to test its feasibility when applied to parents with other cultural backgrounds.

Hong Kong has a culture influenced strongly by Chinese collectivism [33,34], and there seems to be a lot of stigma and shame surrounding children with disabilities and their families [35,36]. Consequently, this could lead parents to withdraw themselves and their children from social situations [37]. Indeed, young children with DD in Hong Kong have been reported to participate less in community activities [6,38], compared to those in other countries [4], and this decreased participation appears to correlate significantly to their parents' parental stress [6,38]. These issues highlight the need for an effective approach that supports parents and their young children with DD and promotes community participation.

The primary aim of this study was to investigate the feasibility of OPC in Hong Kong, with parents of young children (aged < 6 years) with DD, to promote children's community participation and health-related quality of life (HRQOL). Moreover, we also aimed to explore parents' experience of OPC, its effect on their emotions, and their perception of autonomy support from OPC (compared to conventional early intervention services). Specifically, the research questions were: (1) Can OPC lead to improvement in community participation and HRQOL of young children with DD? (2) Can OPC lead to improvement in parents' self-competence, emotional states, and perceived autonomy support? and (3) What are parents' experiences of being coached with OPC?

2. Materials and Methods

2.1. Study Design

A mixed-methods case study design was used to examine the feasibility of applying OPC to Hong Kong parents of young children with DD. Both quantitative and qualitative methods were used to collect and analyze case study data. Quantitatively, pre-post intervention measures were used to describe children's community participation and HRQOL. Parents' goal performance and satisfaction, self-competence, emotional states, and perceived autonomy support were also measured quantitatively. The qualitative approach utilized a semi-structured interview to explore parents' experience of OPC after the intervention. Ethical approval for the study was granted by the Human Subjects Ethics Sub-committee at The Hong Kong Polytechnic University (number: HSEARS20190114005).

2.2. Participants

Parent-child dyads were recruited, via convenience sampling, from three local non-governmental organizations that provided early intervention services to preschool-aged children with DD. Inclusion criteria were: (1) the child had been diagnosed with developmental delay, autism spectrum disorder, intellectual disability, or attention deficit/hyperactivity disorder, by local multidisciplinary child assessment centers; (2) the child was aged between two and five years (inclusive); (3) parents were able to read Chinese; and (4) parent(s) were the main caregiver(s) of the eligible child. Children with comorbidities of specific physical impairment (e.g., cerebral palsy or amputation), blindness, or deafness, were excluded from the study. This is because children with physical/visual/hearing constraints might need more complex environmental modifications or provision of assisting devices for participation in community activities, which were tentatively excluded from the present study. Written consent was obtained from the parents prior to research participation.

2.3. Instruments

2.3.1. Parent-Identified Community Participation Priorities

The Chinese version of the Canadian Occupational Performance Measure (COPM) [39] was used to measure parents' perceptions of children's community participation. The COPM identifies individualized problems in participation in occupations through a semi-structured interview. A two-point or larger difference in COPM scores between pre-post interventions is considered clinically important [39]. The COPM has adequate test-retest reliability [40] and internal consistency (Cronbach's alpha = 0.73–0.88) [41].

Parents were asked to identify goals related to their child's participation, and to rate the child's performance and their satisfaction with current performance on a 10-point Likert scale (1 = not good/satisfied at all, and 10 = optimal performance/satisfaction). Consistent with COPM and OPC, parents were invited to identify goals related to any life areas. In addition to COPM protocol, parents were invited to identify at least one goal for their child's community participation.

2.3.2. Parent-Reported Community Participation in Children

The community section of the Young Children's Participation and Environment Measure (YC-PEM) [4], a caregiver-report questionnaire, was used to evaluate the extent of children's participation in various community activities. Parents were asked to complete 10 items regarding community activities such as outings, class and group activities, community events, and recreational/leisure activities. For each item, parents evaluated three dimensions of child participation: (a) the frequency of participation, using an eight-point Likert scale (never = 0, and once or more each day = 7); (b) the degree of involvement, using a five-point Likert scale (not very involved = 1, and very involved = 5); and (c) whether the caregivers want a change in their child's participation (yes or no, if yes, specify the type(s) of desired change). Three types of participation summary scores (frequency, involvement, and desire for change) can thus be generated, and the score calculation was detailed in Khetani et al.'s study [4]. We analyzed the frequency and involvement dimensions because they are two important aspects representing children's participation patterns [20].

The community section of the YC-PEM has adequate test-retest reliability (interclass correlation coefficients (ICC) = 0.84–89) [6]. Minimal detectable change (MDC) values of 0.7 points were also established for both the frequency and involvement scales [6]. Internal consistency of the YC-PEM was acceptable for the frequency (Cronbach's alpha = 0.64–0.68) and involvement (Cronbach's alpha = 0.77–0.96) scales in its community section [4,6].

2.3.3. Parent-Reported HRQOL in Children

The parent-report version of the Kiddy-KINDL questionnaire was used to measure HRQOL in children aged three to six years. The Kiddy-KINDL comprises 24 items that assess parents' perceptions of their child's HRQOL across six dimensions: physical wellbeing, emotional wellbeing, self-esteem, family, social contacts, and school functioning. The recall period was pre-set as the last month in this study, and each item is rated using a five-point Likert scale (0 = never, and 4 = all the time). Item scores were summed up to indicate dimension scores, and these were summed up to indicate an overall score. Raw dimension and overall scores were subsequently transformed into a scale of 0–100 to facilitate interpretation [42]. The Kiddy-KINDL has demonstrated acceptable internal consistency (Cronbach's alpha = 0.70–0.89) [43,44].

2.3.4. Parenting Self-Competence in Parents

The Parenting Sense of Competence Scale (PSOC) [45] comprises 16 items, and was used to obtain parents' perception of their parenting role in the two dimensions of efficacy and satisfaction. Parents were asked to rate each item on a six-point Likert scale (6 = strongly disagree, and 1 = strongly agree). Total scores were generated by summing all items in each subscale (after reversing the negatively worded items). The PSOC has demonstrated good test-retest reliability (ICCs = 0.82–85) and internal consistency (Cronbach's alpha = 0.77–0.80) [45].

2.3.5. Self-Reported Emotional States in Parents

The Depression, Anxiety and Stress Scale-21 (DASS-21) [46] was used to measure parents' negative emotional states of depression, anxiety, and stress. It is a self-report questionnaire and includes 21 items (7 items for each subscale of depression, anxiety, and stress). Each item is rated on a four-point Likert scale (0 = did not apply to me at all, and 3 = applied to me very much or most of time). Total scores were generated by summing all items in each subscale and multiplying by two. Good internal consistency (Cronbach's alpha = 0.77–0.87) of the DASS-21 has been reported [46].

2.3.6. Parents' Perceived Autonomy Support from Health Care Practitioners

The Health Care Climate Questionnaire (HCCQ) [47] was used to measure the degree to which parents perceived how their health care practitioners encouraged their autonomy. In this study, the term "health care practitioners" was changed to their child's occupational therapists at pre-intervention, and to OPC coach at post-intervention for comparison. Parents were asked to respond to 15 items regarding their relationship with the occupational therapist (OPC coach), on a seven-point Likert scale (1 = strongly disagree, and 7 = strongly agree). Mean of the 15 items was calculated to create the HCCQ index. Good internal consistency (Cronbach's alpha = 0.95) of the HCCQ has been reported [47,48].

2.3.7. Demographic Information

A parent-reported questionnaire was designed to collect demographic information such as child age and gender, family structure, family income, and both parents' age, occupation, and education. During telephone screening, parents were also asked to report the type(s) of clinical diagnosis their child had obtained from the reports of child assessment centers, and rate the severity of their child's disability as a whole, using a four-point Likert scale (1 = very mild, and 4 = severe). In addition, participants' names were collected but replaced by the numbers in this study, allowing for confidentiality when reported.

2.3.8. Parents' Experience of OPC Intervention

A semi-structured guide was developed to elicit parents' experience of OPC. This interview guide included a list of open-ended questions, as well as related probes, allowing direct questions with flexibility when pertinent information emerged during the interview. We designed the guide to explore multiple aspects of parents' interview experience regarding their perceptions, satisfaction, perceived effects, process, and suggestions on OPC intervention. Appendix A details the guiding questions used in the interview.

2.4. Procedure

Research invitations were distributed to eligible participants through occupational therapists working in non-governmental rehabilitation services. Parents who were interested in participating contacted a research assistant, and were screened for eligibility during a telephone conversation. Following signed consent and enrolment in the study, pre-intervention measures (the YC-PEM, Kiddy-KINDL, PSOC, DASS-21, HCCQ and demographic questionnaire) were posted to parents, two weeks before intervention. During the goal setting session, the COPM was administered, by the first author (Chi-Wen Chien), at a location of the parents' choice.

Subsequently, parents attended a maximum of eight weekly sessions of OPC (each for one hour at most). OPC sessions were delivered through several modes, including face-to-face at a location of the parents' choice, or through Zoom video communications (Zoom, San Jose, CA, USA). Consistent with OPC guidance [25], children's attendance at the coaching sessions was at the parents' discretion. During the study period, either parents, their child, or both, continued pre-existing service engagement.

One week after the completion of the OPC sessions, the parents repeated all outcome measures. The COPM was completed with the research assistant, who was blind to the treatment content. The research assistant also conducted the post-intervention interview of the parents' experience of OPC. All interviews lasted 20–40 min, and were conducted via Zoom and audio-recorded. At the two month follow-up, all measures except for the HCCQ were repeated a third time.

2.5. OPC Intervention

OPC was delivered by the first author (Chi-Wen Chien), who is an occupational therapist and researcher. He attended a three-day training workshop conducted by the last author (Fiona Graham), the OPC developer. Prior to the study, he practiced with five parents of children with and without disabilities (achieving the fidelity ratings at an average of 84.4%), and received ongoing guidance from the OPC developer to ensure his fidelity of OPC.

The OPC sessions involved techniques comprising the three enabling domains described by Graham et al. [25]: connect, structure, and share. Connect refers to building parents' trust in the therapist, by using verbal and nonverbal strategies such as mindful listening, empathizing, and partnering, to help parents shift from an emotional (reactive) to a solution-focused (proactive) orientation. Structure alludes to building parents' competence, by guiding them through a problem-solving framework of setting goals, exploring options, planning action, carrying out plans, checking performance, and generalizing. Share refers to optimizing parents' autonomy, by emphasizing and building on parents existing knowledge, skills, and resources.

In the first OPC session, parent(s) and the therapist identified one goal that was currently important to the parent(s), regardless of the performance and satisfaction ratings provided in the COPM. The therapist engaged parents in collaborative performance analysis of that goal, by following the four steps to: (a) identify parents' perception of what currently happened, (b) identify what parents would like to happen, (c) explore barriers and bridges to the desired performance, and (d) identify their needs for taking actions to achieve goals. Each session ended with clarification of the action plan for the following week. In subsequent sessions, parents were prompted to review the usefulness of planned actions to achieve goals. When strategies were useful, the therapist guided parents to generalize their application to other aspects of life. Unsuccessful strategies became discussion points to review goals, knowledge, and alternative ways of engaging in goal activities.

2.6. Data Analysis

Case descriptions were developed to characterize participating children and parents, specify parents' goals, and describe the progress of OPC sessions. Quantitative data were next analyzed using descriptive statistics such as mean, standard deviation, and proportion, and were reported in table forms. No inference statistical analysis was performed because of the nature of the descriptive case study design with a small sample size.

For qualitative data, audio-recorded interviews were transcribed verbatim. Conventional content analysis was used to analyze the interview data [49,50]. Specifically, the first author (Chi-Wen Chien) initially read the transcripts to obtain a general sense of the content. The analysis of manifest content was followed by open coding process independently done by the two coders. In the process, they generated the codes inductively, and read transcripts again to refine and condense codes into extended meaning units, before placing similar codes together where they fitted under an emerging category or sub-category. Once preliminary categories and sub-categories, if needed, were generated, the two coders met and reviewed the coded data to determine if each category/sub-category formed apparently coherent patterns with sufficient supporting data. Discrepancy was discussed and the final list of categories and sub-categories was determined through consensus among the coders.

3. Results

3.1. Case Descriptions

Initially, six parents participated in this study, completed pre-intervention questionnaires, and attended the goal setting sessions (see Table 1). Cases consisted of five boys and one girl, ranging from 4–5.5 years of age. Most of the children had been diagnosed with either DD, autism, or both, and the parent-perceived severity of child disability was reported as mild or moderate.

Table 1. Details of demographic characteristics of participants and the OPC sessions delivered.

Characteristics	Case 1	Case 2	Case 3	Case 4	Case 5	Case 6
Age (years)	5.25	4.00	5.50	5.25	5.33	5.25
Gender	Boy	Boy	Boy	Girl	Boy	Boy
Diagnosis	Autism and DD	Autism	Autism and DD	DD	DD and dyslexia	Autism and DD
Parent-reported severity of disability	Mild	Moderate	Moderate	Moderate	Mild	Mild
Father/mother's age (years)	50/40	45/43	33/36	38/37	44/43	45/32
Father/mother's educational qualification	Bachelor/Bachelor	Form 5/Form 5	Bachelor/Bachelor	Postgraduate/Bachelor	Postgraduate/Postgraduate	A-level/Bachelor
Parent(s) being coached	Father and mother	Mother *	Mother	Mother *	Mother	Father †
Number of coaching sessions received	6 ‡	1	8	1	6 ‡	3 ‡
Number of weeks	10	1	11	1	7	5
Delivery mode	Internet	Face-to-face	Internet	Internet	Face-to-face	Face-to-face

* Two parents withdrew from the study after attending the first session. † The mother joined the second coaching session with the father once. ‡ Coaching was terminated earlier owing to the outbreak of COVID-19. The parent(s) received face-to-face coaching in the first session but chose internet-based coaching for the remaining sessions. Abbreviation: DD, developmental delay.

Each parent identified five to eight goals (mean = 6.7; SD = 1.0) and, of those goals, between one and three (mean = 1.8; SD = 0.8) were related specifically to the child's community participation (see Table 2 for details). Coached participants included one pair of parents, four mothers, and one father. After the first OPC session, two mothers withdrew from the study due to child illness ($n = 1$), and preference for an expert-directed approach ($n = 1$). The remaining four participants are included in the analyses. Parents received three to eight coaching sessions (mean = 5.8 and SD = 2.1), across 5–11 weeks (mean = 8.3; SD = 2.8), dependent on goal achievement. Detailed information on coaching sessions and delivery modes is provided in Table 1. Appendix B provides narrative descriptions of OPC intervention processes and goal achievement in each session.

Table 2. COPM scores for parent-identified goals for their children and themselves.

	Goals	Performance			Satisfaction		
		Pre	Post	FU	Pre	Post	FU
Case 1	Demonstrates stable emotion when talking to the parents or his old brother	5	7	8	6	7	8
	Completes homework with concentration at home	6	6	8	6	7	8
	Participates in school activities with concentration and cooperation	6	8	7	6	8	7
	Shows friendly and good interaction with classmates at school	5	7	7	5	7	7
	* Engages in and keeps focused on the activities during the group's interest classes	5	7	8	6	8	8
	* Shows kindness and does not affect other children outside the home	5	6	7	6	7	7
	Parents learn about the child's emotions and know to deal with his emotional changes	3	7	8	4	7	8
Case 2	Eats the dinner at home on his own by sitting on his chair and has more attempts to try different kinds of food	4	-	-	6	-	-
	Feels acceptable when having haircut at home or at hair salon	5	-	-	4	-	-
	* Eats the meals outside home with more concentration and not watching iPhone or iPad all the time	3	-	-	3	-	-
	* Feels more comfortable when taking public transportation (e.g., MTR, bus, or taxi) for outings	4	-	-	5	-	-
	Wears different clothes and shoes before going outside	4	-	-	6	-	-
	Completes the homework at home by sitting well on the chair	5	-	-	4	-	-
	* Parent finds suitable ways/approaches/strategies to bring the child outside when taking public/private transportation	6	-	-	5	-	-
Case 3	*Regulates himself when getting excited*	3	4	5	2	5	6
	Plays appropriately during his free time at home	3	3	4	2	3	4
	Expresses himself and gets adults' approval before going somewhere outside	5	7	7	7	8	7
	* Goes out to join activities with other kids and has more interactions	2	4	3	6	6	7
	* Performs appropriate interaction behaviors when meeting people/children	6	8	7	2	8	8
	Parent sets up daily routines between family and work to bring the child go out to park or do home training programs	4	7	8	3	6	8
Case 4	Eats meals at home independently and keeps the body and table clean	4	-	-	2	-	-
	Puts on clothes independently	5	-	-	4	-	-
	Does and revises homework with concentration at home	5	-	-	3	-	-
	Engages in games by herself for 15 min at home	4	-	-	4	-	-
	* Performs appropriate social behaviors when playing with other kids at the playground or party in the community	3	-	-	4	-	-
	Brushes teeth routinely with adults' assistance	3	-	-	4	-	-
	Controls emotion when things do not fall in with her wishes	3	-	-	5	-	-

Table 2. Cont.

	Goals	Performance			Satisfaction		
		Pre	Post	FU	Pre	Post	FU
Case 5	Goes to bed by 9:30 p.m. and has the story time completed before that	1	6	4	1	7	5
	Knows the name of tools and uses them in appropriate ways at home	3	5	5	3	6	5
	Tidies up personal belongings at home	7	7	6	5	7	6
	Completes homework with motivation to learn the stroke sequence at home	6	6	6	5	6	6
	Plays toys with his little sister	4	7	5	3	7	6
	Interacts with other siblings during the reading time at home	5	8	6	4	6	6
	* Joins other kids' plays by asking first at clubhouse or church	1	4	5	2	4	5
	Parent incorporates school activities in the child's learning activities at home	1	6	4	1	6	4
Case 6	Does homework with concentration for 30 min at home	2	6	2	1	6	1
	* Plays with other kids appropriately at playground or friends' social events	5	5	6	2	6	5
	* Communicates with other kids or adults appropriately during play/daily life	3	8	7	2	9	5
	Pays attention to put on socks on his own	4	9	7	3	9	8
	Plays games and responds appropriately when losing the games in play	1	6	3	1	7	2

Italicized goals indicate that they were dealt in the OPC sessions. * indicates the goals related to children's community participation. Abbreviation: FU, follow-up.

3.2. Quantitative Results

For parent-identified goals as measured by the COPM, the differences between pre- and post-intervention were greater than or equal to two points in the performance and satisfaction of 19 (73.1%) of 26 goals, and for 5 (71.4%) of 7 goals specific to community participation (see Table 2). Goal performance and satisfaction decreased slightly at two months follow up, but were maintained beyond clinically important levels in terms of the average among the four parents (see Table 3).

Table 3. Aggregated scores of outcome measures related to goals and community participation over time.

Outcome Measures (Score Range)	Pre Mean (SD)	Post Mean (SD)	FU Mean (SD)	Difference across Time		
				Pre vs. Post Mean (SD)	Post vs. FU Mean (SD)	Pre vs. FU Mean (SD)
COPM for all goals						
Child performance (range 0–10)	3.83 (0.85)	6.32 (0.66)	5.85 (1.21)	2.50 (0.95) *	−0.48 (1.13)	2.02 (0.42) *
Parents' satisfaction (range 0–10)	3.55 (1.59)	6.58 (0.93)	5.73 (1.41)	3.03 (1.84) *	−0.85 (1.63)	2.18 (0.26) *
COPM for goals specific to community participation						
Child performance (range 0–10)	3.50 (1.73)	5.75 (1.19)	6.03 (1.27)	2.25 (0.65)	0.28 (0.98)	2.52 (1.23)
Parents' satisfaction (range 0–10)	3.50 (1.91)	6.50 (1.68)	6.25 (1.44)	3.00 (1.78)	−0.25 (1.55)	2.75 (0.87)
YC-PEM						
Frequency (range 0–7)	3.30 (0.42)	3.20 (0.31)	2.25 (0.51)	−0.09 (0.31)	−0.95 (0.58) *	−1.05 (0.47) *
Involvement (range 1–5)	3.34 (0.45)	3.94 (0.51)	3.75 (0.48)	0.60 (0.49)	−0.19 (0.23)	0.40 (0.59)

* indicates the change scores beyond clinically important change of 2 points in parent-identified goal performance and satisfaction or beyond the minimal detectable change value of 0.7 points in children's community participation frequency and involvement. Abbreviations: COPM, Canadian Occupational Performance Measure; YC-PEM, Young Children's Participation and Environment Measure.

For children's community participation, as measured by the YC-PEM, there was a trend of positive changes in all four children's involvement. The average change scores were 0.6 and 0.4 between pre- and post-intervention, and between pre-intervention and follow-up, respectively. However, the magnitude of the average change scores did not exceed the MDC value of 0.7 points of the YC-PEM [6]. On the contrary, there was a trend of a small decrease in the participation frequency scores of half the children, between pre- and post-intervention. The magnitude of the decrease in the children's participation frequency between post-intervention and follow-up and between pre-intervention and follow-up (see Table 3) was larger than the MDC value of 0.7 points, indicating a true decrease beyond the random measurement error.

Table 4 shows the results of outcome measures in relation to children's HRQOL and parent-related outcome. For HRQOL as measured by the Kiddy-KINDL, two to four children were reported by their parents as having a tendency to experience a positive increase in physical wellbeing (mean change = 12.50), family (mean change = 4.69), and school functioning (mean change = 4.69) after OPC intervention, compared to their baseline status. However, except for self-esteem, all aspects of HRQOL tended to decrease negatively between post-intervention and follow-up. By considering the entire study period between pre-intervention and follow-up, only the physical wellbeing had a positive increasing trend (mean = 7.81) in all the four children.

Table 4. Aggregated scores of outcome measures related to children's HRQOL and parents' mental health and parenting competence over time.

Outcome Measures (Score Range)	Pre Mean (SD)	Post Mean (SD)	FU Mean (SD)	Difference across Time		
				Pre vs. Post Mean (SD)	Post vs. FU Mean (SD)	Pre vs. FU Mean (SD)
Kiddy-KINDL (range 0–100)						
Total	57.03 (5.85)	60.42 (1.90)	55.47 (5.13)	3.39 (4.28)	−4.94 (3.93)	−1.56 (3.24)
Physical wellbeing	67.19 (5.98)	79.69 (5.98)	75.00 (8.84)	12.50 (5.10)	−4.69 (11.83)	7.81 (7.86)
Emotional wellbeing	65.63 (6.25)	64.38 (6.25)	63.75 (6.25)	−1.25 (0)	−0.63 (0)	−1.88 (0)
Self-esteem	54.69 (7.86)	51.56 (10.67)	53.13 (8.07)	−3.13 (3.61)	1.56 (9.38)	−1.56 (7.86)
Family	57.81 (9.37)	62.50 (5.10)	53.13 (16.54)	4.69 (10.67)	−9.38 (13.01)	−4.68 (16.44)
Social contacts	43.75 (10.21)	43.75 (11.41)	39.06 (5.98)	0 (16.93)	−4.69 (9.38)	−4.68 (13.86)
School functioning	53.13 (15.73)	57.81 (5.98)	51.56 (18.66)	4.69 (10.67)	−6.25 (15.31)	−1.56 (10.67)
DASS-21 (range 0–42)						
Stress	11.50 (8.39)	10.50 (7.19)	10.50 (4.12)	−1.00 (2.00)	0 (5.89)	1.00 (6.63)
Anxiety	3.50 (3.00)	2.50 (2.51)	3.00 (2.00)	−1.00 (2.00)	0.50 (1.00)	0.50 (2.51)
Depression	5.50 (5.00)	3.00 (2.58)	4.50 (1.91)	−2.50 (4.43)	1.50 (2.51)	1.00 (3.46)
PSOC						
Satisfaction (range 9–54)	30.00 (5.29)	30.75 (8.30)	28.50 (4.79)	0.75 (4.50)	−2.25 (5.80)	−1.50 (1.73)
Efficacy (range 7–42)	25.25 (6.18)	26.50 (2.88)	27.20 (3.77)	1.25 (4.03)	0.75 (6.02)	2.00 (7.83)
HCCQ (range 1–7)	5.70 (0.91)	6.43 (0.58)	-	0.73 (0.37)	-	-

Abbreviations: DASS-21, Depression, Anxiety and Stress Scale-21; PSOC, Parenting Sense of Competence Scale; HCCQ, Health Care Climate Questionnaire.

A similar pattern was observed in the parents' emotional states and parenting competence. That is, the parents' emotional problems, especially depressive symptoms as measured by the DASS-21, tended to improve after OPC intervention, but deteriorate at follow-up when compared to pre- or post-intervention (see Table 4). For parenting competence as measured by the PSOC, the change in parents' satisfaction tended to increase at post-intervention, but decrease at follow-up. One exception was the parenting efficacy which tended to improve gradually at both post-intervention and follow-up period (mean change = 1.25 and 0.75, respectively). In addition, there was a trend that all four parents reported higher HCCQ scores for the OPC therapist's autonomy-supportive behaviors, in comparison with their child's occupational therapist (mean difference = 0.73).

3.3. Qualitative Results

Four major categories (with 12 sub-categories in total) in relation to the parents' experience of OPC intervention were identified from the coding of their post-intervention interviews. These included: (1) increased insight and learning, (2) experiencing changes in their child, (3) positive coach-parent relationship, and (4) factors affecting coaching experience and suggestions. Table 5 shows a summary of the four categories and 12 sub-categories, and illustrative quotations under each sub-category are provided in Appendix C.

Table 5. Categories and sub-categories for parents' experience of OPC.

Category	Sub-Categories with Examples
Increased insight and learning	Sub-category 1: New insight into child's difficulties • The parents understood which time slot in the day that the child had the best emotional status. Sub-category 2: New insight into parents' needs • The parents gained an insight into how they are supposed to train with the child properly. Sub-category 3: Learning new strategies, skills, or thinking models • The parents learnt techniques that could be applied to see how time could be arranged for the child's activities. • The parents could think about what is the most ideal way to solve the child's problem slowly.
Experiencing changes in their child	Sub-category 1: Increased participation in home activities • The child completed homework within a reasonable time frame. • The child read more stories and did housework together with the parents and siblings. Sub-category 2: Increased emotion or confidence • The number of times the child lost their temper dropped. • The child built confidence in school life.
Positive coach-parent relationship	Sub-category 1: Felt supported or encouraged • The parents felt that the coach gave good advice. • The parents were encouraged to keep working towards the target. Sub-category 2: Felt understood • The parents felt that the coach understood their difficulties and the situation in Hong Kong.
Factors affecting coaching experience and suggestions	Sub-category 1: Disturbed by social issues or seasonal holidays • Schools were closed owing to social unrest, and the child's whole routine was messed up. Sub-category 2: Delivery mode and location of coaching • Some parents preferred face-to-face coaching and some parents preferred internet-based coaching to show their home environment to the coach. Sub-category 3: Number of coaching sessions • The parents wanted more coaching sessions to achieve their goals or build better habits to train their child. Sub-category 4: Frequency of coaching sessions • The parents wanted more than one week to observe the child's improvement or have more time to apply the strategies. Sub-category 5: Additional suggestions • The parents suggested that the coach could provide access to a resource book, email/mobile message reminders, or parents' education before or during OPC.

3.3.1. Increased Insight and Learning

All parents considered their coaching experience to have contributed to an increased insight of their and their child's needs. For example, the mother of Case 3 realized that her lack of time-management skills hindered the implementation of effective strategies to her child's morning routine. Shifting her focus to her own time management led to goal progress. The other three parents reported an increased understanding of their child's emotions or learning styles, which allowed them to explore or adjust strategies to meet the child's needs. Most parents reported that access to strategies, skills, or thinking models during OPC, enabled them to facilitate their child's activity participation.

3.3.2. Experiencing Changes in Their Child

Three of the four parents reported their children participated more in home activities, following the OPC, for example, children were more engaged in doing homework or playing with siblings at home. The parents also observed changes in their child's emotions or confidence at home, at school, or in the community. However, when asked about whether OPC had helped with their child's participation in community activities, no to little improvement was reported.

3.3.3. Positive Coach-Parent Relationship

Positive partnership between the therapist and parents was a major category, which contributed to parents' perceptions of how OPC had helped to facilitate their child's participation. Those parents felt supported by the therapist to guide the solution-focused thinking process, or felt encouraged to focus on goal achievement, with constant experimentation of suitable strategies. The parents also felt understood and accepted by the therapist.

3.3.4. Factors Affecting Coaching Experience and Suggestions

The parents expressed a consistently high level of satisfaction regarding the coaching process. For example, the mother of Case 5 said *"The parent-coaching process is very good. The 1-h meeting drove us to be very focused."* The most common word to describe their perceptions of the OPC process was *"satisfied"*. However, the parents commented that their experience of coaching had been compromised either by the social unrest, seasonal holidays, or both, particularly when their child was unable to go to school as usual. Two parents (Cases 5 and 6) also preferred the face-to-face coaching mode, but the father of Case 6, who had had coaching in his car due to it being the quietest option, was displeased with the lack of formality. On the other hand, the parents of Cases 1 and 3 enjoyed the advantage of having internet-based coaching.

In addition, the parents provided several suggestions regarding the application of OPC in Hong Kong, for example, an increase in the total number of coaching sessions but a decrease in their frequency, would give the parents more time to try the planned strategies, or see the improvement, especially during seasonal holidays. Access to a resource book, email/mobile message reminders, or parents' education before or during OPC, were some of the other suggestions.

4. Discussion

The case studies evaluated the feasibility of OPC with Hong Kong parents, to promote community participation and HRQOL of their young children with DD. Overall, quantitative results indicated clinically meaningful gains in the performance and satisfaction of parents' identified goals regarding children's community participation after OPC intervention. A trend for the post-intervention gains were also revealed in children's participation involvement in community activities, although only a relatively small improvement in the children's HRQOL was observed after OPC. Most parents tended to experience an increase in their parenting self-competence and perceived autonomy support. This concurred with qualitative findings that parents engaged in the OPC process positively, gained insights about their child and themselves, learnt new skills/mindsets, and felt supported. The parents' positive engagement and learning in the OPC process might help them in facilitating children's participation and emotions. Additionally, parents provided several suggestions on the OPC process in Hong Kong, which warrant consideration for future studies.

Coaching has been increasingly used as the core approach in several interventions that have been found to promote children's community participation [51–53]. Similarly, our case studies also support the use of OPC to achieve parents' aspirations regarding children's participation in community activities. Nevertheless, in this study, not all community-related goals were addressed during OPC sessions. According to post-intervention interviews, parents perceived change in their child's participation mostly at home. We thus think that the increase in children's community participation may have resulted from the generalization effect of OPC, as reported in previous studies [28,31,54]. This is because, during OPC, parents' generalization of successful strategies is encouraged by explicitly asking them about other areas to which the strategies might apply [25]. For example, the mother of Case 1 reported that her child became cooperative in his extracurricular piano lessons, after she shared the strategy with the teacher that had helped motivating her child to do homework. Parents also reported a range of enhancements to their capacity, and showed an increase in their parenting efficacy and autonomy. These findings reflect the possibility of changing parents' mindsets or behaviors, empowering them to be active in supporting their child's involvement in community activities.

Contrary to the trend of the increased involvement in community activities after OPC, no increase in the frequency of community activities among children was observed from the results of the YC-PEM. The different nature of community activities may be one possible reason for the finding. For example, some community activities occur regularly (e.g., weekly extracurricular lessons), whereas others are held on specific occasions (e.g., summer overnight trips, parades). Furthermore, preschool children, as they are young, tend to have regular daily routines [55], making little room for them to take part in community activities more often. Maul and Singer [56] found that some types of community activities (e.g., going to crowded places or shopping malls) were avoided by parents of young children with disabilities. Additionally, during 2019–2020, protests against the extradition bill took place over the weekends in Hong Kong [57], when the case studies were carried out. This also coincided with the outbreak of Coronavirus Disease 2019 (COVID-19) in early 2020, which rendered children and people to self-isolate and, in turn, might affect the primary outcome of the present study (i.e., frequency of community activities).

Improved parent-identified goal performance using OPC appeared to be translated into increased HRQOL of children, even though the increase was small, domain-specific, and of unclear clinical significance. We found a trend that some children had higher physical wellbeing and family and school functioning after OPC, perhaps because their parents developed increased insights about the child, and learnt handling skills/strategies. Those parents might know how to arrange activities and optimize their child's vitality, manage conflict between the child and themselves, and enable the child to complete homework. On the contrary, no improvement, or even a decreasing trend for the children's psychosocial aspects of HRQOL (i.e., emotional wellbeing, self-esteem, and social contacts with friends) was noted. This could be explained by the systematic impact of social unrest, as mentioned above, causing the families to stay at home and feel unhappy [58,59]. The trend of decreased emotional wellbeing and self-esteem, however, was somewhat contradictory to the findings of some parents' post-intervention interviews, where OPC was indicated to benefit the child's emotions and confidence. We speculated that such improvement could be specific to certain contexts, which may not be reflected by comprehensive HRQOL measures. Given that the finding is preliminary at the case-study level, continued studies are warranted to clarify the effect of OPC on children's HRQOL.

Consistent with previous findings of OPC [31,32], the parents in this study tended to show improvements in their sense of efficacy in parenting. We also found that those parents felt supported and understood by the OPC therapist, and perceived the therapist as more supportive of their autonomy, compared to their child's occupational therapist. This might be because traditional early intervention tends to focus directly on children, whereas coaching is a highly collaborative approach highlighting close partnership with the family [22,60]. In OPC, parents can identify goals meaningful to them, create their own strategies, and plan with the coach when to implement such strategies in practice. Furthermore, some parents in this study tended to report a small reduction of their stress, anxiety, and depression at post-intervention. This suggests that the tendency for their improved emotional wellbeing may be related to that for either their increased self-efficacy, autonomy support, or both, gained from OPC. This is consistent with the findings of Dunn et al.'s study [61] which used similar coaching approaches, and parents reported increased parental efficiency but decreased distress. Thus, coaching may lead to improvements, in not only child-related, but also parent-related outcomes, including self-efficacy, autonomy, or even emotional states [60].

The parents in this study generally expressed satisfaction with the OPC process but, inevitably, their experience was compromised by the social unrest, which impacted on the delivery mode and locations of intervention. From post-intervention interviews, we noticed that the parents of Cases 1 and 3 enjoyed having internet-coaching in their homes, while the other two parents favored face-to-face modalities, either at home or in a formal location. This suggests that, regardless of the coaching mode used, parents seem to prefer interventions that focus on the home environment, as this could be more useful to their child. As the comparative influence of remote versus face-to-face use of OPC is not yet fully understood [28], it might be preferable to use one or the other in a consistent manner, while tending to each participant's preferences and needs.

All parents suggested the necessity of having either more sessions, time between the sessions, or both. These suggestions were expected, as three of the four participants had merely three or six sessions, owing to the impact of COVID-19. There were also unforeseen variations in family schedules during seasonal holidays, or school suspension caused by the social unrest. Parents thus needed to cope with the variations immediately, and were unable to try out the planned action agreed upon during each OPC session. To accommodate such situations, and allow for more time to implement the plan, we decided to reduce the frequency of the sessions from weekly to weekly/fortnightly in future interventions. The total number of eight sessions, however, will be kept the same, given that the coaching frequency has been reduced, and the entire coaching period is lengthened. We think that the parents' additional suggestions (e.g., providing handbooks, reminders, or parental education) are more relevant to parent's training, where therapists tend to instruct parents and demonstrate how to apply strategies in a straightforward manner. According to Akhbari Ziegler and Hadders-Algra [62], these are unlikely to fit into approaches like OPC, where the focus is on empowering and supporting parents in the process of decision making regarding strategies specific to their child's participation in daily life activities.

Limitations of this study include the small number of case studies, the inclusion of all boys as the child participants and, especially, the influence of the social unrest and COVID-19 on study progress and outcome. For example, the parents attributed the lack of change in their child's community participation to the fact that they had not gone out often between June and December 2019, when the social unrest was persistent. Furthermore, the fact that all participating children continued receiving their usual early intervention services during the study period might have acted as a confounding factor. Future studies, with larger samples of a balanced gender proportion, and using a randomized controlled trial design, with children assigned to either the OPC and usual care group, or usual care only, are warranted to evaluate additional contribution of OPC, and to confirm the findings of this study.

5. Conclusions

This study provides preliminary support for the use of OPC in parents of young children with DD in Hong Kong. We found a trend that OPC may have a positive effect both on children's involvement in community activities and on specific aspects of quality of life. OPC can also assist parents in developing insight, skills, autonomy, and self-efficacy which, in turn, may benefit their emotional state. While satisfaction with OPC was high among the parents, some suggestions were useful to adjust the intervention to fit with local needs. These findings could help inform further planning of either a pilot, feasibility randomized controlled trial, or both, to establish evidence supporting the effectiveness of OPC when being applied in Hong Kong.

Author Contributions: Conceptualization, C.-W.C., Y.Y.C.L., C.-Y.L., and F.G.; methodology, Y.Y.C.L., C.-Y.L., and F.G.; formal analysis, C.-W.C.; resources, C.-W.C., Y.Y.C.L., and F.G.; data curation, C.-W.C.; writing—original draft preparation, C.-W.C., Y.Y.C.L., C.-Y.L., and F.G.; writing—review and editing, C.-W.C.; project administration, C.-W.C.; funding acquisition, C.-W.C., Y.Y.C.L., C.-Y.L., and F.G. All authors have read and agreed to the published version of the manuscript.

Funding: This research was funded by the Food and Health Bureau under Health Care and Promotion Scheme, Health and Medical Research Fund (grant reference number: 02180358).

Acknowledgments: We express our gratitude to all the parents that participated in this study as well as Heep Hong Society, Hong Kong Christian Service, and SAHK that assisted in data collection. We also thank Ms Pauline Cheung for her assistance in project coordination, post-intervention assessments, and qualitative analysis as the research assistant in this project.

Conflicts of Interest: The authors declare no conflict of interest.

Appendix A. Guiding Questions Used in Semi-Structured Interview of Parents, after OPC Intervention

1. What was your overall experience of the parent-coaching training?

    Probe Q1: What have you learnt during the parent-coaching period?
    Probe Q2: What did you like most (or least) during the parent-coaching period?
    Probe Q3: During the parent-coaching period, what difficulties did you encounter?
    Probe Q4: How closely did this parent-coaching meet your expectations?
    Probe Q5: How would you describe your relationship with the coach?

2. How did the parent-coaching training help you or your child?

    Probe Q1: How has the parent-coaching training helped your child to engage in home activities?
    Probe Q2: How has the parent-coaching training helped your child to engage in community activities?
    Probe Q3: How has the parent-coaching training helped to improve your child's psychosocial health?
    Probe Q4: How has the parent-coaching training affected your psychosocial health?

3. During the study period, how satisfied were you with the parenting-coaching process?

    Probe Q1: What did you think about the coaching schedule? Or what did you think of the maximum number of sessions being eight? Or what did you think about the sessions being once a week?
    Probe Q2: What did you think about each sessions being one hour long?
    Probe Q3: What did you think about the delivery method (face-to-face or internet-based)? What did you think if we deliver the parent-coaching training through (internet-based or face-to-face)?

4. Would you recommend the parent-coaching training to other parents in need? If yes, how would you explain the intervention to them? (If no, why would you not recommend it?)
5. Lastly, what improvements to the parent-coaching training would you suggest, if it was to be applied in Hong Kong in the future?

Appendix B. Narrative Description of OPC Sessions and Goal Achievement of Each Participant

1. Case 1 (a boy with autism and developmental delay, aged 5.25 years)

    Both parents of Case 1 were coached for six sessions. During the first session, the parents considered that concentrating on completing homework within 30 min after school, while remaining emotionally stable, was the most important goal for their child. They reported many concerns regarding the child's emotional stability, and the impact of his engagement in academic tasks. The OPC coach directed the parents' focus to the days on which the child could complete the homework timely. During the solution-focused talk, the mother noted that the child might be more obedient if he was told about what to do one day before. The father also mentioned that the use of iPad/television as a reward after homework completion worked sometimes. The OPC coach instructed the parents to notice the timing and details around using those strategies in their daily routine, to which the parents agreed.

The second session was postponed for one week, due to school suspension as a result of the social unrest happening at the time. In the session, the parents reported an improvement in the child's performance in completing homework, but they were unable to continue implementing the strategies during the school suspension period. The parents also had concerns about the child's slow pace in writing Chinese words with complex strokes, and the over-use of iPad/television as the reward. The parents were encouraged to explore other strategies to write the complex words efficiently (e.g., breaking down the words or completing the same word in a row), and alternative rewards (e.g., allowing playtime with his brother) that could support the child's performance.

In the third session, the parents reported further improvement in the child's performance. They also identified the best timing for the child to engage in Chinese homework (e.g., good quality sleep the night before). Subsequently, a new goal emerged from the parents' concern regarding the child's emotion and disruptive behavior during piano lessons. After eliciting the parents' knowledge, the mother decided to use a similar strategy, in other words, to let the child know what the piano teacher would teach in the next lesson. The mother would also practice with the child, letting him familiarize himself with the learning topics.

The fourth session was held two weeks later, as the mother had work commitments. In the session, the parents reported that the child became more cooperative and, in fact, the mother had not told him about the teaching content of the next lesson in advance. Instead, she had modified the strategy and asked the piano teacher to tell the child directly about what she would teach him at the beginning of the piano lesson. This modified strategy did enhance the child's emotion and cooperation successfully.

During the remaining sessions (fourth, fifth, and sixth), the parents shifted their focus to another goal, which was that the child could complete homework during Christmas and Chinese New Year holidays. However, they struggled to identify successful strategies every time, because their holiday schedules were varied. The OPC coach shared several ideas (e.g., sorting out types of homework based on difficulty, offering breaks for lengthy homework), and invited the parents' comments on the ideas. The parents decided to let the child complete difficult homework when he was emotionally stable, and shift to easy/interesting homework when he was tired. The plan was modified twice over the fifth and sixth sessions, when the child felt distressed and unsettled. For example, in the sixth session, the mother reported that the child suddenly stopped doing the homework after being asked to correct a wrong stroke sequence of a Chinese word. The OPC coach led the parents to think about what they observed at that moment, and how they could maintain the child's motivation for homework completion. Additional strategies were further generated from the parents' reflection; those were, to allow the child to make mistakes, but guide him to find and correct mistakes after the completion through game-playing approaches. These strategies were used depending on the child's emotional status.

In the fifth session, the father reported an incident that had impacted on the child's emotional state. The child had bit his brother's arm when the brother did not want to share the new toy with him. The OPC coach facilitated the parents' reflection on their understanding of their child's behavior, and identification of possible strategies to prevent or deal with the behavior in the future (e.g., educating the child and reaching an agreement before playing with new toys, or using a timer to take turns to play). Similarly, in the sixth session, the mother reported an occasion where the child had suddenly started to cry and refused to eat lunch at home. Through the OPC coach's guidance, the parents concluded that this incident might have been caused by the differences in the child's routine, as they usually had lunch outside on the weekends. The mother further reported that she made use of the timer and gave the child time to calm himself down. Surprisingly, these strategies worked. The parents planned to continue using these strategies to help the child calm down when needed, as well as teach him to count down and take deep breaths as a self-soothing strategy.

In summary, three out of the seven goals were addressed in the six sessions (see Table 2). One goal was particularly related to the child's community participation. Unfortunately, the remaining OPC sessions were terminated because of the outbreak of COVID-19, and the post-intervention measures were completed immediately. The parents also completed the follow-up measures two months after post-intervention.

2. Case 2 (a boy with autism, aged 4.00 years)

The mother of Case 2 was coached for one session only. During the session, it emerged that the mother's priority was that her son followed her instructions during the morning routine, and left for school on time. The mother used a problem-oriented narrative to describe her son's stubborn tendency, in other words, her son would cry and require time to calm down if things did not go the way he wanted. This would delay the arrival time at school in the morning. The OPC coach guided the mother to think about what happened in a good morning, and explore possible strategies. The mother reported that she used candy/seaweed as the reward to motivate her son, or used pictures to explain things along the road, which sometimes worked. Furthermore, if the iPad or iPhone were used as the reward, the child would comply. However, the mother hesitated to reward her son with the iPad/iPhone, as she was afraid that people would think that she was not a good mother. The OPC coach elicited her to reflect on the reasons behind this fear. The mother proposed to give her son the opportunity to watch the iPad or iPhone for ten minutes whenever they arrived at school on time (rather than along the way to school) as the reward. Unfortunately, the second session was postponed for one week because of the social unrest and, later, the child was ill and required hospitalization, resulting in the mother's decision to withdraw from the research. Thus, no post-intervention or follow-up measures were completed.

3. Case 3 (a boy with autism and developmental delay, aged 5.50 years)

The mother of Case 3 was coached for the whole eight sessions. In the first session, the mother reported that the most important thing for her son was to have a regular morning routine, in order to get ready for school without any conflict. The OPC coach guided the mother to think about what she would like to happen in her son's morning routine, and to explore strategies that might work. For example, her son was a visual learner, so the mother, as a casual architect, decided to use her skills to make a series of visual cards that could be shown to her son, letting him know what he needed to do in the morning. She also planned to use verbal prompts and reward, to encourage her son to complete the morning routine. The mother agreed to try the plan one morning in the following week. She would generate the visual cards, one day before executing the plan, and set the alarm in order to get up earlier.

In the second session, however, the mother reported that she only made some of the visual cards. Her son understood the steps of the cards, but was slow and felt unmotivated to complete the morning routine. He required a lot of verbal prompts from the mother, and ended up upset and crying. The OPC coach supported the mother and they worked together to explore alternative strategies (e.g., encouragement-oriented prompting, aiding in completing difficult steps, or using sensory play as the reward). However, the following week was affected by the social unrest, postponing the third session for one week.

During the third session, the mother reported that the plan had not been successfully implemented, as the school had re-opened for two days and their morning was very rushed. She also disclosed that she was tired from the previous night because she had spent time sorting her son's toys and tidying up the home, and had gone to sleep late. This impacted on her energy level and she did not feel up to try the entire plan. Later she recognized the organization of her timetable as being important, in order for her to have sufficient energy. The mother identified that setting an alarm to go to bed by 12 a.m. could be a workable strategy, and she also planned to use a timer and visual cards to prompt her son to tidy up his toys after free play in the afternoon.

In the fourth session, the mother reported that she was unable to manage her time and went to bed by 12 a.m. Her sleep was also disrupted a few times by her second son at night. The original morning routine plan was missed out completely, and became less important for her. Instead she wanted to manage her time in order to organize the home (i.e., tidying up all her son's toys and sorting them into lockers). Strategies were identified, through the OPC coach's guiding questions, and included involving her son and husband in putting the toys away. At the same time, she put forward the idea of involving her husband in part of her son's morning routine (i.e., taking charge in playing warm-up games or jumping on the trampoline with her son).

In the fifth session, the mother reported that she had had an unexpectedly busy week at work, and did only a little sorting and planning. Through guided reflection, the mother expressed that she had a perfectionist tendency, which made her want to sort out everything at once and, if not, she would feel that she could not do anything next. The OPC coach worked with her to narrow down the goal, and develop a step-by-step plan that began with two categories of toy sorting. Furthermore, the mother reported that her son had enjoyed playing matching games and trampoline with her husband in the morning, and she would continue with the plan. Meanwhile, her son had received a therapeutic listening program, requiring him to wear a special headphone for 30 min in the morning. The child seemed more calm and willing to follow instructions in the morning, according to the mother's observation.

In the sixth session, the mother had managed to complete almost all of the domestic chores the night before. She planned to continue packing her son's toys into the lockers, by narrowing the task down and labeling the items. When asked what the most important thing for her at that moment was, the mother returned to the previously unfinished goal regarding her son's morning routine, and revealed that she wanted it to be extended to his after-school routine at home. The OPC coach guided her to think about what she wanted, and she created five-step morning and after-school routines for her son. The mother would use the visual cards to let her son know the steps and try out the routine plans for two days in the coming week. However, in the seventh session, the mother explained that the routine plans had not been implemented due to the busy holiday preparation. She had only been able to organize the house, but she felt comfortable with her time schedule and routine, and ready to implement the activities in the after-school routine with her son. In addition, while he still wore diapers at home, she had noticed that her son had started telling her when he needed the toilet. So, she created another goal for her child, which involved him going to the toilet every 45 min, without wearing diapers at home or when he expressed the need. Through collaborative performance analysis, she devised a reward system, to be trialed for half a day in the coming week, and an electronic alarm would be used as a reminder for her son to go to toilet regularly.

In the last session, the mother reported that she had modified the types of reward (originally collecting five points to get a chocolate croissant at the end) from small and instant ones (i.e., candy) to big and delayed ones (i.e., going to a theme park). The child was able to express the need to go to the toilet on two occasions. However, the mother did not use the system consistently, owing to the sickness of the child over the previous week. The OPC coach guided the mother to apply the successful reward system to other daily routines. The mother thought about behavior at the dinner table and homework compliance, and planned to extend the reward system to these areas.

In summary, two of the six goals were addressed in the eight sessions (see Table 2). None of the two goals were related to the child's community participation. Since the number of sessions had reached the maximum, the OPC intervention was concluded. The mother completed the post-intervention and follow-up measures.

4. Case 4 (a girl with developmental delay, aged 5.25 years)

The mother of Case 4 was coached for one session only. During the initial stage of the session, the mother specified that she wanted her daughter to be more motivated to engage in academic-learning activities, for 30 min at home, during weekday evenings. The OPC coach used collaborative performance analysis to guide the mother to think about a preferred future and, through solution-focused conversation, to identify strategies that could support her daughter's performance. Some strategies that were identified as being useful sometimes included having enough sleep the night before, incorporating motor activities that did not require sitting, using snacks as the reward after completion, or reducing the time of the activities. When the OPC coach moved it forward to action identification, the mother's mobile phone had no battery charge, and the session ended abruptly. After the participant's phone was recharged, she sent a text-message to the OPC coach, enquiring why she had been asked to identify solutions by herself, rather than receiving advice from the coach. As she preferred an expert-directed approach, she decided to withdraw from the study. No post-intervention or follow-up measures were completed.

5. Case 5 (a boy with developmental delay and dyslexia, aged 5.33 years)

The mother of Case 5 was coached for six sessions. In the first session, the mother identified the two most important things for her son. One was to complete the morning routine without bargaining behaviors, and the other was to complete the bed-time routine by 9 p.m. and go to bed by 9:30 p.m. For the morning routine, the mother was encouraged to identify a strategy that could motivate her three children (including the target child) to follow the rules. Strategies included processes around breakfast preparation, for example, asking the children what foods they would like to eat, preparing the necessary materials, and making breakfast in the morning. For the bed-time routine, the mother identified that watching television until bedtime could be a good motivator, provided that the children had showered, eaten, and completed their homework on time. The mother agreed to implement the two plans in the following week.

In the second session, the mother reported that the strategy for the morning routine had worked very well with her children, and they were now able to complete it smoothly. However, for the bed-time routine, watching television as a reward had only been successful on specific days, in other words, when the child did not receive intervention training and was back home at 5 p.m. When the child had to attend intervention after school he arrived home around 7 p.m., and by then was tired and just wanted to have free play. Furthermore, the child's father usually came back home around that time, and had dinner together with the children. Before/after dinner, the children played with their father, or watched television, which delayed the bed-time routine. Through the mother's reflection and knowledge elicited by the OPC coach, she put forward two strategies to be trialed in the coming week. One was to prepare different foods for her children (children's favorite meals) and husband (ordinary meals), to incentivize the children to eat quicker. The other was to involve her husband in the bed-time routine by reading books to the children (instead of watching television) after dinner.

In the third session, the mother seemed frustrated as her son was still going to bed around 10 p.m. on the days when he had the intervention. The strategy of separate meals for her children and husband had been successful, but her husband did not feel comfortable reading books to the children. The mother reflected that it was understandable as her husband was not good at reading books and was also tired after work. The mother decided to create a schedule, and educate the children about the evening routine by using a whiteboard. In addition, the children were allowed to watch television if they completed the evening routine on time. The mother also relaxed the bedtime from 9:30 p.m. to 10 p.m., on those days the child came back late, to allow room for a buffer. In addition, during story time, the mother wanted to encourage her son to read more books and express his ideas, to reinforce his learning from school. She discovered who to approach at the school, in order to find out the school themes in advance, and where she could borrow similar books. She also planned to facilitate a story sharing time among her children during the weekends.

In the fourth session, the mother reported that her children did not get the meaning of the evening routine written on the whiteboard. Therefore, she had decided to put up pictures to assist their understanding of what they needed to follow in the evening routine for the next week's plan. The mother was able to obtain the school theme from the teacher and incorporated it into the bedtime reading. Meanwhile, the mother reported that she had recently taken her child to the playground near the school, or to the clubhouse after school. Her son was able to invite his classmates or other kids to play together, by sharing snacks with them. Since this was one of the mother's goals identified in the goal setting session, the OPC coach encouraged her to continue the initiative. For the remaining time, the mother expressed a need for her son to complete Chinese homework with a proper sitting posture at home. The OPC coach guided her to review her son's current sitting posture and elicited her knowledge about the ideal one. Soon, the mother realized that the height of the chair was relatively lower than the table, so that her son had to lean his body toward the table, and sometimes the hand he used for writing was not placed on the table. The mother showed willingness to address this issue.

In the fifth session, the mother reported that she had managed to get her children to go to bed around 9:30 p.m. by following the previously discussed strategies on the days her son had the intervention. The child started to express his ideas, and interacted with his little sister during the story-time. The mother also went to the library to borrow books with similar themes to the ones being learned at school, to reinforce learning. Additionally, it was unexpected by the OPC coach that the mother asked her husband to share her workload and help with the child's homework. Since her husband appeared to accept this duty, the mother would continue it. The mother also reported that the chair, after the height adjustment, improved the child's sitting posture and performance in writing Chinese. She also adjusted the height of the chairs for her other two children. For the remaining time, the mother raised a concern about her son's poor performance in using scissors to cut lines/shapes accurately for homework. Several strategies were generated to enhance his performance, for example, to widen the lines by using color markers to easily trace lines while cutting, and to place direction signs in each turn to remind her son to turn the paper while cutting. The mother planned to apply these strategies while sharing a fun project with the child, such as making a Chinese New Year card.

In the sixth session, the mother reported that the child was able to accurately cut the straight lines that were highlighted in red using the marker, and to turn the paper using the non-dominant hand while cutting. However, he needed constant reminders to place his elbow on the table and maintain good sitting posture. He also did not enjoy making the card and stopped it after cutting six pieces. After the OPC coach-guided reflection, the mother realized that the paper for making the cards seemed too thick for the child to cut. Thus, she planned to organize a Chinese lantern making activity in the coming weeks, as this was usually a homework task for the Lantern Festival. The mother would prepare different sets of materials for the child and his older sister, divide the task into smaller portions, and complete some portions daily. Highlighting with color markers and reminders for the posture were continued, and the mother also thought that cutting straight (not curve) lines was most suitable for her son's ability at that moment.

Unfortunately, the remaining OPC sessions were terminated because of the same reason (i.e., the impact of COVID-19) mentioned previously for Case 1. In summary, four of the eight goals were addressed in the six sessions (see Table 2). One goal that was dealt with was related to the child's community participation. The mother completed the post-intervention measures immediately and the follow-up measures two months later.

6. Case 6 (a boy with autism and developmental delay, aged 5.25 years)

The father of Case 6 was coached for three sessions. In the first session, he considered his son's completion of homework within one hour to be the most important goal to achieve. The father reported that the child was constantly asking for assistance or refusing to do the homework, especially when the subject was Chinese. After prompting for the father's reflection, he reasoned that his son might not know how to write Chinese words, particularly within the grids. Since the child's Chinese homework was supervised by his wife, the father agreed to invite his wife to join the next OPC session. In addition, the father identified several strategies that he planned to try out for enhancing his son's compliance with homework completion. These included watching television as the reward, and physical demonstration of how to write simple Chinese words (within 4 strokes).

Both mother and father attended the second session. The father reported that his son had shown some improvement, after he had been instructed on how to break down the Chinese for writing, and was also more willing to complete the homework that contained less complicated Chinese words on his own. However, the mother reported that the child was still unable to write Chinese words with complicated structures, even though she had taught him the stroke sequence twice. Through the OPC coach's guidance, the mother reflected that she, at times would get very angry if the stroke sequence made by the child was wrong, and would require 5–10 min to calm herself down. In the meantime, the child would be offered a break to watch television before continuing the homework. The parents identified the inconsistency in their parenting styles, especially regarding the use of television as a reward, in other words, at the end (father's style), or as a break in-between (mother's style). The break was important for the mother, as it helped her to calm down, however she agreed to use it as little as possible. The OPC coach shared his view about breaking down complicated Chinese words into small parts, given that the child was able to write simple Chinese words. The mother considered it as a possible strategy, and agreed to try it out. Regarding the reward for homework completion, after being prompted for an alternative, the father suggested taking his son out to the playground.

In the third session, the mother was not available. The father reported that the plan for taking the child to the playground as the reward had worked only for school days but not for holidays. He reasoned that there was not much homework over Chinese New Year holidays, and his son wanted to watch television as the reward. He would continue the playground plan after the holiday period. He also did not know whether breaking down Chinese words supported the child's performance. This plan would be reviewed when his wife attended the session later. For the remaining time, the father prioritized that he wanted his son to play with other children with no fighting, and demonstrate appropriate behaviors when visiting friends or engaging in the community. He noticed that the child behaved differently (i.e., more uncooperative) when he was present, compared to when his wife was present (more obedient). Through guided reflection, the father mentioned that he usually acted as a friend of his son, which could explain the difference in behavior. He felt it was necessary for him to change this, and to show his son that he would not be manipulated easily. The father proposed a punishment system, which involved reducing the time spent watching television if the child had a fight with other children, as well as removing his son from the conflict situation immediately to allow him to calm down. Afterward, he would listen to his son and educate him about appropriate behavior when playing with other children.

Owing to the impact of COVID-19 starting in March 2020, the father agreed to stop the OPC intervention earlier. In summary, two out of the five goals were addressed in the three sessions (see Table 2). One of the goals that was addressed referred to the child's community participation. The father completed the post-intervention measures immediately and the follow-up measures two months later.

Appendix C. Illustrative Quotations of Each Identified Sub-Category for Parents' Experience of OPC

Table A1. Quotations of Identified Sub-Categories for Parents' Experience of OPC

Category and Sub-Categories	Quotations
Increased insight and learning	
Sub-category 1: New insight on child's difficulties	• Need to know, need us more to understand which time slot in a day that he (the child) has the best emotional status. Then I will make use of that time, enabling him to complete the things that I want him to do. (Case 1's mother) • I never been that kind of coaching. Sometimes it is hard for parents to see the blind spot, how we interact with our kids, or how we teach our kids. We just use the way how we learnt, and then teach the kid. Maybe my son is not learning with the same method as me. (Case 5's mother) • By taking these classes, it does give me more patience and understanding of my son's problems. (Case 6's father)
Sub-category 2: New insight on parents' needs	• I guess it (what I like most during the coaching period) is the space, I don't feel so pressured which I feel more comfortable in terms of doing it but I, like again, it's really depends on the self-discipline. So it's, it's good that I have a coach. (Case 3's mother) • Give me an insight of, you know, how you suppose to train properly with the kid. In fact, the things we actually give a lot of rewards on TV time, and sometimes, me and my wife is (not consistent), because I have my style of teaching kids, and my wife has another style of teaching the kid. And that's our problem. Because we won't be consistent. (Case 6's father)
Sub-category 3: Learning new strategies, skills, or thinking models	• I learnt some techniques, those are, he (the coach) shared some treasured experience that we could try to apply to see how much the child could improve or how we arrange time (for the child's activities). Overall, it helps the parents and the child. (Case 1's father) • I learnt to look at, I think I learnt some sort of thinking model that, if I hit a problem, I would think what is the most ideal way that I wanted. And I try to think from that angle, and do it slowly … Like what would be ideal, and how do I achieve it. And then, and then, I also learnt to start small, start slow. (Case 3's mother) • I remember there were occasions I failed. The first one was … The second one was making an environmental-friendly lantern my son would bring it to school. I planned to do it with my son during the 6th meeting. I did not make good use of the holiday and failed. Even, I failed to make the lantern with my son. I learnt skills from the coaching sessions. (Case 5's mother)
Experiencing changes in their child	
Sub-category 1: Increased participation in home activities	• Maybe for doing the homework. He (the coach) told us how to do to make the child feel interested to do homework. Using different techniques to communicate with him (the child), I think this aspect (doing homework) improved. (Case 1's mother) • My son talks with us more and he plays less by himself. Before joining the parent coaching, if we don't stop him, he will keep playing the train with himself for more than 1 h. After the coaching, we start to interrupt him and invite him to play with others … We read more stories together and do the housework together, from 0 to once or twice a week. (Case 5's mother) • It (coaching) helps a little bit with writing, and helps a little bit with putting on the socks. (Case 6's father)

Table A1. *Cont.*

Category and Sub-Categories	Quotations
Sub-category 2: Increased emotion or confidence	• Even in the interest class he (the child) takes, the teacher also faced the situation where the child has a bad mood. When not good, he (the coach) told us that, actually, we could tell the teacher directly and ask her to give advanced announcement (about what she would teach) … improved, improved a lot actually for the emotion … that is he (the coach) had taught us some techniques and we tried how to communicate with our child to control his emotion. That is the emotional responses at home, and the number of losing his temper was dropped. (Case 1's mother) • My son is very shy and afraid to express his feelings. He does not know how to ask help or raise questions … I let him practice by staying behind after school and enforce his learning in our conversation. He (the coach) provided a lot of suggestions and possibilities to help my son to build confidence in his school life. (Case 5's mother)
Positive coach-parent relationship	
Sub-category 1: Felt supported or encouraged	• I feel like (the coach is) a very experienced person who is very willing to share his experience, so as to let us know how to consider in every aspect, or in the aspect of arranging time, difficulty of challenge (of tasks), etc. That means, giving us a lot of treasured experience. (Case 1's father) • I'm happy not because of the process of the coaching but it's because of everything else, like because of the talking, because of the sharing session, and maybe the guiding of my own thinking process. So he (the coach) gives guidance and he also gives really good advice. (Case 3's mother) • First, being encouraged is most important. Second one is receiving very detailed suggestions that are very practical. As I have 3 kids, the time constraint is bigger for me, it is harder for me to take care them at the same time. I need detailed suggestions to execute my plan smoothly. He (the coach) had been encouraging me to keep going to my target. (Case 5's mother)
Sub-category 2: Felt understood	• Because he (the coach) is very professional. He understands the difficulties of parents. And he understands the situation in Hong Kong. (Case 5's mother) • He (the coach) is funny, he is willing to teach, and you know, I think we have a good relationship, understanding of, you know, his techniques and he understands mine, you know, situation. He is really listening. (Case 6's father)
Factors affecting coaching experience and suggestions	
Sub-category 1: Disturbed by social issues or seasonal holidays	• I think, (it) is to do with the whole situation. It was first school holidays, a lot of, yes, so it's just because of the social situation that schools stop. And because I have 2 kids at home, and when they don't go to school, it's, the whole routine messed up. And I'm at the moment of building my routine. And if it got messed up, it's adding difficulties to build things. (Case 3's mother) • Um, yes, the holidays didn't work as well. Because a lot of training require, you know, like, the repetition but let's say, during Christmas holidays, we suppose to train him repetition, but a lot of time we have to go to other peers, other parties, and you know, when we go to the parties, you cannot, you cannot train him as well as at home, because there's no more writing, there's no more guidance, there's no more rules. You know, everything went out the door, will be training. (Case 6's father)

Table A1. *Cont.*

Category and Sub-Categories	Quotations
Sub-category 2: Delivery mode and location of coaching	• I think that both have their advantages. Because, for internet, I can arrange the time. Going to the university takes us a few hours for return, just only for the transportation. If conducted through internet, it saves time. However, for face-to-face, we think there is a need to take the child to visit the coach at the first session, and so let him (the coach) observe the child's conditions ... Maybe, when there is chance in the future, maybe half-half, that is, half for the training conducted through face-to-face and half through internet. (Case 1's father) • It's fine for me. Like meeting in person would be good, but, I don't see there's any difference if I have to do it on internet ... Because, while I was at home, I was able to show my home environment to the coach, and he's able to see something that I've done over the past week. So in that regard, online meeting is better. (Case 3's mother) • The face-to-face method is very useful. He (the coach) and my family live in the same district ... I am so glad he does not mind coming to my home ... I think it would still be good enough now. The coronavirus stopped us from meeting. It would be better to have face-to-face coaching at the beginning. After building trust and understanding the concept, we would move to internet-based methods such as Zoom. (Case 5's mother) • What do I like least? ... Maybe the training area, because the university was, you know, disrupted. We have to do everything in the car. So maybe that I like least, but, you know, that is the problem of it ... Face-to-face is actually better than anything else. (Case 6's father)
Sub-category 3: Number of coaching sessions	• I will definitely want more (sessions) because, like I said before, I feel it's going slightly slow ... I always refer it as a snowball. So I think that everything to begin with is slow ... So if you have to build something, the foundation is always taking longer. So, I think, for anything to get built up or achieve, or snowballing, and, this time so far isn't quite enough to make a base. So I think it needs, it needs longer. (Case 3's mother) • With longer coaching time, I will build better habits to train my son. It would be much easier for parents to enforce what we had learnt if there are 10 coaching sessions. (Case 5's mother)
Sub-category 4: Frequency of coaching sessions	• Maybe one to two weeks will be better for observing his improvement. It is because sometimes there are holidays, school suspension, maybe, slightly extending the frequency of the training during these periods. (Case 1's father) • I think maybe twice every 3 weeks, maybe more ideal for me. (Case 3's mother) • If possible, it would be better to meet every 2 weeks in the first and second period of the coaching. It would allow me to have more time to apply what he (the coach) is coaching. I mean the duration ... My son will have more time to do the preparation. (Case 5's mother)
Sub-category 5: Additional suggestions	• Designing a handbook about "the most common 100 problems and solutions for coping with the difficulties faced by children". In addition to every meeting, we can have this handbook and refer to it, to understand the guidance of using the techniques, and so let us to make the reference, to practice, to see whether it (the technique) can help the child. (Case 1's father) • Receiving an email or WhatsApp message between 2 weeks gap will be more helpful for the parent. The reminder would refresh key points which were discussed with the coach. (Case 5's mother) • I think my recommendation is to train the parents first, with a class of 2, and then, be go on, on the, focus on the kids instead. (Case 6's father)

References

1. Law, M. Participation in the occupations of everyday life. *Am. J. Occup. Ther.* **2002**, *56*, 640–649. [CrossRef] [PubMed]
2. King, G.; Law, M.; King, S.; Rosenbaum, P.; Kertoy, M.K.; Young, N.L. A conceptual model of the factors affecting the recreation and leisure participation of children with disabilities. *Phys. Occup. Ther. Pediatr.* **2003**, *23*, 63–90. [CrossRef] [PubMed]
3. Hoogsteen, L.; Woodgate, R.L. Can I play? A concept analysis of participation in children with disabilities. *Phys. Occup. Ther. Pediatr.* **2010**, *30*, 325–339. [CrossRef] [PubMed]
4. Khetani, M.A.; Graham, J.E.; Davies, P.L.; Law, M.C.; Simeonsson, R.J. Psychometric properties of the Young Children's Participation and Environment Measure. *Arch. Phys. Med. Rehabil.* **2015**, *96*, 307–316. [CrossRef]
5. Lim, C.Y.; Law, M.; Khetani, M.; Pollock, N.; Rosenbaum, P. Participation in out-of-home environments for young children with and without developmental disabilities. *OTJR Occup. Particip. Health* **2016**, *36*, 112–125. [CrossRef]
6. Chien, C.W.; Leung, C.; Schoeb, V.; Au, A. A Chinese version of the Young Children's Participation and Environment Measure: Psychometric evaluation in a Hong Kong sample. *Disabil. Rehabil.* **2020**, (in press). [CrossRef]
7. Bornstein, M.H.; Hendricks, C. Screening for developmental disabilities in developing countries. *Soc. Sci. Med.* **2013**, *97*, 307–315. [CrossRef]
8. Rice, C.; Schendel, D.; Cunniff, C.; Doernberg, N. Public health monitoring of developmental disabilities with a focus on the autism spectrum disorders. *Am. J. Med. Genet. C Semin. Med. Genet.* **2004**, *125*, 22–27. [CrossRef]
9. Larson, R.W.; Verma, S. How children and adolescents spend their time across the world: Work, play, and developmental opportunities. *Psychol. Bull.* **1999**, *125*, 701–736. [CrossRef]
10. Zeng, N.; Ayyub, M.; Sun, H.; Wen, X.; Xiang, P.; Gao, Z. Effects of physical activity on motor skills and cognitive development in early childhood: A systematic review. *Biomed. Res. Int.* **2017**, *2017*, 2760716. [CrossRef]
11. Powrie, B.; Kolehmainen, N.; Turpin, M.; Ziviani, J.; Copley, J. The meaning of leisure for children and young people with physical disabilities: A systematic evidence synthesis. *Dev. Med. Child Neurol.* **2015**, *57*, 993–1010. [CrossRef] [PubMed]
12. Holder, M.D.; Coleman, B.; Sehn, Z.L. The contribution of active and passive leisure to children's well-being. *J. Health Psychol.* **2009**, *14*, 378–386. [CrossRef] [PubMed]
13. Schiavone, N.; Szczepanik, D.; Koutras, J.; Pfeiffer, B.; Slugg, L. Caregiver strategies to enhance participation in children with autism spectrum disorder. *OTJR Occup. Particip. Health* **2018**, *38*, 235–244. [CrossRef] [PubMed]
14. Anaby, D.; Pozniak, K. Participation-based intervention in childhood disability: A family-centred approach. *Dev. Med. Child Neurol.* **2019**, *61*, 502. [CrossRef] [PubMed]
15. Andrews, J.; Falkmer, M.; Girdler, S. Community participation interventions for children and adolescents with a neurodevelopmental intellectual disability: A systematic review. *Disabil. Rehabil.* **2015**, *37*, 825–833. [CrossRef]
16. Novak, I.; Honan, I. Effectiveness of paediatric occupational therapy for children with disabilities: A systematic review. *Aust. Occup. Ther. J.* **2019**, *66*, 258–273. [CrossRef]
17. Adair, B.; Ullenhag, A.; Keen, D.; Granlund, M.; Imms, C. The effect of interventions aimed at improving participation outcomes for children with disabilities: A systematic review. *Dev. Med. Child Neurol.* **2015**, *57*, 1093–1104. [CrossRef]
18. Reedman, S.; Boyd, R.N.; Sakzewski, L. The efficacy of interventions to increase physical activity participation of children with cerebral palsy: A systematic review and meta-analysis. *Dev. Med. Child Neurol.* **2017**, *59*, 1011–1018. [CrossRef]
19. Kang, L.J.; Palisano, R.J.; King, G.A.; Chiarello, L.A. A multidimensional model of optimal participation of children with physical disabilities. *Disabil. Rehabil.* **2014**, *36*, 1735–1741. [CrossRef]
20. Imms, C.; Granlund, M.; Wilson, P.H.; Steenbergen, B.; Rosenbaum, P.L.; Gordon, A.M. Participation, both a means and an end: A conceptual analysis of processes and outcomes in childhood disability. *Dev. Med. Child Neurol.* **2017**, *59*, 16–25. [CrossRef]

21. Kessler, D.; Graham, F. The use of coaching in occupational therapy: An integrative review. *Aust. Occup. Ther. J.* **2015**, *62*, 160–176. [CrossRef] [PubMed]
22. Bachmann, C.J.; Hofer, J.; Kamp-Becker, I.; Poustka, L.; Roessner, V.; Stroth, S.; Wolff, N.; Hoffmann, F. Affiliate stigma in caregivers of children and adolescents with autism spectrum disorder in Germany. *Psychiatry Res.* **2020**, *284*, 112483. [CrossRef] [PubMed]
23. International Coaching Federation. ICF Definition of Coaching. Available online: https://coachfederation.org/about (accessed on 17 September 2020).
24. Rush, D.D.; Shelden, M.L.L. *The Early Childhood Coaching Handbook*, 2nd ed.; Paul H. Brookes Publishing Co.: Baltimore, MD, USA, 2020.
25. Graham, F.; Kennedy-Behr, A.; Ziviani, J. *Occupational Performance Coaching (OPC): A Manual for Practitioners and Researchers*; Routledge: England, UK, 2020; pp. 1–222.
26. Graham, F.; Rodger, S.; Kennedy-Behr, A. Occupational Performance Coaching (OPC): Enabling caregivers' and children's occupational performance. In *Occupation-Centred Practice with Children: A Practical Guide for Occupational Therapists*, 2nd ed.; Rodger, S., Kennedy-Behr, A., Eds.; Wiley-Blackwell: Oxford, UK, 2017; pp. 209–231.
27. Graham, F.; Rodger, S.; Ziviani, J. Coaching parents to enable children's participation: An approach for working with parents and their children. *Aust. Occup. Ther. J.* **2009**, *56*, 16–23. [CrossRef]
28. Graham, F.; Rodger, S.; Ziviani, J. Enabling occupational performance of children through coaching parents: Three case reports. *Phys. Occup. Ther. Pediatr.* **2010**, *30*, 4–15. [CrossRef] [PubMed]
29. Hui, C.; Snider, L.; Couture, M. Self-regulation workshop and Occupational Performance Coaching with teachers: A pilot study. *Can. J. Occup. Ther.* **2016**, *83*, 115–125. [CrossRef] [PubMed]
30. Kennedy-Behr, A.; Rodger, S.; Graham, F.; Mickan, S. Creating enabling environments at preschool for children with developmental coordination disorder. *J. Occup. Ther. Sch. Early Interv.* **2013**, *6*, 301–313. [CrossRef]
31. Graham, F.; Rodger, S.; Ziviani, J. Effectiveness of occupational performance coaching in improving children's and mothers' performance and mothers' self-competence. *Am. J. Occup. Ther.* **2013**, *67*, 10–18. [CrossRef]
32. Kahjoogh, M.A.; Kessler, D.; Hosseini, S.A.; Rassafiani, M.; Akbarfahimi, N.; Khanheh, H.R.; Biglarian, A. Randomized controlled trial of occupational performance coaching for mothers of children with cerebral palsy. *Br. J. Occup. Ther.* **2019**, *82*, 213–219. [CrossRef]
33. Kim, U.; Triandis, H.C.; Kâğitçibaşi, Ç.; Choi, S.-C.; Yoon, G. *Individualism and Collectivism: Theory, Method, and Applications*; Sage Publications, Inc.: Los Angeles, CA, USA, 1994; pp. 1–348.
34. Bond, M.H.; Hwang, K.K. The social psychology of Chinese people. In *The Psychology of the Chinese People*; Bond, M.H., Ed.; Oxford University Press: Hong Kong, China, 1986; pp. 213–266.
35. Sue, D.; Sue, S. Cultural factors in the clinical assessment of Asian Americans. *J. Consult. Clin. Psychol.* **1987**, *55*, 479–487. [CrossRef]
36. Mak, W.W.S.; Kwok, Y.T.Y. Internalization of stigma for parents of children with autism spectrum disorder in Hong Kong. *Soc. Sci. Med.* **2010**, *70*, 2045–2051. [CrossRef]
37. Ng, C.K.M.; Lam, S.H.F.; Tsang, S.T.K.; Yuen, C.M.C.; Chien, C.W. The relationship between affiliate stigma in parents of children with autism spectrum disorder and their children's activity participation. *Int. J. Environ. Res. Public Health* **2020**, *17*, 1799. [CrossRef]
38. Lam, S.F.; Wong, B.P.; Leung, D.; Ho, D.; Au-Yeung, P. How parents perceive and feel about participation in community activities. The comparison between parents of preschoolers with and without Autism Spectrum Disorders. *Autism* **2010**, *14*, 359–377. [CrossRef]
39. Law, M.; Baptiste, S.; McColl, M.; Carswell, A.; Polatajko, H.; Pollock, N. *Canadian Occupational Performance Measure*; CAOT Publications ACE: Ottawa, ON, Canada, 2004; pp. 1–34.
40. McColl, M.A.; Carswell, A.; Law, M.; Pollock, N.; Baptiste, S.; Polatajko, H. *Research on the Canadian Occupational Performance Measure: An Annotated Bibliography*; CAOT Publications ACE: Ottawa, ON, Canada, 2006.
41. Cusick, A.; Lannin, N.A.; Lowe, K. Adapting the Canadian Occupational Performance Measure for use in a paediatric clinical trial. *Disabil. Rehabil.* **2007**, *29*, 761–766. [CrossRef] [PubMed]
42. Hunsberger, M.; Lehtinen-Jacks, S.; Mehlig, K.; Gwozdz, W.; Russo, P.; Michels, N.; Bammann, K.; Pigeot, I.; Fernandez-Alvira, J.M.; Thumann, B.F.; et al. Bidirectional associations between psychosocial well-being and body mass index in European children: Longitudinal findings from the IDEFICS study. *BMC Public Health* **2016**, *16*, 949. [CrossRef] [PubMed]

43. Pakpour, A.H.; Chen, C.Y.; Lin, C.Y.; Strong, C.; Tsai, M.C.; Lin, Y.C. The relationship between children's overweight and quality of life: A comparison of Sizing Me Up, PedsQL and Kid-KINDL. *Int. J. Clin. Health Psychol.* **2019**, *19*, 49–56. [CrossRef]
44. Ravens-Sieberer, U.; Bullinger, M. *KINDL Questionnaire for Measuring Health-Related Quality of Life in Children and Adolescents Revised Version*; Manual, KINDL Group: Hamburg, Germany, 2000.
45. Ngai, F.W.; Wai-Chi Chan, S.; Holroyd, E. Translation and validation of a Chinese version of the parenting sense of competence scale in Chinese mothers. *Nurs. Res.* **2007**, *56*, 348–354. [CrossRef] [PubMed]
46. Taouk, M.; Lovibond, P.F.; Laube, R. *Psychometric Properties of A Chinese version of the Short Depression Anxiety Stress Scales (DASS21)*; Cumberland Hospital: Sydney, NSW, Australia, 2001; pp. 1–29.
47. Williams, G.C.; Grow, V.M.; Freedman, Z.R.; Ryan, R.M.; Deci, E.L. Motivational predictors of weight loss and weight-loss maintenance. *J. Pers. Soc. Psychol.* **1996**, *70*, 115–126. [CrossRef]
48. Chan, D.K.; Lonsdale, C.; Ho, P.Y.; Yung, P.S.; Chan, K.M. Patient motivation and adherence to postsurgery rehabilitation exercise recommendations: The influence of physiotherapists' autonomy-supportive behaviors. *Arch. Phys. Med. Rehabil.* **2009**, *90*, 1977–1982. [CrossRef]
49. Elo, S.; Kyngas, H. The qualitative content analysis process. *J. Adv. Nurs.* **2008**, *62*, 107–115. [CrossRef]
50. Krippendorf, K. *Content Analysis: An Introduction to Its Methodology*; Sage: Thousand Oaks, CA, USA, 2013.
51. King, G.; Schwellnus, H.; Servais, M.; Baldwin, P. Solution-focused coaching in pediatric rehabilitation: Investigating transformative experiences and outcomes for families. *Phys. Occup. Ther. Pediatr.* **2019**, *39*, 16–32. [CrossRef]
52. Law, M.; Anaby, D.; Imms, C.; Teplicky, R.; Turner, L. Improving the participation of youth with physical disabilities in community activities: An interrupted time series design. *Aust. Occup. Ther. J.* **2015**, *62*, 105–115. [CrossRef] [PubMed]
53. Little, L.M.; Pope, E.; Wallisch, A.; Dunn, W. Occupation-based coaching by means of telehealth for families of young children with autism spectrum disorder. *Am. J. Occup. Ther.* **2018**, *72*, 7202205020. [CrossRef] [PubMed]
54. Graham, F.; Rodger, S.; Ziviani, J. Mothers' experiences of engaging in Occupational Performance Coaching. *Br. J. Occup. Ther.* **2014**, *77*, 189–197. [CrossRef]
55. Dunst, C.J.; Hamby, D.; Trivette, C.M.; Raab, M.; Bruder, M.B. Young children's participation in everyday family and community activity. *Psychol. Rep.* **2002**, *91*, 875–897. [CrossRef] [PubMed]
56. Maul, C.A.; Singer, G.H.S. "Just good different things": Specific accommodations families make to positively adapt to their children with developmental disabilities. *Top. Early Child. Spec. Educ.* **2009**, *29*, 155–170. [CrossRef]
57. Shek, D.T.L. Protests in Hong Kong (2019–2020): A perspective based on quality of life and well-being. *Appl. Res. Qual. Life* **2020**, *15*, 619–635. [CrossRef]
58. Ni, M.Y.; Yao, X.I.; Leung, K.S.M.; Yau, C.; Leung, C.M.C.; Lun, P.; Flores, F.P.; Chang, W.C.; Cowling, B.J.; Leung, G.M. Depression and post-traumatic stress during major social unrest in Hong Kong: A 10-year prospective cohort study. *Lancet* **2020**, *395*, 273–284. [CrossRef]
59. Ng, R.M.K. Mental health crisis in Hong Kong: Its Current Status and Collective Responses from Mental Health Professionals in Hong Kong. Available online: www.psychiatrictimes.com/mental-health/mental-health-crisis-hong-kong (accessed on 18 September 2020).
60. Ogourtsova, T.; O'Donnell, M.; De Souza Silva, W.; Majnemer, A. Health coaching for parents of children with developmental disabilities: A systematic review. *Dev. Med. Child Neurol.* **2019**, *61*, 1259–1265. [CrossRef]
61. Dunn, W.; Cox, J.; Foster, L.; Mische-Lawson, L.; Tanquary, J. Impact of a contextual intervention on child participation and parent competence among children with autism spectrum disorders: A pretest-posttest repeated-measures design. *Am. J. Occup. Ther.* **2012**, *66*, 520–528. [CrossRef]
62. Akhbari Ziegler, S.; Hadders-Algra, M. Coaching approaches in early intervention and paediatric rehabilitation. *Dev. Med. Child Neurol.* **2020**, *62*, 569–574. [CrossRef]

Publisher's Note: MDPI stays neutral with regard to jurisdictional claims in published maps and institutional affiliations.

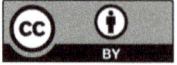

© 2020 by the authors. Licensee MDPI, Basel, Switzerland. This article is an open access article distributed under the terms and conditions of the Creative Commons Attribution (CC BY) license (http://creativecommons.org/licenses/by/4.0/).

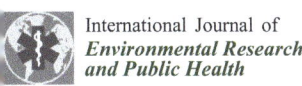

International Journal of *Environmental Research and Public Health*

Article

Cross-Cultural Adaptation and Evaluation of the Participation and Environment Measure for Children and Youth to the Indian Context—A Mixed-Methods Study

Roopa Srinivasan [1,*], Vrushali Kulkarni [1], Sana Smriti [2], Rachel Teplicky [3] and Dana Anaby [4]

1. Ummeed Child Development Center, Department of Developmental Pediatrics and Occupational Therapy, Mumbai 400011, Maharashtra, India; vrushali.kulkarni@ummeed.org
2. Butterflies Child Development Centre, Hyderabad 500081, Telangana, India; drsanasmriti@gmail.com
3. CanChild Center for Childhood Disability Research, McMaster University, Hamilton, ON L8S 4L8, Canada; teplicr@mcmaster.ca
4. School of Physical and Occupational Therapy, McGill University, Montreal, QC H3G 1Y5, Canada; dana.anaby@mcgill.ca
* Correspondence: roopa.srinivasan@ummeed.org; Tel.: +91-9930495210

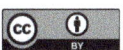

Citation: Srinivasan, R.; Kulkarni, V.; Smriti, S.; Teplicky, R.; Anaby, D. Cross Cultural Adaptation and Evaluation of the Participation and Environment Measure for Children and Youth to the Indian Context—A Mixed-Methods Study. *Int. J. Environ. Res. Public Health* **2021**, *18*, 1514. https://doi.org/10.3390/ijerph18041514

Academic Editor: Paul B. Tchounwou
Received: 30 December 2020
Accepted: 25 January 2021
Published: 5 February 2021

Publisher's Note: MDPI stays neutral with regard to jurisdictional claims in published maps and institutional affiliations.

Copyright: © 2021 by the authors. Licensee MDPI, Basel, Switzerland. This article is an open access article distributed under the terms and conditions of the Creative Commons Attribution (CC BY) license (https://creativecommons.org/licenses/by/4.0/).

Abstract: Culturally appropriate measures enable knowledge transfer and quality improvement of rehabilitation services in diverse contexts. The Applied Cultural Equivalence Framework (ACEF) was used in a two-phased mixed methods study to adapt and evaluate the Participation and Environment Measure-Children and Youth (PEM-CY) in India. Cognitive interviews with caregivers of children with disabilities ($n = 15$) aged 5–17 years established conceptual, item, semantic, and operational equivalence of the Indian PEM-CY. Construct validity was assessed by comparing PEM-CY scores of children with and without disabilities ($n = 130$) using a case-control design. Cognitive interviews resulted in operational (60.3%), semantic (26.4%), and item-level (13.2%) modifications in the PEM-CY with no changes at the conceptual level. Internal consistency ($n = 130$) was acceptable to excellent (0.61–0.87) on most scales. Test–retest reliability ($n = 30$) was good to excellent (ICC $\geq$ 0.75, Kappa 0.6–1.0) for most scales. Significant differences in all PEM-CY summary scores were found between children with and without disabilities, except for environmental supports. Children with disabilities had lower scores on frequency and involvement in activities across all settings; their caregivers desired greater change in participation and reported experiencing more environmental barriers across settings. Findings suggest the adapted PEM-CY is a valid and reliable measure for assessing the participation of Indian children.

Keywords: rehabilitation; PEM-CY; participation; cultural adaptation; India

1. Introduction

Participation in daily activities that one wants to and/or is expected to be engaged in is globally recognized as an indicator of health and as one of the most important outcomes of rehabilitation interventions [1,2]. The International Classification of Functioning, Disability, and Health (ICF) framework [3], endorsed by the World Health Organization, emphasizes the role of environmental factors in positively or negatively affecting an individual's participation. Indeed, previous research demonstrated that participation is a highly individualized, multidimensional concept that is dependent on environmental factors such as the physical (e.g., built environment), social (e.g., family and peer support), cultural (e.g., attitudes and values), and institutional (e.g., availability of program, services, and inclusive policies) aspects of the environment [4,5]. Researchers recommend that the ICF framework and participation-related research should guide the development of measures for children's participation [6–8]. The Participation and Environment Measures (PEM) are examples of such measures that uniquely look at both participation and environmental barriers and facilitators for children and youth with and without disabilities across home, school, and community settings [9,10]. The PEM also assesses key elements of participation; attendance ("being there") and involvement ("being in the moment") [5], making them one of the most comprehensive tools available. Specifically, the Participation and Environment Measure—Children and Youth version (PEM-CY), developed in North America, is a psychometrically sound parent-report assessment intended for children aged 5–17-years-old [6]; however, it has yet to be adapted to the unique context of low-resource countries.

Low and middle-income countries such as India are home to 95% of the world's children with disabilities under the age of five years [11]. Global estimates for older children with disabilities, though unavailable, are likely to follow a similar trend and very little information is available on the participation and well-being of these children [12,13]. While resources and services for children with disabilities have been steadily increasing, the caregivers face several challenges while accessing them. Services infrequently consider psychosocial factors and their influence on a person with a disability or their family [14]. Societal stigma and cultural beliefs may often force caregivers to seek "fixes" and cures for their child's disability [14]. Low caregiver literacy levels limit access to information about disabilities and available services [15]. Policies and laws that are supportive of children with disabilities are often poorly utilized on account of poor awareness and weak regulatory mechanisms [15]. Cultural preferences and inadequacy of formal supports for interventions prompt caregivers in under-resourced contexts to seek informal sources of supports within the family and the community [13]. The opportunity to leverage these supports for child and caregiver well-being is often missed by providers because of the focus on finding a fix for the disabilities. The availability of a measure like the PEM-CY would provide an opportunity for measuring children's participation, the impact of the environment on the child's participation, and evaluating the outcomes of rehabilitation services in low resource contexts.

Objectives

To culturally adapt and evaluate PEM-CY to the Indian context using the Applied Cultural Equivalence Framework (ACEF). Specifically, we aimed to (1) adapt the content of the PEM-CY and its administration to the Indian culture (phase 1) and (2) examine the psychometric properties of the adapted version in terms of reliability (internal consistency and test-retest) and construct validity (phase 2).

2. Materials and Methods
2.1. Study Design

A two-phase mixed-method design [16] was used to culturally adapt and test the English and Hindi PEM-CY among parents living in India. This process was guided by the five criteria outlined in the Applied Cultural Equivalence Framework (ACEF) [17–19] as shown in Table 1. In phase 1, the conceptual, item, semantic, and operational criteria of the ACEF were used to adapt the measure to the local context after considering the influence of the local culture, language, and interpretation of the construct. The inclusion of operational criterion is unique to this framework, which helps to evaluate not just the content of the instrument, but also its administration. This is critical considering the diversity in educational background and familiarity with self-administered instruments in the study setting. The ACEF framework has been used previously for cultural adaptation for various participation instruments [17].

Table 1. Adapted version of Applied Cross-Cultural Equivalence Framework (ACEF) [17].

	Equivalence Criteria	Definition of Criteria
Phase 1: Qualitative focus	Conceptual	The relevance of the underlying domain
	Item	Acceptability of items
	Semantic	Consistency of the meaning in the local language
	Operational	Suitability of instructions, administration, formatting, design
Phase 2: Quantitative focus	Measurement	Equivalence in the psychometric properties

This study included two phases, as shown in Figure 1.

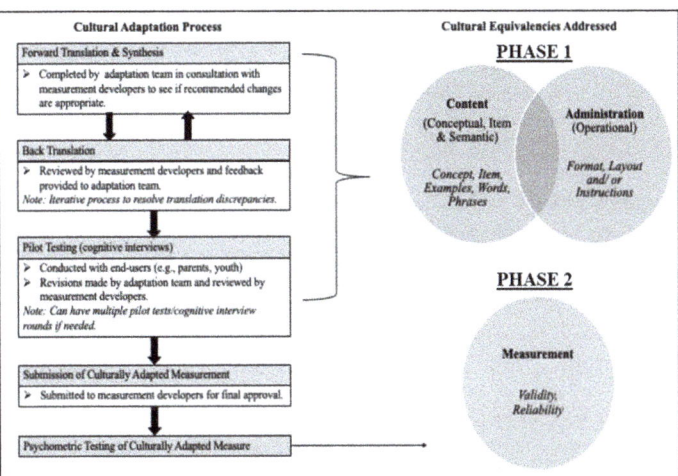

Figure 1. The adaptation process to achieve cultural equivalency for pediatric participation measures [20].

2.2. Procedure

The study was conducted at a large, not-for-profit organization serving children with disabilities between 0 and 18 years of age, during September 2018–July 2019. Ethics committee approval was obtained from an Institutional Review Board (Approval ID 01/2019) on 20th of April, 2019. Informed consent was obtained from the caregivers in both parts of the study.

Phase 1: PEM-CY was forward and backward translated in Hindi and English respectively by research assistants who were proficient in both languages and unfamiliar with the measure as per guidelines suggested by Beaton and colleagues [21]. A conceptual strategy [22] was used for the translation, where the significance of the items and instructions was preserved, rather than aiming for a direct text translation. Descriptive phrases were used when an equivalent word in Hindi was unavailable. Widely understood English words were retained where applicable. The backward translated English version of the PEM-CY was compared with the original PEM-CY to verify the accuracy and consistency of translation by the authors and developers of the measure.

Two rounds of cognitive interviews were used to establish the conceptual, item level, operational, and semantic equivalence of the translated version of the PEM-CY. To ensure diversity of perspectives, an important principle of cognitive interviews, 15 caregivers (10 for the Hindi version and 5 for the English version) of children with disabilities between the ages of 5–17 years were purposefully recruited, as recommended by Peterson et al. [23]. Caregivers were asked to choose either the original English PEM-CY or the translated Hindi version based on their comfort with reading, understanding, and completing a questionnaire in either of these languages. An open-ended interview guide was developed (based on the ACEF criteria) to conduct semi structured cognitive interviews using the Think Aloud and Verbal Probes approach in the first and second round of cognitive interviews respectively [23–25]. In the Think Aloud approach, the caregivers are encouraged to verbalize their thought processes with the interviewer performing the role of listening and using minimal prompts to avoid interruption in thinking (e.g., what made you choose this response?) [23]. In the Verbal Probes approach, specific pre decided probes are used immediately after the caregivers responded to the item (e.g., what did you understand by the example given here?) to confirm that the modifications made were helpful and enquire if additional modifications were needed [23]. The second round involved five caregivers who had not completed high school education. Modifications recommended by this group of caregivers (round 2) were hypothesized to be acceptable to caregivers with higher levels of education.

Phase 2 of the study assessed the psychometric properties of the PEM-CY after modifications made in Phase 1. The scores generated by the modified PEM-CY was used to assess our hypothesis regarding significant differences in participation between children with and without disabilities. A case-control study design was employed including caregivers of children with (n = 65) and without disabilities (n = 65) who were matched by the respondents' educational level and child's age and sex [26]. Caregivers of children were included in the study if (1) they had a child with or without disabilities between the ages of 5–17 years; (2) they could read and understand English or Hindi; (3) they lived in Mumbai; and (4) provided written consent to participate in the study. Internal consistency was examined in this cohort (n = 130) and test–retest reliability was assessed among a subsample of 30 parents at two-time points with a delay of 2–4 weeks [6,27]. Image 1 illustrates the procedure of the study.

Caregivers of children with disabilities in both phases (who participated in the second round of cognitive interviews and Phase 2 of the study) rated the feasibility and understandability of the instrument. Additionally, in phase 2, research assistants documented the type of assistance needed by caregivers of children with and without disabilities in completing the Indian-PEM-CY using the following criteria: redirecting caregivers to survey guidelines, prompts that included reading assistance and reminders to think about their everyday experiences and discussions to help caregivers connect their everyday experiences with the items in the measure (Appendix A).

All data was deidentified in both phases with restricted access to the research team. In Phase 1, the audio/video recording of the cognitive interviews was used to transcribe and translate the interviews. The transcripts were saved securely in a password-protected folder and thumb drive. In Phase 2, data from the completed PEM-CY paper forms was entered on MS Excel software (Microsoft Excel Macro Enabled Worksheet, Mumbai, Maharashtra).

2.3. Measurements

The PEM-CY, a caregiver-report measure, was used to assess the participation patterns of children and youth, aged 5–17, and the impact of the environment of their participation [6]. It includes 25 items focused on participation in broad types of activities at home (10 items), school (5 items), and community (10 items) settings. For each item, the caregiver reports on three dimensions of the child's participation: (1) frequency (8-point scale, from never (0) to daily (7)); (2) level of involvement (5-point scale, from minimally involved (1) to very involved (5)); and (3) the caregiver's desire for change in the child's participation (yes or no; if yes, the parent can select whether he or she desires a change in frequency, level of involvement, and/or broader variety). For each setting, the parent also reports on whether various environmental features or resources impact their child's participation. There are 12 environmental items in the home setting, 17 for school, and 16 for the community. The PEM-CY has moderate to very good internal consistency (0.59–0.91) and moderate to good test–retest reliability for all participation and environment sections when assessed within a 4-week period after the completion of first round (ICC 5 0.58–0.95) [6]. The validity was established as PEM-CY detected a significant effect of disability on child's participation across all settings and variables [6]. Recommendations provided in the manual were used to calculate summary scores to facilitate comparisons among groups [28]. Four mean scores were calculated to illustrate participation patterns in each setting: number of activities participated (in percentages), frequency (mean score ranging from 1 to 7), involvement (mean score ranging from 1 to 5), and desire for change (number of activities in which parented wanted to see changed, presented in percentages). Two additional scores per setting were calculated to describe the number of the environment supports and barriers, in percentages. Thus, six average group summary scores in each of the three settings (overall 18 scores) were derived.

Caregiver perceptions about the feasibility of the use of the instrument, understandability, relevance of items, and examples for home, school, and community were measured using several Visual Analogue Scales (VAS) [29,30]. The VAS included a 10 cm scale with 0 being "Not understandable and irrelevant" and 10 being "understandable and relevant". Overall, three VAS mean scores were generated for each of the three settings, and one overall score to assess caregivers' perception about the relevance and feasibility of use of the measure resulting in a total of 10 scores ranging from 0 to 10. Further, caregivers participating in phase 2 completed 4 questions related to the overall relevance, whether the PEM-CY should be used in the intervention, its understandability, and time taken to complete the measure with a simple "Yes" or "No" response. These were reported as the absolute number of responses and percentages.

Child and family characteristics, such as the caregiver's relationship with the child, age, and education levels, were collected using a standard demographic questionnaire. Information about the child including their age, gender, diagnosis, and functional limitations was also reported by the caregivers. Parents reported the diagnoses (up to 3) and functional limitations using a scale [31]. The diagnoses involved developmental disabilities like Autism Spectrum Disorder, Learning Disability, Developmental Delay, and Intellectual Disability and health conditions like asthma, cardiac problems, and epilepsy. The diagnoses for children with disabilities receiving services at our center was made by Developmental Pediatricians using the Diagnostic and Statistical Manual (DSM) V criteria [32]. When caregivers could not report the diagnoses, it was retrieved from patient records. The severity of the child's condition in terms of the number of functional limitations was reported by the caregivers by indicating whether a functional skill was "not a problem", a "little problem" or a "big problem" using a checklist of 11 functional areas. The number of functional issues was tallied. This checklist was found effective in explaining levels of participation among children and youth across different disabilities [6].

2.4. Data Analysis

Phase 1—Cultural adaptation of the PEM-CY to the Indian context (ACEF criteria for content and administration):

To analyze information gathered by the sequential rounds of cognitive interview, a deductive coding approach [33] was used to organize findings according to the first four criteria of the ACEF for all three settings home, school, and community section. In each round of cognitive interviews, similar modifications were grouped and counted as one, to avoid duplication in counting. Two of the authors independently reviewed the coding and the appropriateness of their listing under each of the ACEF criteria and any discrepancies were resolved by discussion. A summary report of these findings across the 15 interviews was sent to the codevelopers of the original measure. The proposed changes were reviewed, discussed, and any divergence of opinion reconciled by consensus of all the authors.

Phase 2—Testing the psychometric properties of the adapted PEM-CY (ACEF criteria measurement):

To examine construct validity, we assessed the extent to which the scores of the adapted PEM-CY was consistent with our hypothesis about difference in participation, involvement, change desired, environmental supports, and barriers between children with and without disabilities [34]. An unpaired t-test was used if the data was normally distributed, whereas the Mann–Whitney U test was used if the data failed the "Normality" test, as determined by the Shapiro–Wilks test [35]. A p-value of less than or equal to 0.05 was considered as a cut-off for the failure of the normality test. Effect sizes were calculated using Cohen's d where $d = 0.2$ is considered a small effect, $d = 0.5$ is medium, and $d = 0.8$ is large [36]. Reliability (i.e., internal consistency and test–retest reliability) was assessed using the Cronbach Alpha, Intraclass Correlation (ICC), and the Kappa Agreement test, respectively. The test–retest pairs for each individual Likert scale item in each of the three settings were analyzed using Intraclass Correlation [37] and when the scores were dichotomous, the simple Kappa Agreement was used [38]. Kappa scores ranging from 0 to 1 were interpreted using Landis and Koch guidelines [39]. ICC values less than 0.5 are indicative of poor reliability, values between 0.5 and 0.75 indicate moderate reliability, values between 0.75 and 0.9 indicate good reliability, and values greater than 0.90 indicate excellent reliability [40]. Values of $p < 0.05$ were used as the cut-off for statistical significance. IBM PSPP version 1.0.1 was used to analyze data recorded in MS EXCEL (Microsoft Excel Macro Enabled Worksheet, Mumbai, Maharashtra).

3. Results

3.1. Phase 1—Caregiver and Child Characteristics

The sociodemographic profile of the 10 caregivers in the 1st round (Hindi and English) and the 5 caregivers from the 2nd round of cognitive interviews along with information about their children is presented in Table 2. Thirteen mothers and two fathers of children with disabilities participated in this study. All caregivers resided in the Mumbai Metropolitan Region.

Table 2. Sociodemographic table of caregivers and children in Phase 1 ($n = 15$).

	Round 1 ($n = 10$)	Round 2 ($n = 5$)
Caregivers		
Fathers	1	1
Mothers	9	4
Caregiver education		
Up to High school	2	5
Graduation	6	0
Postgraduation	2	0
Employment status		
Employed	4	2
Unemployed	6	3
Monthly Family Income		
Below Minimum Wage (INR 10,000)	2	3
Above Minimum Wage (INR 10,000)	8	2
Children		
Sex		
Males	7	3
Females	3	2
Age		
5–8 years	7	1
8.1–12 years	2	4
12.1–17 years	1	0

Table 2. *Cont.*

	Round 1 (*n* = 10)	Round 2 (*n* = 5)
Diagnosis		
Autism Spectrum Disorder	3	0
Autism Spectrum Disorder and Global Developmental Delay	1	0
Autism Spectrum Disorder and Intellectual Disability	1	0
Cerebral Palsy	1	0
Cerebral Palsy with Global Developmental Delay, Vision Impairment and Hearing Impairment	0	1
Global Developmental Delay	0	1
Global Developmental Delay and Learning Disability	1	0
Global Developmental Delay and Cerebral Palsy	1	0
Attention Deficit Hyperactivity Disorder	1	0
Language Disorder	1	0
Learning Disability	0	2
Intellectual Disability	0	1

Modifications in English and Hindi PEM-CY

The majority of the changes were operational in nature (60.3%), followed by semantic (26.4%) and item-level changes (13.2%). No conceptual changes were required in either round of the cognitive interviews. As the second round of cognitive interviews was conducted with caregivers who completed the Hindi PEM-CY there were no modifications that were unique to the English PEM-CY after this round. There were fewer item-level modifications needed in the second round (16.6% vs. 9.8%), similar operational modifications in both rounds (61.6% vs. 59%), and a higher number of semantic changes that were needed in round 2 (21.6% vs. 31.1%). The lower education levels of the caregivers participating in the 2nd round of cognitive interviews may have led to the increased numbers of semantic and operational changes in the second round of the cognitive interviews overall. Overall, the modifications proposed remained the same in both rounds of cognitive interviews.

While the caregivers did not perceive the need for any changes at a concept level, 13 out of 15 caregivers needed reminders that "involvement" is about attention, concentration, and emotional engagement in activities and not about "independence". This was especially seen in the home section of the PEM-CY. Once reminders were given parents were able to complete and relate to these questions and therefore this was listed under operational modifications. Caregivers tended to focus on the child's difficulties and impairment rather than on environmental barriers or supports. They required an additional set of instructions and examples to understand this concept.

For the item-related modifications, contextually relevant examples made the items easier for the caregivers to understand. For example, adding "mobile" to the item "Computer and Video games" in the home setting. Caregivers could relate to cultural programs organized in their residential area or apartment during religious festivals and public holidays and therefore we modified the item "Programs in Community" to "Programs organized by the apartment/ building". The word "etcetera" was added to encourage caregivers to think more broadly about the type of activities that could be considered within an item as, at times, they felt constrained by the examples provided. Fewer item-level modifications were needed in Round 2 of cognitive interviews.

In terms of semantic modifications, two types of changes were made in both the English and Hindi PEM-CY. In the Hindi PEM-CY, English words like "puzzles", "craft", and "class" were retained as they were more commonly used and better understood. Colloquial words and descriptive phrases in Hindi were preferred over a literal and poorly understood Hindi translation; for example, "support" was replaced by "help", phrases were used to explain words or phrases such as "community", "organized physical activities", and "unstructured physical activities". For example, "community" was replaced by "locality and nearby area", and "organized physical activities" was modified to "physical sports organized in a private class". All the semantic modifications made to the Hindi PEM-CY after the second round of cognitive interviews were replicated in the English PEM-CY. Additionally, in the English PEM-CY, words like "field trips" and "dress up games" were replaced by "picnic" and "dress up with saree or dupatta" respectively. The words "Survey Instruction" was replaced by "Survey Guide", "independence" was replaced by "child's abilities", and "cognitive demands" of the activity by "brain/thinking demands".

Operational modifications were often required; the majority (61.6% in Round 1 and 59% in Round 2) of the changes were operational and involved changes to the layout and the administration of the questionnaire. The interviewers observed challenges faced (skipping a column) or strategies used by the caregiver (using their finger to keep track of rows) while completing the instrument. Caregivers recommended modifications that involved clarifications of survey instructions, formatting changes, and highlighting key transition points within the PEM CY.

- Clarifying Survey Instructions included providing explanations for concepts such as "involvement" and pictorial examples for completing the participation and environment sections. A sample of a completed PEM-CY question with clear instructions for entering responses was added to the survey instructions (see Figure 2). Specific pointers such as "For question B on Involvement" were used instead of the less specific term "important" that was part of the original survey instructions. The stem questions and response options were elaborated and made more self-explanatory after Round 2. For example, the question "What do you do to support your child's participation?" was modified to "What do you do to support your child's participation at present?" to make the question easier to understand and respond to. Contextually relatable examples were used for environmental supports that could be made available to enhance the child's participation (e.g., In the survey guidelines-wheelchair to support mobility was used as an example of environmental support).
- Reformatting of the questionnaire was also required. Specifically, modifications such as increased font size, color coding, italicizing, underlining, the spacing between items, and columns were used to draw the attention of the caregiver to important instructions and steps in both rounds of interviews.
- Help with transitions within the PEM-CY sections was also needed. Transition boxes were added between the participation and environment section to alert the caregiver to the change in section.

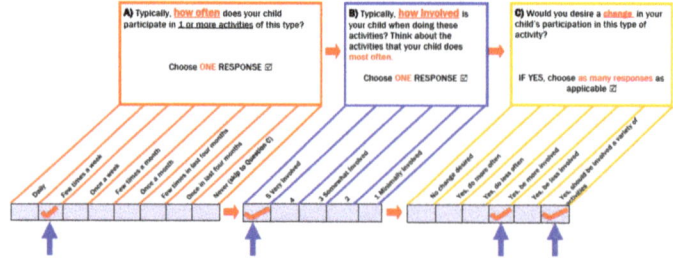

Figure 2. Clarifying survey instruction; (**A**), (**B**) and (**C**) subparts of the question on participation in a given setting elicit information about Frequency, Level of Involvement and Caregivers' desire for change in frequency, involvement and variety of activities in which the child participates respectively.

Results of the VAS questions indicated a relatively high level of understandability and relevance of items and relevance of examples from the modified PEM CY in the community (8.8, 9, and 9.4 out of 10, respectively), followed by the school (8, 8.2, and 8.8 out of 10) and the home setting (6.6, 8.6, and 9.4 out of 10). On a maximum score of 10, the caregivers rated the feasibility of PEM-CY at 8.8 on average.

3.2. Phase 2

3.2.1. Caregiver Characteristics ($n = 130$)

Initially, 73 caregivers of children with disabilities (case group) completed the modified PEM-CY questionnaires. This sample was matched with caregivers of children without disabilities (control group). Responses from 65/73 caregivers were complete with less than 20% missing data and could be included in the final data set for analysis. The sociodemographic profile of the case ($n = 65$) and control group ($n = 65$) was included in Table 3. A nearly equal number of caregivers in the case and control group completed the Hindi and the modified English PEM CY. From among the functional issues, most of the caregivers, 66% (43/65), reported issues in 4–9 (Median 5) functional areas. The most common functional issues included difficulty in "paying attention" (78%), "communication" (66%), "managing emotions" (60%), "remembering information" (58%), and "controlling behaviors" (57%) in that order. On the lower end, 25 (38%) reported difficulties in moving around, 16 (25%) in use of hands, 9 (12%) in vision, and 8 (13%) in hearing.

Table 3. Sociodemographic details of caregivers and children.

Variable	Cases ($n = 65$) n	%	Controls ($n = 65$) n	%
Child Gender				
Male	37	57%	40	62%
Female	28	43%	25	38%
Child Age (Mean = 8.7 years)				
5–8	27	42%	27	41%
8.1–12	21	32%	21	32%
12.1–15	15	23%	13	20%
15.1 to 18	2	3%	4	6%
Autism Spectrum Disorder	21	32%	-	-
Specific Learning Disability	17	26%	-	-
Attention Deficit Hyperactivity Disorder	16	25%	-	-
Global Developmental Delay	16	25%	-	-
Child—Number of health conditions				
1	30	46%	-	-
2	11	17%	-	-
3	18	28%	-	-
0	6	9%	-	-
Child—Number of functional limitations				
1–3	16	25%	-	-
4–6	26	40%	-	-
7–9	19	29%	-	-
10–11	4	6%	-	-
Respondent relationship to the child				
Mother	49	75%	55	85%
Father	16	25%	6	9%
Other	0	0%	4	6%

Table 3. Cont.

Variable	Cases (n = 65) n%		Controls (n = 65) n%	
Respondent age (years)				
18–29	3	5%	9	14%
30–39	36	55%	35	53%
40–55	24	37%	20	31%
Missing	2	3%	1	2%
Respondent education				
High School Education or lower	26	40%	26	40%
Graduate/Diploma/technical training	25	38%	27	42%
Postgraduate	14	22%	12	18%
Family income *				
Above Minimum Wage (INR 10,000/136.5 USD)	47	72%	50	76.9%
Below Minimum Wage (INR 10,000/136.5 USD)	17	26%	10	15.3%
Language of PEM-CY				
English	32	49%	37	57%
Hindi	33	51%	28	43%

* Minimum wages of Maharashtra State is 10,000 INR.

3.2.2. Psychometric Properties

Construct Validity of the Adapted PEM-CY

Significant differences, with moderate to large effect sizes, in participation frequency and involvement were found between children with disabilities and their typically developing counterparts across all settings: home, school, and within the community (see Table 4). As expected, children with disabilities participated less often and were less involved in activities at the home, school, and the community. In addition, a significantly greater number of caregivers (with a large effect size) of children with disabilities desired change in participation in all three settings. There was no statistically significant difference in the diversity of activities at home, school, and community. Children with disabilities were like their typically developing counterparts in viewing television, socialization using technology and participation in classroom work. They participated less frequently in indoor games, household chores, preparing for school, socializing with peers at home and school, and in all community-based activities. Caregivers of children with disabilities identified significantly more (with a large effect size) environmental barriers for their children's participation across settings as compared to caregivers of children without disabilities. Social demands of activities, inadequate money, supplies, services, and information were identified as barriers to participation at home by caregivers of children with disabilities. Cognitive and social demands along with inadequate money, services, supplies, transportation, policies and procedures were considered as barriers to participation in school and community. Differences in the perceived environmental support were evident descriptively (lower number of supports reported among those with disabilities), yet no statistical significance across any of the settings was observed.

Reliability of the Adapted PEM-CY

Estimates of internal consistency of items pertaining to all the scores across settings, examined among the entire cohort (n = 130), were acceptable to very good (0.61–0.87), as shown in Table 4 The test–retest reliability was examined among a subsample of 30 caregivers who participated; most of them had education levels above graduation (26/30) and earned more than minimum wage (29/30). Estimates of intraclass correlation were greater than 0.75, considered good to excellent in more than 80% of the items in most scales and Kappa was between 0.6 and 1.0 (good-excellent) for activities to which parents desired change in the home, school, and community settings.

On questions related to relevance, understandability, and time consumed for completing the PEM-CY, 94% (61/65) caregivers of children with disabilities reported that PEM-CY should be used in the intervention, 95% (62/65) found it relevant, 71% (46/65) found it easy to understand, and 58.4% (38/65) did not find it time-consuming to complete the measure. Twenty-seven percent (35/129) sought help for the participation sections and 39.5% (51/129) in the environmental sections. Thirty percent (27/129) participants needed assistance in both the participation and environment sections. Including the overlap between both these sections, a total of 57 percent (74/129) of caregivers needed assistance overall with various aspects of the instrument like with reading, understanding the items, and reflecting and correlating it with their personal experience.

Table 4. Group summary scores of children with (cases) and without disabilities (controls).

	Cases (n = 65)				Controls (n = 65)				n = 130	n = 130
	Home									
	Min	Max	Mean	Sd	Mean	Sd	Z/T value *	p-value	Internal consistency (Cronbach's alpha)	Effect size (Cohen's d)
Average frequency of home Participation	4.17	7	6.05	0.63	6.32	0.54	−2.649	0.008	0.7103	0.5759
Percentage of activities at home	10%	100%	87.23%	19.73%	92.92%	9.14%	−0.939	0.347		0.2419
Average of involvements at home	1	5	3.56	0.79	4.04	0.74	−3.716	<0.001	0.7158	0.7036
Home-percentage of change desired	0%	100%	77.28%	25.89%	54.91%	27.77%	−4.613	<<0.001	0.8161	0.8157
Home environment-score 3 (Support)	0	66.7%	27.692%	16.345%	32.692%	18.768%	−1.695	0.090	0.8303	1.2377 (HE)
Home environment-score 1 (Barriers)	0	66.6%	16.154%	16.853%	2.820%	6.633%	−5.837	<<0.001		
	School									
	Min	Max	Mean	Sd	Mean	Sd	Z/T value *	p-value	Internal consistency (Cronbach's alpha)	Effect size (Cohen's d)
Average of school frequency **	1	7	4.73	1.32 (IQR: 1.70)	5.42	1.00 (IQR: 1.65)	−3.272	0.0013	0.6079	0.9225
Percentage of activities at school	20%	100%	68%	26%	83%	20%	−3.257	0.001		0.3038

Table 4. Cont.

			Cases (n = 65)		Controls (n = 65)				n = 130	n = 130
Average of involvements at school	1	5	3.12	1.28	4.11	0.86	−4.457	<<0.001	0.7041	0.871
School percentage of change desired	0	100	78.65%	30.86%	45.47%	38.25%	−4.960	<<0.001	0.8535	1.0339
School environment-score 3 (Support)	0	94%	35.93%	21.57%	39.71%	18.98%	−1.195	0.232	0.8647	1.1139 (SE)
School environment-score 1 (Barriers)	0	70.5%	15.20%	19.28%	2.85%	5.55%	−4.618	<<0.001		

Community										
	Min	Max	Mean	Sd	Mean	Sd	Z/T value *	p-value	Internal consistency (Cronbach's alpha)	Effect size (Cohen's d)
Average of community frequency **	1.83	6.80	4.27	1.07 (IQR: 1.47)	4.81	1.17 (IQR: 1.44)	−2.724	0.0073	0.7355	0.8076
Percentage of activities at community	0	10%	54%	21%	66%	19%	−3.486	<0.001		0.0543
Average of involvements at community	1	5	3.13	1.12	3.87	0.91	−3.486	<0.001	0.7929	0.525
Community percentage of change desired	0	100%	73.18%	28.98%	49.74%	34.00%	−4.006	<<0.001	0.8626	0.7774
Community environment-score 3 (Support)	0	93.7%	28.17%	18.95%	30.19%	18.51%	−0.710	0.478	0.8768	1.0235 (CE)
Community environment-score 1 (Barriers)	0	81.25%	21.83%	22.78%	8.56%	13.05%	−3.876	<0.001		

* Z-value replaced with T-Value where an unpaired t-test was applied. ** Unpaired t-test was applied to the average school frequency and community frequency; IQR: Interquartile range; SD: Standard Deviation; HE: Home environment; SE: School environment; CE: Community environment; p-value of ≤ 0.05 was used as the cutoff for statistical significance.

4. Discussion

The ACEF framework provides a systematic method to culturally adapt and evaluate the PEM-CY in diverse contexts. Findings from our study suggest that the adapted version of the PEM-CY, modified based on in-depth interviews with caregivers, is a valid and reliable tool for assessing the participation of children and youth living in India.

The development of the original PEM-CY (content and layout) involved in-depth interviews and focus groups with parents/caregivers of children with and without disabilities living in North America, the end-users of these measures [9]. This has likely contributed to the widespread acceptability of the construct of participation across cultures and may explain why no modifications at the level of the "concept" were required. Caregivers of children with disabilities participating in our study too agreed that participation was a relevant construct and a measure like the Indian PEM-CY should be used in practice. Among certain cultures, parents associate successful participation with independence and autonomy in family life and the larger community [41]. Similarly, we observed that caregivers in our study initially tended to focus on the child's abilities and independence while responding to questions related to the frequency and involvement or environment sections in various activities. In addition to this, having a deficit-based approach might be contributing to difficulties in understanding the contribution of the environment to a child's ability to participate. However, the use of reminders and repeating instructions, as part of "operational" modifications, assisted in overcoming this challenge. In this sense, the PEM-CY provides a structured method and opportunity to discuss participation and factors that influence it thereby creating a shift towards a strengths-based, participation-focused approach to disabilities from a provider and caregiver perspective.

Further, we found that operational modifications were the most common in a low resource setting such as ours and studies conducted in other high resource contexts [17,42,43]. The need for operational modifications in high and low resource settings alike underscores the importance of health literacy in the caregiver respondents across settings [44]. Cognitive interviews were critical in establishing item, semantic, and operational equivalencies and identifying the need for a dual-mode of administration of the measure (self and provider administered).

Overall, the psychometric equivalencies including construct validity, test–retest reliability, and internal consistency of adapted PEM CY were adequate. The test–retest reliability was relatively lower on a few scales such as school frequency and community environment. This could be explained by the caregivers' report on having less information and control over the child's participation in school and some community settings during the cognitive interviews. As anticipated, this PEM-CY was able to identify the discrepancies between frequency and involvement in the participation of children with and without disabilities, supporting its construct validity. In addition, caregivers of children with disabilities desired change in participation more often and experienced more environmental barriers, as expected. While caregivers of children with disabilities perceived money, time, information, and supplies as being supports to a lesser extent than caregivers of children without disabilities these differences were not statistically significant. The physical, social, cognitive, or sensory demands of activity were not considered as supports by both groups. This is perhaps because caregivers in India are found to rely on informal social supports for enhancing the diversity of their child's participation and to improve their well-being [13].

Participation is a relatively new construct for caregivers of children in the Indian context [14]. The use of the PEM-CY provides an opportunity to engage caregivers and children in identifying and utilizing formal and informal social supports that can improve participation. Such information can inform tailored intervention plans that address environmental barriers and supports identified by parents.

Limitations and Future Directions

The diversity of the education level of caregivers participating in our study is not representative of the education levels of caregivers from rural India. Further, there are likely to be differences in environmental supports and barriers between urban and rural India. For these reasons, the Indian PEM-CY may be better suited for use in urban India. Caregivers who participated in our study endorsed the relevance, utility, and feasibility of the Indian PEM-CY. The PEM-CY has the potential to evaluate programmatic outcomes.

Facilitators, barriers, and feasibility of such an exercise from a providers' perspective needs to be examined in further studies.

5. Conclusions

The Indian PEM-CY is a reliable and valid measure that can be used in an urban context. The availability of a culturally adapted measure for evaluating the participation of children with disabilities offers a unique opportunity. At an individual level, it has the potential to reorient the child, caregiver, and health care provider focus on participation and environmental supports and barriers. Using parent interviews as a mode of administration offers service providers an important opportunity to dialogue with and influence the thinking about participation and the impact of the environment in resource-poor settings like ours.

Author Contributions: Conceptualization, R.S., R.T. and D.A.; methodology, R.T. and D.A.; validation, R.T. and D.A.; formal analysis, R.S. and V.K.; data curation, R.S., V.K. and S.S.; writing—original draft preparation, R.S., V.K. and S.S.; writing—review and editing, R.S., R.T. and D.A.; supervision, V.K.; project administration, R.S.; funding acquisition, R.S. All authors have read and agreed to the published version of the manuscript.

Funding: This study was funded by Corporate Social Responsibility (CSR) Grant from Bajaj Finance Ltd. for expenses towards research work (Grant ID: 0959/BFL).

Institutional Review Board Statement: The study was conducted according to the guidelines of the Declaration of Helsinki and approved by the Institutional Review Board (or Ethics Committee) of KASTURBA HOSPITAL OF INFECTIOUS DISEASES- Approval ID 01/2019.

Informed Consent Statement: Informed consent was obtained from all subjects involved in the study.

Data Availability Statement: The data presented in this study are openly available in Fig-share at https://doi.org/10.6084/m9.figshare.13455110.v1.

Acknowledgments: We would like to acknowledge Linaila D'souza, Occupational Therapist and Research Assistant who was involved in the data collection process for the phase 2 of this study. We also would like to acknowledge our colleagues at the child development center who supported us to conduct this study. Lastly, this study would not have been possible without the caregivers who participated in it.

Conflicts of Interest: The authors declare no conflict of interest. The funders had no role in the design of the study; in the collection, analyses, or interpretation of data; in the writing of the manuscript, or in the decision to publish the results.

Appendix A

Table A1. Likert Scale for Level of Assistance.

Level of Assistance	Type of Assistance
Level 1	Redirecting them to the survey guidelines (Formatting issues, reminding to reread survey guidelines).
Level 2	Prompts like reading out the items and asking questions like "what opportunities are available in your context?" (reading with them and encouraging them to think of examples related to their context).
Level 3	Discussion over an item and then filling up the question (explaining the item to them, giving them examples, talking about understanding, and relating to their context).

References

1. Law, M. Participation in the Occupations of Everyday Life. *Am. J. Occup. Ther.* **2002**, 640–649. [CrossRef] [PubMed]
2. World Health Organization. Towards a Common Language for Functioning, Disability and Health: ICF. *Int. Classif.* **2002**, *1149*, 1–22.
3. World Health Organization. *How to Use the ICF: A Practical Manual for Using the International Classification of Functioning, Disability and Health (ICF). Exposure Draft for Comment*; WHO: Geneva, Switzerland, 2013.
4. Law, M.; Anaby, D.; Teplicky, R.; Khetani, M.A.; Coster, W.; Bedell, G. Participation in the Home Environment among Children and Youth with and without Disabilities. *Br. J. Occup. Ther.* **2013**, *76*, 58–66. [CrossRef]
5. Imms, C.; Adair, B.; Keen, D.; Ullenhag, A.; Rosenbaum, P.; Granlund, M. "Participation": A Systematic Review of Language, Definitions, and Constructs Used in Intervention Research with Children with Disabilities. *Dev. Med. Child Neurol.* **2016**, *58*, 29–38. [CrossRef] [PubMed]
6. Coster, W.; Bedell, G.; Law, M.; Khetani, M.A.; Teplicky, R.; Liljenquist, K.; Gleason, K.; Kao, Y.C. Psychometric Evaluation of the Participation and Environment Measure for Children and Youth. *Dev. Med. Child Neurol.* **2011**, *53*, 1030–1037. [CrossRef] [PubMed]
7. Adair, B.; Ullenhag, A.; Rosenbaum, P.; Granlund, M.; Keen, D.; Imms, C. Measures Used to Quantify Participation in Childhood Disability and Their Alignment with the Family of Participation-Related Constructs: A Systematic Review. *Dev. Med. Child Neurol.* **2018**, *60*, 1101–1116. [CrossRef] [PubMed]
8. Resch, C.; Van Kruijsbergen, M.; Ketelaar, M.; Hurks, P.; Adair, B.; Imms, C.; De Kloet, A.; Piskur, B.; Van Heugten, C. Assessing Participation of Children with Acquired Brain Injury and Cerebral Palsy: A Systematic Review of Measurement Properties. *Dev. Med. Child Neurol.* **2020**, *62*, 434–444. [CrossRef]
9. Bedell, G.M.; Khetani, M.A.; Cousins, M.A.; Coster, W.J.; Law, M.C. Parent Perspectives to Inform Development of Measures of Children's Participation and Environment. *Arch. Phys. Med. Rehabil.* **2011**, *92*, 765–773. [CrossRef] [PubMed]
10. Khetani, M. Psychometric Evaluation of the Young Children's Participation and Environment Measure (YC–PEM). *Am. J. Occup. Ther.* **2015**, *69*, 6911500184p1. [CrossRef]
11. Olusanya, B.O.; Davis, A.C.; Wertlieb, D.; Boo, N.Y.; Nair, M.K.C.; Halpern, R.; Kuper, H.; Breinbauer, C.; de Vries, P.J.; Gladstone, M.; et al. Developmental Disabilities among Children Younger than 5 Years in 195 Countries and Territories, 1990–2016: A Systematic Analysis for the Global Burden of Disease Study 2016. *Lancet Glob. Health* **2018**, *6*, e1100–e1121. [CrossRef]
12. Schlebusch, L.; Huus, K.; Samuels, A.; Granlund, M.; Dada, S. Participation of Young People with Disabilities and/or Chronic Conditions in Low- and Middle-Income Countries: A Scoping Review. *Dev. Med. Child Neurol.* **2020**, *62*, 1259–1265. [CrossRef] [PubMed]
13. Dada, S.; Bastable, K.; Halder, S. The Role of Social Support in Participation Perspectives of Caregivers of Children with Intellectual Disabilities in India and South Africa. *Int. J. Environ. Res. Public Health* **2020**, *17*, 6644. [CrossRef] [PubMed]
14. Jindal, P.; MacDermid, J.C.; Rosenbaum, P.; DiRezze, B.; Narayan, A. Perspectives on Rehabilitation of Children with Cerebral Palsy: Exploring a Cross-Cultural View of Parents from India and Canada Using the International Classification of Functioning, Disability and Health. *Disabil. Rehabil.* **2018**, *40*, 2745–2755. [CrossRef] [PubMed]
15. Kumar, S.G.; Roy, G.; Kar, S.S. Disability and Rehabilitation Services in India: Issues and Challenges. *J. Fam. Med. Prim. care* **2012**, *1*, 69–73. [CrossRef]
16. Creswell, J. *Research Design: Qualitative, Quantitative, and Mixed Methods Approaches*, 4th ed.; SAGE Publications, Inc.: Thousand Oaks, CA, USA, 2014; Volume 71. [CrossRef]
17. Lim, C.Y.; Law, M.; Khetani, M.; Pollock, N.; Rosenbaum, P. Establishing the Cultural Equivalence of the Young Children's Participation and Environment Measure (YC-PEM) for Use in Singapore. *Phys. Occup. Ther. Pediatr.* **2016**, *36*, 422–439. [CrossRef]
18. Stevelink, S.A.M.; Van Brakel, W.H. The Cross-Cultural Equivalence of Participation Instruments: A Systematic Review. *Disabil. Rehabil.* **2013**, *35*, 1256–1268. [CrossRef]
19. Terwee, C.B.; Bot, S.D.M.; de Boer, M.R.; van der Windt, D.A.W.M.; Knol, D.L.; Dekker, J.; Bouter, L.M.; de Vet, H.C.W. Quality Criteria Were Proposed for Measurement Properties of Health Status Questionnaires. *J. Clin. Epidemiol.* **2007**, *60*, 34–42. [CrossRef]
20. Tomas, V.; Srinivasan, R.; Kulkarni, V.; Teplicky, R.; Anaby, D.; Khetani, M. A Guiding Process for Culturally Adapting Assessments for Participation-Focused Pediatric Practice: The Case of the Participation and Environment Measures (PEM). *Disabil. Rehabil.* **2020**. Under review.
21. Beaton, D.E.; Claire, B.; Guillemin, F.; Ferraz, M.B. Guidelines for the Process of Cross-Cultural Adaptation of Self-Report Measures. *Spine* **1976**, *25*, 3186–3191. [CrossRef]
22. Bowden, A.; Fox-Rushby, J.A. A Systematic and Critical Review of the Process of Translation and Adaptation of Generic Health-Related Quality of Life Measures in Africa, Asia, Eastern Europe, the Middle East, South America. *Soc. Sci. Med.* **2003**, *57*, 1289–1306. [CrossRef]
23. Peterson, C.H.; Peterson, N.A.; Powell, K.G. Cognitive Interviewing for Item Development: Validity Evidence Based on Content and Response Processes. *Meas. Eval. Couns. Dev.* **2017**, *50*, 217–223. [CrossRef]
24. Patrick, D.L.; Burke, L.B.; Gwaltney, C.J.; Leidy, N.K.; Martin, M.L.; Molsen, E.; Ring, L. Content Validity-Establishing and Reporting the Evidence in Newly Developed Patient-Reported Outcomes (PRO) Instruments for Medical Product Evaluation: ISPOR PRO Good Research Practices Task Force Report: Part 2-Assessing Respondent Understanding. *Value Health* **2011**, *14*, 978–988. [CrossRef] [PubMed]

25. Charters, E. The Use of Think-Aloud Methods in Qualitative Research An Introduction to Think-Aloud Methods. *Brock Educ. J.* **2003**, *12*. [CrossRef]
26. Chow, S.C.; Shao, J.; Wang, H. *Sample Size Calculations in Clinical Research*, 2nd ed.; Chapman & Hall: New York, NY, USA, 2008.
27. Streiner, D.L.; Norman, G.R. *Health Measurement Scales: A Practical Guide to Their Development and Use*, 5th ed.; Oxford University Press: Oxford, UK, 2008. [CrossRef]
28. Coster, W.; Law, M.; Bedell, G.; Anaby, D.; Khetani, M.; Teplicky, R. *PEM-CY User's Guide*; Version 1.1; CanChild Centre for Childhood Disability Research McMaster University: Hamilton, ON, Canada, 2014.
29. McCormack, H.M.; Horne, D.J.d.L.; Sheather, S. Clinical Applications of Visual Analogue Scales: A Critical Review. *Psychol. Med.* **1988**, *18*, 1007–1019. [CrossRef] [PubMed]
30. Paul-Dauphin, A.; Guillemin, F.; Virion, J.M.; Briançon, S. Bias and Precision in Visual Analogue Scales: A Randomized Controlled Trial. *Am. J. Epidemiol.* **1999**, *150*, 1117–1127. [CrossRef] [PubMed]
31. Anaby, D.; Law, M.; Coster, W.; Bedell, G.; Khetani, M.; Avery, L.; Teplicky, R. The Mediating Role of the Environment in Explaining Participation of Children and Youth with and without Disabilities across Home, School, and Community. *Arch. Phys. Med. Rehabil.* **2014**, *95*, 908–917. [CrossRef]
32. American Psychiatric Association. *Diagnostic and Statistical Manual of Mental Disorders*, 5th ed.; American Psychiatric Publishing: Arlington, VA, USA, 2013.
33. Knafl, K.; Deatrick, J.; Gallo, A.; Holcombe, G.; Bakitas, M.; Dixon, J.; Grey, M. The Analysis and Interpretation of Cognitive Interviews for Instrument Development. *Res. Nurs. Health* **2007**, *30*, 224–234. [CrossRef]
34. Mokkink, L.B.; Terwee, C.B.; Knol, D.L.; Stratford, P.W.; Alonso, J.; Patrick, D.L.; Bouter, L.M.; De Vet, H.C. The COSMIN Checklist for Evaluating the Methodological Quality of Studies on Measurement Properties: A Clarification of Its Content. *BMC Med. Res. Methodol.* **2010**, *10*. [CrossRef]
35. Shapiro, A.S.S.; Wilk, M.B. An Analysis of Variance Test for Normality. *Biometrika* **1965**, *52*, 591–611. [CrossRef]
36. Cohen, J. *Statistical Power Analysis for the Behavioral Sciences*, 2nd ed.; Lawrence Erlbaum Associates: New York, NY, USA, 1988.
37. Shrout, P.E.; Fleiss, J.L. Intraclass Correlations: Uses in Assessing Rater Reliability. *Psychol. Bull.* **1979**, *86*, 420–428. [CrossRef]
38. Cohen, J. A Coefficient of Agreement for Nominal Scales. *Educ. Psychol. Meas.* **1960**, *20*, 37–46. [CrossRef]
39. Landis, J.R.; Koch, G.G. Landis Amd Koch1977_agreement of Categorical Data. *Biometrics* **1977**, *33*, 159–174. [CrossRef] [PubMed]
40. Portney, L.G.; Watkins, M.P. *Foundations of Clinical Research: Applications to Practice*, 2nd ed.; Pearson/Prentice Hall: Upper Saddle River, NJ, USA, 2000.
41. Munyi, C.W. Past and Present Perceptions Towards Disability: A Historical Perspective. *Disabil. Stud. Q.* **2012**, *32*. [CrossRef]
42. Krieger, B.; Schulze, C.; Boyd, J.; Amann, R.; Piškur, B.; Beurskens, A.; Teplicky, R.; Moser, A. Cross-Cultural Adaptation of the Participation and Environment Measure for Children and Youth (PEM-CY) into German: A Qualitative Study in Three Countries. *BMC Pediatr.* **2020**, 1–32. [CrossRef] [PubMed]
43. Jeong, Y.; Law, M.; Stratford, P.; DeMatteo, C.; Kim, H. Cross-Cultural Validation and Psychometric Evaluation of the Participation and Environment Measure for Children and Youth in Korea. *Disabil. Rehabil.* **2016**, *38*, 2217–2228. [CrossRef] [PubMed]
44. Nutbeam, D. Health Literacy as a Public Health Goal: A Challenge for Contemporary Health Education and Communication Strategies into the 21st Century. *Health Promot. Int.* **2000**, *15*, 259–267. [CrossRef]

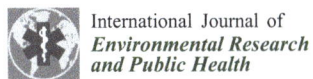

Article

The Participation of Children with Intellectual Disabilities: Including the Voices of Children and Their Caregivers in India and South Africa

Shakila Dada [1,*], Kirsty Bastable [1], Liezl Schlebusch [1] and Santoshi Halder [2]

[1] Centre for Augmentative and Alternative Communication, University of Pretoria, Pretoria 0001, South Africa; kgb0071978@gmail.com (K.B.); liezl@treesofhope.co.za (L.S.)
[2] Department of Education, University of Calcutta, Kolkata 700078, India; santoshi_halder@yahoo.com
* Correspondence: shakila.dada@up.ac.za

Received: 14 August 2020; Accepted: 10 September 2020; Published: 15 September 2020

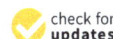

Abstract: There is a shortage of research on the participation of children with intellectual disabilities from middle-income countries. Also, most child assessments measure either the child's or the caregiver's perceptions of participation. Participation, however, is an amalgamation of both perspectives, as caregivers play a significant role in both accessing and facilitating opportunities for children's participation. This paper reports on both perceptions—those of children with intellectual disabilities and those of their caregiver, in India and South Africa. A quantitative group comparison was conducted using the Children's Assessment of Participation and Enjoyment (CAPE) that was translated into Bengali and four South African languages. One hundred child–caregiver dyads from India and 123 pairs from South Africa participated in the study. The results revealed interesting similarities and differences in participation patterns, both between countries and between children and their caregivers. Differences between countries were mostly related to the intensity of participation, with whom, and where participation occurred. Caregiver and child reports differed significantly regarding participation and the enjoyment of activities. This study emphasises the need for consideration of cultural differences when examining participation and suggests that a combined caregiver-and-child-reported approach may provide the broadest perspective on children's participation.

Keywords: participation; intellectual disabilities; low- and middle-income country; self-report; proxy report; India; South Africa

---

1. Introduction

The right of individuals with disabilities to "full and effective participation and inclusion in society" [1] (p. 6) is enshrined in the United Nations convention on the rights of people with disabilities. As a result, participation is often highlighted as an intervention goal for children who have disabilities. However, the measurement and implementation of this goal have been challenging as participation is bi-directional. That is, participation is both the mechanism for, and the outcome of development [2]. Where children's development is typical, they participate in activities using behaviours or skills, the complexity of which is fostered and increased within the activities until the skills are mastered [2,3]. For children with disabilities, however, barriers to participation may arise both from individual and environmental factors. As such, the child may be prevented from participating or from participating at the required level for their skills to develop and grow. The barriers experienced by children with disabilities have been described in studies that compared the participation of children with disabilities to that of their peers who were typically developing. These studies identified decreased attendance (or diversity) in active physical, academic, and social activities [4–6], and decreased intensity (or frequency) of participation in formal activities outside of school [4,5] for children with disabilities.

In addition to the challenges identified in the research for children with disabilities, several gaps have been identified in the literature on participation. First, the majority of research has been conducted among children with cerebral palsy, while research on other disabilities has been limited [7–13]. This is despite evidence that intellectual disability has been ranked as one of the most severe and commonly occurring disabilities in children worldwide [14]. Intellectual disability is a pervasive and lifelong condition characterised by significant limitations in both intellectual functioning and adaptive behaviour originating before the age of 18 years [15]. A recent systematic review of the participation of children with intellectual disabilities identified only four studies [16], while a further four studies not included in the review were subsequently also identified [4,17–19]. These studies noted more limited participation in active physical and skills-based activities for children with intellectual disabilities [4,16–20] than for typically developing children, and found that participation occurred more frequently in the home setting with adults, rather than in the community with peers [4,19,21].

A second challenge specifically related to children with intellectual disabilities is that the tools used to obtain participation data have thus far been founded on the premise that children's participation is best understood from their own perspective [4,22]. Hence, assessments of participation rely on only information from the child. However, as described by Nilsson et al. (2015), including the perspectives of adults/children in research is not an either/or scenario but rather a continuum, and the use of only one component on the continuum can limit the depth of the research [23]. For children with intellectual disabilities in particular, the requirement for self-reporting participation can introduce barriers associated with cognitive, linguistic, and communication difficulties [4], which can affect the results reported. Hence, obtaining participation data on a continuum that includes both adult and child input may be beneficial. This position is supported in the ICF-CY where the role of adults in the participation of children who are younger or who have disabilities is described as "integral to understanding participation" [24] (pp. xvi.). This is because for these children, participation opportunities are more likely to be identified by parents or caregivers than by the child themselves [24–26].

A third challenge in the literature is that both the development of tools to measure participation and studies on the participation of children have been primarily implemented in high-income countries [27–29]. Although the Picture my Participation tool [29] has been developed and validated specifically for use in low-and middle-income countries, as yet no comparative data from this has been published. A lack of research from low- and middle-income countries introduces complexity to the evaluation of participation, as low- and middle-income countries are culturally and economically different from high-income countries [30]. Furthermore, as participation requires the measurement of culturally relevant activities [2], cultural differences may affect the results obtained in respect of participation measures and limit the generalisability of findings.

A fourth concern relating to the dearth of participation research in low- and middle-income countries is evidence that worldwide up to 94.5% of children with epilepsy, intellectual disabilities, vision, or hearing loss live in low and middle-income countries [14,30]. Hence, the data on the participation of children with intellectual disabilities is limited both in extent (research among children with intellectual disabilities) and context (research in low- and middle-income countries).

Although the field of participation research has grown since the introduction of the ICF-CY [24], significant gaps in knowledge remain around children with intellectual disabilities and children from low- and middle-income countries. The current study sought to describe and compare the participation of children with intellectual disabilities from two middle-income countries, India (lower-middle-income) and South Africa (upper-middle-income) [31]. Due to the challenges experienced by children with intellectual disabilities in self-reporting, the data on participation was collected using both caregiver and child reports of participation, which enabled a comparison of the child and caregiver reports to compare the two perspectives for similarities and differences.

The countries for the study were selected because India has one of the highest (≈6%), and South Africa has one of the lowest (≈2.25%) reported prevalence of intellectual disability among middle-income countries [14]. In addition, India and South Africa both have cultures that differ from those of high-income countries. Culture is described as the combination of collective norms, values, experiences and histories of a particular group, which emerges from daily activities in which families and communities are connected [32]. Culture is reported to shape the day-to-day activities that are most important to families and communities [33–35]. Both India and South Africa tend towards a collectivist culture in which the individual is an integral component of the community, while high-income countries tend towards a more individualistic culture in which the individual remains conceptually separate from the community [35–38]. Although India and South Africa are considered collectivist cultures, one of the differences between the two cultures is the presence of the class system that is socially maintained in India. At the same time, South Africa is divided primarily by racial group and economic class [36]. Furthermore, India has a much higher gender gap than South Africa, but South Africa reports higher poverty rates [31,39]. Comparing India and South Africa may provide insight into differences in participation not only between high- and middle-income countries, but also between middle-income countries with different cultures.

2. Materials and Methods

2.1. Aims

The current research study aimed to (a) describe the participation of children with intellectual disabilities from India and South Africa; (b) compare the participation results between groups (India and South Africa) and respondents (children and caregivers).

2.2. Design

The study made use of a multi-factor design, firstly to describe the participation of children with intellectual disabilities, and secondly to compare self- and proxy-reported and country-specific participation data.

2.3. Sampling and Participant Selection

Participants for this study were selected using convenience sampling in schools and centres that catered for children who have intellectual disabilities. To participate in the study, children had to be between the ages of six and 21 and scored as having a mild to moderate intellectual disability on the Kaufman Brief Intelligence Test (KBIT) [40]. The children's home language had to be Bengali, English, Afrikaans, isiZulu, or isiXhosa, as these were the languages into which the Children's Assessment of Participation and Enjoyment (CAPE) [41] had been translated. If a child's home language was not the same as the language in which the CAPE [41] was to be administered at their school, then the child needed to have been schooled in the language of the CAPE [41] for at least $1\frac{1}{2}$ years to be included in the study. Caregivers were required to be literate in Bengali, English, Afrikaans, isiZulu, or isiXhosa.

2.4. Ethics

India: Ethics approval for the study was obtained from the Ethics Committee of the University of Calcutta, and the appropriate departments and heads of schools or organisations. Participants were recruited from twelve government and non-government associations or schools.

South Africa: Ethics approval was obtained from the Research Committee of the University of Pretoria (GW20160409HS), and permission was obtained from the Department of Education in six provinces in South Africa. Additionally, permission was obtained from school principals or school governing bodies. Participants were recruited from 15 schools (11 government/public schools and four non-government/private schools).

2.5. Participants

A total of 100 caregiver-child dyads from India and 123 dyads from South Africa took part in the study. The children ranged in age from five to 18 years (mean = 12.3); 61.3% of them were male, and 38.7% female. Caregivers reporting on their child's participation were primarily mothers (73.6%), but fathers (15.6%) and other caregivers (10.8%) also responded. Most caregivers had not completed high school and earned less than R4500.00 (approximately €220.00) per month.

Respondents reported their home language as Bengali (37.1%), English (17.2%), Afrikaans (13.6), isiZulu (9.3%), isiXhosa (6.7%), and other languages (16.1%), while the survey was completed in Bengali (43.1%), English (37.1%), Afrikaans (9.5%), isiZulu (5.2%) and isiXhosa (5.2%). The summarised demographic data of the participants is represented in Table 1.

Table 1. Demographic data of participants from India and South Africa.

	India	South Africa	Combined Data	Equivalence [1] p-Value
Caregiver-child dyads	n = 100	n = 132	232	
Child age (years)	mean = 11.9 (SD: 2.5)	mean = 12.7 (SD: 2.6)	mean = 12.3	0.000 [2]
Sex				
Male	66.0	57.8	61.3	0.44 [4]
Female	34.0	42.2	38.7	
Additional impairments (%) [3]	12.6	13.0	25.6	0.17 [4]
Home language				
	Bengali: 37.1 Hindi: 5.2 Other: 2.0	English: 17.2 Afrikaans: 13.6 isiZulu: 9.3 isixhosa: 6.7 SiSwati: 1.3 Sesotho: 2.6 Sepedi: 2.6 Other: 2.3 Setswana: 1.7		
Survey language (%) [3]				
Bengali	43.1			
English		37.1		
Afrikaans		9.5		
isiZulu		5.2		
isiXhosa		5.2		
Caregiver respondent (%) [3]				
Mother	33.8	39.8	73.6	
Father	6.1	9.5	15.6	0.129 [4]
Other	3.5	7.4	10.8	
Caregiver education (%) [3]				
Grade 11 or less	23.1	17.8	40.9	
Grade 12	7.1	17.8	24.9	0.000 [2]
Degree	12.0	8.9	20.9	
Other	2.2	11.1	13.3	
Household income (%) [3]				
<R4500 (≈€220)/month	1.8	26.2	28.0	
R4501-R12500 (≈€600)/month	4.4	12.4	16.9	
R12501-R30000 (≈€1500)/month	11.6	7.6	19.1	
R30001-R52000 (≈€2500)/month	5.8	3.6	9.3	0.000 [2]
R52001-R70000 (≈€3370)/month	6.2	3.1	9.3	
>R70001 (≈€3370)/month	14.7	2.7	17.3	

Notes: [1] Group equivalence between India and South Africa; [2] Pearson chi-square $p < 0.05$; [3] Percentages may not add up to 100 due to rounding; [4] Fisher's exact test—one-sided.

2.6. Materials

Data on participation for this study was obtained by administering the Children's Assessment of Participation and Enjoyment (CAPE) [41]. The CAPE [41] is a self-report questionnaire that has been developed for use with children (with and without disabilities) between the ages of 6–21 years. The CAPE [41] considers 55 activities grouped into eight activity domains: (1) overall; (2) informal activities; (3) formal activities; (4) recreational activities; (5) active physical activities; (6) social activities; (7) skills-based activities; and (8) self-improvement. For each activity domain, five dimensions of participation were measured: (1) diversity; (2) intensity; (3) companionship; (4) location; and (5) enjoyment. The CAPE [41] is typically administered in an interview with the child and takes 45 min to complete [41].

The CAPE [41] was developed and has been shown to have adequate validity and reliability in English [42–44]. Internal consistency and test-retest reliability have been confirmed in Dutch [45], Greek [46], Spanish [47,48], Swedish [49], Chinese [50] and Norwegian [51]. However, the need for cultural validation (in addition to translation) has been highlighted by various authors [48–50,52]. For this study, permission was obtained by the publishers to translate the CAPE [41] for use in India and South Africa. For India it was translated into Bengali and for South Africa into Afrikaans, isiXhosa and isiZulu. Translation included forward and backward translation as well as the consideration of linguistic, functional and cultural equivalence [53].

For this study, the proxy report version of the CAPE [41] was developed with permission from the publishers, and it was translated following the same procedures as the child's version [52]. The caregiver version of the CAPE [41] was modified so that the subject of all questions was the caregiver's child and not the caregiver. The caregiver version was a pen-and-paper version of the CAPE [41].

2.7. Data Collection

Caregivers received an information pack from their child's school. The language of the information pack was based on feedback from the school. Included in the information pack were an information letter about the study, a consent form for caregivers to complete, and the proxy version of the CAPE [41]. Caregivers had to give consent for themselves and their children to be involved in the study. Caregivers independently completed and returned the consent form and proxy version of the CAPE [41] to the school. Children were asked to provide assent to participate in the study on the day of data collection. The researcher administered the CAPE [41] to the children individually at school. The child was asked the questions and their answers were recorded using the methods and visual supports recommended in the manual. The CAPE [41] was administered to the children in the language of the school, and participants were provided with a small token of appreciation for their help (a ruler and an eraser). The researchers were fluent in the language in which they administered the CAPE [41].

2.8. Data Analysis

The data for this study was analysed using IBM SPSS version 26 [54]. Demographic data was described statistically using means (reported in percentages). The distribution of the data was assessed and found to be non-normally distributed. Hence, further assessments were non-parametric (Pearson Chi-squared, Fisher's exact test) to test for group equivalence. Participation data for each participant was summed, while data on intensity, with whom, where and enjoyment was calculated as the mean of all activities participated in. The CAPE [41] data was assessed for internal consistency using Cronbach's alpha. Between-group statistical correlation of the participation data was conducted using an independent samples Kruskal–Wallis test with a post hoc pairwise comparison using the Bonferroni correction for multiple tests.

3. Results

The results of this study are presented below. The internal consistency of items on the CAPE [41] is presented first. This is followed by the self- and caregiver-reported participation of children with intellectual disabilities for India and South Africa. The reported data is then compared across children and caregivers and India and South Africa. Participation is reported overall, in the formal and informal domains, the five activity groups, and the five participation dimensions.

3.1. Internal Consistency of the CAPE Data from India and South Africa

The analysis of the data from the CAPE [41] from India and South Africa indicated that the internal consistency of the data was excellent across all domains, for both children and caregivers ($0.923 < \alpha > 0.993$) [55].

3.2. Participation of Children with Intellectual Disabilities

Significant differences were evident in the reported participation of children in India and South Africa, and as reported by children or their caregivers in all areas except participation in self-improvement.

3.2.1. Self-Reported Participation

The self-reported participation of children with intellectual disabilities averaged 27 activities in India and South Africa. Children from India were most likely to participate in activities two to three times a week, with their families, at a relative's house. In South Africa, however, children were most likely to participate in activities once a week, with other relatives, and at a relative's house. Children from both countries enjoyed participating in activities "very much". Participation results across all domains, and dimensions are presented in Table 2.

Table 2. Self-reported and caregiver-reported participation of children with intellectual disabilities in India and South Africa (Mean).

	India		South Africa		All Participants		Significance [†]
	Child	Caregiver	Child	Caregiver	Child	Caregiver	$p < 0.05$
	Participation domains and activities [1]						
Overall [i]	27.02	23.98 [a]	26.77	28.36	26.88	26.47 [b]	0.001
Informal [ii]	20.70	19.57	22.01	23.04	21.44	21.54 [b]	0.000
Formal [iii]	6.32	4.50 [a]	4.91	5.44	5.53 [b]	5.04	0.000
Recreational [iv]	6.86	6.25	8.21	8.33	7.63 [b]	7.43 [b]	0.000
Active physical [v]	5.45	4.01 [a]	4.36	4.95	4.84 [b]	4.54	0.000
Social [vi]	6.52	6.94	6.23	6.97 [a]	6.35	6.96	0.008
Skills-based [vi]	3.70	2.43 [a]	3.33	3.53	3.49	3.06 [b]	0.000
Self-improvement [vi]	4.71	4.61	5.11	5.06	4.94	4.87	0.084
	Intensity of participation [2]						
Overall [i]	5.92	5.94	4.98	4.98	5.38 [b]	5.40 [b]	0.000
Informal [ii]	5.93	5.89	5.01	5.02	5.41 [b]	5.39 [b]	0.000
Formal [iii]	5.92	6.30	4.97	4.83	5.39 [b]	5.46 [b]	0.000
Recreational [iv]	6.33	6.33	5.48	5.34	5.85 [b]	5.77 [b]	0.000
Active physical [v]	5.82	5.81	4.64	4.86	5.16 [b]	5.28 [b]	0.000
Social [vi]	5.33	5.09	4.38	4.52	4.79 [b]	4.76 [b]	0.000
Skills-based [vi]	6.56	7.29 [a]	5.12	4.82	5.75 [b]	5.88 [b]	0.000
Self-improvement [vi]	6.14	6.32	5.15	5.27	5.58 [b]	5.73 [b]	0.000

Table 2. Cont.

	India		South Africa		All Participants		Significance [†]
	Child	Caregiver	Child	Caregiver	Child	Caregiver	p < 0.05
With whom participation occurred [3]							
Overall [i]	1.68	1.57	2.40	2.62	2.09 [b]	2.16 [b]	0.000
Informal [ii]	1.61	1.51	2.29	2.46	2.00 [b]	2.05 [b]	0.000
Formal [iii]	1.89	1.77	2.90	3.36	2.46 [b]	2.68 [b]	0.000
Recreational [iv]	1.53	1.34	2.26	2.30	1.94 [b]	1.89 [b]	0.000
Active physical [v]	1.67	1.64 [a]	2.83	3.44	2.32 [b]	2.65 [b]	0.000
Social [vi]	1.72	1.65	2.47	2.52	2.15 [b]	2.14 [b]	0.000
Skills-based [vi]	1.88	1.65	2.86	3.34	2.43 [b]	2.61 [b]	0.000
Self-improvement [vi]	1.63	1.58	1.98	2.35	1.83 [b]	2.02 [b]	0.000
Where participation occurred [4]							
Overall [i]	1.79	1.83	2.53	2.43	2.21 [b]	2.18 [b]	0.000
Informal [ii]	1.66	1.71	2.36	2.23	2.06 [b]	2.01 [b]	0.000
Formal [iii]	2.23	2.36	3.49	3.40	2.94 [b]	2.95 [b]	0.000
Recreational [iv]	1.44	1.41	1.87	1.83	1.68 [b]	1.65 [b]	0.000
Active physical [v]	1.89	2.09	2.95	2.97 [a]	2.49 [b]	2.58 [b]	0.000
Social [vi]	2.00	2.11	2.70	2.51	2.40 [b]	2.34 [b]	0.000
Skills-based [vi]	2.25	2.11	2.94	3.11	2.64 [b]	2.67 [b]	0.000
Self-improvement [vi]	1.55	1.59	2.74	2.64	2.22 [b]	2.18 [b]	0.000
Enjoyment of participation [5]							
Overall [i]	4.34	4.23	4.29	3.92 [a]	4.31	4.05 [b]	0.000
Informal [ii]	4.35	4.23	4.28	3.89 [a]	4.31	4.04 [b]	0.000
Formal [iii]	4.32	4.22	4.31	4.04 [a]	4.32	4.12	0.000
Recreational [iv]	4.35	4.20	4.35	3.87 [a]	4.35	4.02 [b]	0.000
Active physical [v]	4.35	4.20	4.35	3.97 [a]	4.35	4.07	0.000
Social [vi]	4.36	4.25	4.43	4.15 [a]	4.40	4.19	0.000
Skills-based [vi]	4.23	4.25 [a]	4.25	3.85	4.25	3.97 [b]	0.000
Self-improvement [vi]	4.32	4.12	3.92	3.39 [a]	4.09 [b]	3.70 [b]	0.000

Notes: [†] Independent Samples Kruskal–Wallis test ($p < 0.05$). Post hoc pairwise comparison with Bonferroni correction for multiple tests ($p < 0.05$): [a] Significant caregiver-child difference; [b] Significant India-South Africa difference; [1] Participation = mean number of activities attended out of [i] 55 activities, [ii] 40 activities, [iii] 15 activities, [iv] 12 activities, [v] 13 activities, [vi] 10 activities; [2] Intensity: 0 = never, 1 = once in 4 months, 2 = twice in 4 months, 3 = once a month, 4 = 2–3 times a month, 5 = once a week, 6 = 2–3 times a week, 7 = once a day; [3] With whom: 1 = alone, 2 = with family (parents, siblings), 3 = with other relatives (grandparents, uncles, cousins, etc.), 4 = with friends, 5 = with others; [4] Where: 1 = at home, 2 = at a relative's house, 3 = in your neighbourhood, 4 = at school, 5 = in your community, 6 = beyond your community; [5] Enjoyment: 1 = not at all, 2 = sort of/somewhat, 3 = pretty much, 4 = very much, 5 = love it!

3.2.2. Caregiver-Reported Participation

Caregivers in India reported that their children with intellectual disabilities participate in 24 activities, compared to 28 activities reported by caregivers in South Africa. Children in India were reported to participate in the activities two to three times a week, while in South Africa, participation once a week was reported. Children in India were reported to participate most often with family, while children in South Africa were reported to participate most often with other relatives. Children in both India and South Africa were most likely to participate in activities at a relative's house and were reported to enjoy participation "pretty much". The full participation results are listed in Table 2.

3.3. Comparing the Self-and Proxy Reported Participation of Children with Intellectual Disabilities in India and South Africa

The self-reported participation of children with intellectual disabilities in India and South Africa was not significantly different overall, in the informal domain, for social, skills-based, or self-improvement activities. However participation in the formal domain and active physical and recreational activities was significantly different. Intensity, with whom and where participation occurred also differed significantly when self-reported by children in India and South Africa, but enjoyment was not significantly different.

Caregivers in India and South Africa reported differences in participation of their children who have intellectual disabilities overall, in the informal domain and in recreational and skills-based activities. Intensity, with whom and where participation occurred also differed significantly as did enjoyment in a number of areas.

Caregivers and children in India provided similar reports on participation in the informal domain, recreational, active physical, social and self-improvement activities. While caregivers and children in South Africa provided similar reports on participation in all areas except for social activities. No significant differences were evident between most child- and caregiver- reports on intensity, with whom and where participation occurred. However, significant differences were evident in the reports of enjoyment of participation between children and their caregivers in South Africa, but not in India.

4. Discussion

This study considered the participation of children with intellectual disabilities in two middle-income countries, India and South Africa. First, the participation in India and South Africa is described (self- and proxy-reported) and considered in relation to results from high income countries. Then the differences between self- and proxy-reports are examined. The discussion concludes with recommendations for practice and future research.

The self-reported participation of children who have intellectual disabilities in India and South Africa shows similarities overall, in the informal domain, social, skills-based and self-improvement activities. These results are also comparable to those from children who have intellectual disabilities in Australia [4], a high-income country. Differences in participation in the formal, recreational, and active physical domains may be associated with culture. These activities fall mostly in the formal domain, and are organised by adults. For example, sports are strongly influenced by the environment and culture. Hence, children in the US are more likely to play baseball and American football, while children in India are more likely to play cricket and hockey, and children in South Africa soccer and rugby. In contrast, socio-emotional development, which is key in informal and social activities has been reported to be similar across different collectivist cultures and individualistic cultures [35], hence the similarities in these areas between India and South Africa are not unexpected.

Differences in the intensity of participation reported between India and South Africa were evident. These differences may be related to where and with whom children participate. In the case of the children from India, a more frequent intensity of participation was reported, but participation also occurred more often at home and with their immediate family. Thus it is plausible that because the child does not have to go anywhere or participate with anyone other than those nearby, participation may occur more frequently. In contrast, the children in South Africa indicated a lower intensity of participation but more often had extended family as participation partners and venues. When compared to results from the study conducted in Australia, participation intensity in South Africa was more similar to that in Australia than that in India. Differences in with whom and where children participate could well relate to cultural or family practices, family support or the availability of resources. It is interesting that in India, where employment rates were significantly higher than in South Africa, participation occurred most often at home, as one might infer that children would attend a daycare or similar while caregivers were at work. This result, however, may suggest a greater level of in home support for caregivers in India, than for caregivers in South Africa.

Enjoyment of participation was similar when self-reported between India and South Africa, except for self-improvement activities. The mean scores for enjoyment indicate that both groups of children enjoyed these activities "very much". These results concur with other studies on participation, which propose that children, regardless of disability, enjoy participating in activities to a high degree [52].

The proxy-reported participation and enjoyment of children differed significantly between India and South Africa in all areas, except for formal, active physical and social activities. The similarities in participation in formal, active-physical, and social activities between caregivers is of interest, as it is in contrast to the differences reported by their children. A possible explanation of these differences may be related to the number of activities that children participated in. Overall caregivers in India reported fewer activities that their children participated in than caregivers in South Africa. If the activities which were not reported as participated in fell into the informal domain or were clustered in recreational, and skills-based activities a decrease in participation in these areas and the measurement of enjoyment in these areas may be seen. An alternative explanation relates to the historic educational contexts of India and South Africa. Both countries were historically British colonies, whose education systems were obligated to follow a British model, features of which are maintained today. As caregivers would have been educated in this model, it is possible that their perceptions of formal, active physical and social activities have been informed by similar constructs within the education systems, while the informal domain has been formed to a greater extent by the local culture.

Caregivers' reports on intensity of participation, with whom and where participation occurred, mirrored those of their children, showing significant differences in each of these areas. The reporting of Enjoyment of participation showed a similar pattern of significant differences to participation.

When the self- and proxy-reported participation data is compared, differences were evident in India for participation overall, in the formal domain, active physical and skill-based activities. In South Africa however only social activities were reported differently. Reasons for the different directions of reporting are not known but could relate to the child's preferences or independence. Caregivers may only perceive participation to be occurring when their child has chosen to participate, or is able to participate independently. In contrast, children may report on "being there", regardless of their choice or role in the activity [56]. In addition, different cultural norms may impact the activities available to children. For example, within Indian culture, a person's position is strongly determined by their caste, and the activities families may access are determined by this social structure [36–38]. In South Africa, on the other hand, the provision of activities is more likely to be linked to an educational or economic opportunity. Other differences not explored in this paper could also be the availability of support from others, the number of children in the household, or the cultural beliefs of the caregivers regarding children with disabilities, their needs, rights and abilities [57,58].

This paper expected to report significant differences in the reporting of enjoyment for self and proxy-reports. This was based on studies that have suggested that proxy reports vary from direct-reports in areas of non-observable functioning, for example emotions [59–62]. Hence, the lack of difference in the reporting of enjoyment of participation between children and caregivers in India requires consideration. It is possible that differences in the expression of enjoyment could be linked to communication styles from India and South Africa. As reported in relation to socioemotional skills, adolescents from South Africa were reported to be more likely to have medium communication skills than counterparts from Malaysia, who were more likely to have high communication skills (an Asian collectivist culture). If this pattern is repeated between India and South Africa, it would suggest that children in India communicate with their caregivers at a different level than do children in South Africa, which could impact the likelihood of emotions, which are not clearly visible being recognised [35] and accurately reported.

Overall, the significant differences in participation from children in India and South Africa highlight the need for increased research from low- and middle-income countries and for an understanding that participation is culturally biased. Hence there is a need for participation assessment and intervention to take cultural norms, values, and differences into account. In addition, there are significant differences in self- and proxy-reports on participation, but the differences do not negate the consideration of either perspective. Instead, if perspective, as described by Nilsson et al. [23], is considered, the combination of child and proxy reports could provide more comprehensive participation information, particularly where children experience difficulty in communicating.

4.1. Limitations

This study is limited by a lack of comparison group of children who have typical development in either country. Without this, it is not possible to ascertain if differences in participation are culturally based or related to the children's disabilities. In addition, it is not possible to determine if the children in India and South Africa who have intellectual disabilities are able to have "full and effective participation and inclusion in society" [1] (p. 6). A further limitation of this study is the lack of comparative data from high-income countries. Although results from Australia are referred to, without the actual data for full analysis, the comparison between the participation of children with intellectual disabilities from middle- and high-income countries remains superficial.

4.2. Recommendations for Practice and Future Research

For interventionists in the field, particularly those working in diverse societies, the participation of children is a key aim. However, the measurement of participation needs careful consideration due to the sensitivity of participation to cultural differences, and the need to include both self- and proxy-reported participation data. Goal setting for intervention needs to be driven by the child's, family such that their own culture is expressed in their child's participation.

Further research on the reasons for the differences between the participation of children in South Africa and India is required, in particular concerning environmental factors such as culture, social support and available resources. Also, further research on participation of children who have typical development in low-income and other middle-income countries would add to the understanding of participation in different cultures. Further research on the validity of the CAPE [41] in low- and middle-income settings is also required.

5. Conclusions

Overall, the patterns of participation of children with intellectual disabilities in India and South Africa showed a number of similarities. However, differences in patterns of participation could be related to cultural differences between the two countries. Caregiver and child reports on participation also showed differences that could be culturally based. The results of this study support the use of proxy reporting for measuring participation as a valid strategy when used in combination with child reporting, specifically of perspectives and emotions. Further research on the participation of children in low- and middle-income countries is recommended.

Author Contributions: Conceptualisation, S.D. and S.H.; methodology, S.D. and S.H.; validation, K.B., S.D. and L.S.; formal analysis, K.B.; investigation, S.D. and S.H.; resources, S.D. and S.H.; data curation, K.B., S.D., S.H., L.S.; writing—original draft preparation, K.B., S.D.; writing—review and editing, K.B., S.D., S.H., L.S.; visualization, K.B. and S.D.; supervision, K.B., S.D.; project administration, S.D., S.H.; funding acquisition, S.D. and S.H. All authors have read and agreed to the published version of the manuscript.

Funding: Funding from the National Institute of Humanities and Social Sciences/Indian Council of Social Science Research is hereby acknowledged. The content of this paper is solely the responsibility of the authors and does not necessarily represent the official views of the funders.

Acknowledgments: The authors would like to acknowledge the assistance of the Masters in Early Childhood Intervention students from who assisted with data collection in South Africa.

Conflicts of Interest: The authors declare no conflict of interest. The funders had no role in the design of the study; in the collection, analysis or interpretation of data; in the writing of the manuscript, or in the decision to publish the results.

References

1. UN. *United Nations Convention on the Rights of Persons with Disabilities*; UN: Genva, Switzerland, 2006; p. 37.
2. Imms, C.; Granlund, M.; Wilson, P.H.; Steenbergen, B.; Rosenbaum, P.L.; Gordon, A.M. Participation, both a means and an end: A conceptual analysis of processes and outcomes in childhood disability. *Dev. Med. Child Neurol.* **2016**, *59*, 16–25. [CrossRef] [PubMed]
3. Bronfenbrenner, U.; Morris, P.A. The Bioecological Model of Human Development. In *Handbook of Child Psychology*; John Wiley & Sons, Inc.: Hoboken, NJ, USA, 2006; pp. 793–828. ISBN 9780470147658.
4. King, M.G.; Shields, N.; Imms, C.; Black, M.; Ardern, C.L. Participation of children with intellectual disability compared with typically developing children. *Res. Dev. Disabil.* **2013**, *34*, 1854–1862. [CrossRef] [PubMed]
5. Law, M.; King, G.; King, S.; Kertoy, M.; Hurley, P.; Rosenbaum, P.; Young, N.; Hanna, S. Patterns of participation in recreational and leisure activities among children with complex physical disabilities. *Dev. Med. Child Neurol.* **2006**, *48*, 337–342. [CrossRef]
6. King, G.; Law, M.; Hurley, P.; Petrenchik, T.; Schwellnus, H. A developmental comparison of the out-of-school recreation and leisure activity participation of boys and girls with and without physical disabilities. *Int. J. Disabil. Dev. Educ.* **2010**, *57*, 77–107. [CrossRef]
7. Imms, C.; Reilly, S.; Carlin, J.; Dodd, K. Diversity of participation in children with cerebral palsy. *Dev. Med. Child Neurol.* **2008**, *50*, 363–369. [CrossRef] [PubMed]
8. Voorman, J.M.; Dallmeijer, A.J.; Schuengel, C.; Knol, D.L.; Lankhorst, G.J.; Becher, J.G. Activities and participation of 9 to 13-year-old children with cerebral palsy. *Clin. Rehabil.* **2006**, *20*, 937–948. [CrossRef] [PubMed]
9. Beckung, E.; Hagberg, G. Neuroimpairments, activity limitations, and participation restrictions in children with cerebral palsy. *Dev. Med. Child Neurol.* **2002**, *44*, 309–316. [CrossRef]
10. Chiarello, L.A.; Palisano, R.J.; Bartlett, D.J.; McCoy, S.W. A multivariate model of determinants of change in gross-motor abilities and engagement in self-care and play of young children with cerebral palsy. *Phys. Occup. Ther. Pediatr.* **2010**, *31*, 150–168. [CrossRef]
11. Bult, M.; Verschuren, O.; Jongmans, M.; Lindeman, E.; Ketelaar, M. What influences participation in leisure activities of children and youth with physical disabilities? A systematic review. *Res. Dev. Disabil.* **2011**, *32*, 1521–1529. [CrossRef]
12. Imms, C. Children with cerebral palsy participate: A review of the literature. *Disabil. Rehabil.* **2008**, *30*, 1867–1884. [CrossRef]
13. Anaby, D.; Hand, C.; Bradley, L.; DiRezze, B.; Forhan, M.; Digiacomo, A.; Law, M. The effect of the environment on participation of children and youth with disabilities: A scoping review. *Disabil. Rehabil.* **2013**, *35*, 1589–1598. [CrossRef] [PubMed]
14. Olusanya, B.O.; Wright, S.M.; Nair, M.; Boo, N.-Y.; Halpern, R.; Kuper, H.; Abubakar, A.A.; Almasri, N.A.; Arabloo, J.; Arora, N.K.; et al. Global burden of childhood epilepsy, intellectual disability, and sensory impairments. *Pediatrics* **2020**, *146*, e20192623. [CrossRef] [PubMed]
15. Schalock, R.L.; Luckasson, R.A.; Shogren, K.A. The renaming of mental retardation: Understanding the change to the term intellectual disability. *Intellect. Dev. Disabil.* **2007**, *45*, 116–124. [CrossRef]
16. Shields, N.; King, M.G.; Corbett, M.; Imms, C. Is participation among children with intellectual disabilities in outside school activities similar to their typically developing peers? A systematic review. *Dev. Neurorehabilit.* **2013**, *17*, 64–71. [CrossRef]
17. Westendorp, M.; Houwen, S.; Hartman, E.; Visscher, C. Are gross motor skills and sports participation related in children with intellectual disabilities? *Res. Dev. Disabil.* **2011**, *32*, 1147–1153. [CrossRef]
18. Dahan-Oliel, N.; Mazer, B.; Riley, P.; Maltais, D.B.; Nadeau, L.; Majnemer, A. Participation and enjoyment of leisure activities in adolescents born at ≤ 29week gestation. *Early Hum. Dev.* **2014**, *90*, 307–314. [CrossRef]
19. Nelson, F.; Masulani-Mwale, C.; Richards, E.; Theobald, S.; Gladstone, M. The meaning of participation for children in Malawi: Insights from children and caregivers. *Child Care Health Dev.* **2016**, *43*, 133–143. [CrossRef]
20. Eguia, K.F.; Capio, C.M.; Simons, J. Object control skills influence the physical activity of children with intellectual disability in a developing country: The Philippines. *J. Intellect. Dev. Disabil.* **2015**, *40*, 265–274. [CrossRef]
21. Solish, A.; Perry, A.; Minnes, P. Participation of children with and without disabilities in social, recreational and leisure activities. *J. Appl. Res. Intellect. Disabil.* **2010**, *23*, 226–236. [CrossRef]

22. Granlund, M.; Arvidsson, P.; Niia, A.; Björck-Åkesson, E.; Simeonsson, R.; Maxwell, G.; Adolfsson, M.; Eriksson-Augustine, L.; Pless, M. Differentiating activity and participation of children and youth with disability in Sweden. *Am. J. Phys. Med. Rehabil.* **2012**, *91*, S84–S96. [CrossRef]
23. Nilsson, S.; Björkman, B.; Almqvist, A.-L.; Almqvist, L.; Björk-Willén, P.; Donohue, D.; Enskär, K.; Granlund, M.; Huus, K.; Hvit, S. Children's voices—Differentiating a child perspective from a child's perspective. *Dev. Neurorehabil.* **2013**, *18*, 162–168. [CrossRef] [PubMed]
24. World Health Organisation. *International Classification of Functioning, Disability and Health—Child and Youth Version (ICF-CY)*; World Health Press: Geneva, Switzerland, 2007; ISBN 9789241547321.
25. Amaral, M.F.D.; Drummond, A.D.F.; Coster, W.J.; Mancini, M.C. Household task participation of children and adolescents with cerebral palsy, Down syndrome and typical development. *Res. Dev. Disabil.* **2014**, *35*, 414–422. [CrossRef] [PubMed]
26. Einfeld, S.; Stancliffe, R.J.; Gray, K.M.; Sofronoff, K.; Rice, L.J.; Emerson, E.; Yasamy, M.T. Interventions provided by parents for children with intellectual disabilities in low and middle income countries. *J. Appl. Res. Intellect. Disabil.* **2012**, *25*, 135–142. [CrossRef] [PubMed]
27. Schlebusch, L.; Huus, K.; Samuels, A.; Granlund, M.; Dada, S. Participation of young people with disabilities and/or chronic conditions in low- and middle-income countries: A scoping review. *Dev. Med. Child Neurol.* **2020**, 1–7. [CrossRef]
28. Rainey, L.; Van Nispen, R.; Van Der Zee, C.; Van Rens, G. Measurement properties of questionnaires assessing participation in children and adolescents with a disability: A systematic review. *Qual. Life Res.* **2014**, *23*, 2793–2808. [CrossRef] [PubMed]
29. Arvidsson, P.; Dada, S.; Granlund, M.; Imms, C.; Bornman, J.; Elliott, C.; Huus, K. Content validity and usefulness of picture my participation for measuring participation in children with and without intellectual disability in South Africa and Sweden. *Scand. J. Occup. Ther.* **2019**, 1–13. [CrossRef]
30. Vawter-Lee, M.; McGann, P.T. The increasing global burden of childhood disability: A call for action. *Pediatrics* **2020**, *146*, e20201119. [CrossRef]
31. The World Bank; IBRD; IBA. World Bank Open Data. Available online: https://data.worldbank.org/ (accessed on 23 October 2019).
32. López, S.R.; Guarnaccia, P.J. Cultural psychopathology: Uncovering the social world of mental illness. *Annu. Rev. Psychol.* **2000**, *51*, 571–598. [CrossRef]
33. Yang, L.H.; Kleinman, A.; Link, B.G.; Phelan, J.C.; Lee, S.; Good, B. Culture and stigma: Adding moral experience to stigma theory. *Soc. Sci. Med.* **2007**, *64*, 1524–1535. [CrossRef]
34. Gallimore, R.; Goldenberg, C.N.; Weisner, T.S. The social construction and subjective reality of activity settings: Implications for community psychology. *Am. J. Community Psychol.* **1993**, *21*, 537–559. [CrossRef]
35. Irava, V.; Pathak, A.; DeRosier, M.; Singh, N.C. Game-based socio-emotional skills assessment: A comparison across three cultures. *J. Educ. Technol. Syst.* **2019**, *48*, 51–71. [CrossRef]
36. Yin, J. Beyond postmodernism: A non-western perspective on identity. *J. Multicult. Discourses* **2018**, *13*, 193–219. [CrossRef]
37. Kubow, P.K. Exploring Western and non-Western epistemological influences in South Africa: Theorising a critical democratic citizenship education. *Comp. A J. Comp. Int. Educ.* **2017**, *48*, 349–361. [CrossRef]
38. Ameka, F.K.; Terkourafi, M. What if ... ? Imagining non-Western perspectives on pragmatic theory and practice. *J. Pragmat.* **2019**, *145*, 72–82. [CrossRef]
39. The World Bank. Poverty and Equity Brief South Asia, Bangladesh. 2018. Available online: http://povertydata.worldbank.org/poverty/country/BGD (accessed on 4 June 2018).
40. Kreutzer, J.S.; De Luca, J.; Caplan, B. Kaufman Brief Intelligence Test. In *Encyclopedia of Clinical Neuropsychology*; Springer: New York, NY, USA, 2011; p. 103. [CrossRef]
41. King, G.; Law, M.; King, S.; Hurley, P.; Rosenbaum, P.; Hanna, S.; Kertoy, M.; Young, N. *Children's Assessment of Participation and Enjoyment & Preferences for Activities of Children*; Pearson: San Antonio, TX, USA, 2004.
42. Imms, C. Review of the children's assessment of participation and enjoyment and the preferences for activity of children. *Phys. Occup. Ther. Pediatr.* **2008**, *28*, 389–404. [CrossRef]
43. Phillips, R.; Olds, T.; Boshoff, K.; Lane, A.E. Measuring activity and participation in children and adolescents with disabilities: A literature review of available instruments. *Aust. Occup. Ther. J.* **2013**, *60*, 288–300. [CrossRef]

44. King, G.A.; Law, M.; King, S.; Hurley, P.; Hanna, S.; Kertoy, M.; Rosenbaum, P. Measuring children's participation in recreation and leisure activities: Construct validation of the CAPE and PAC. *Child Care Health Dev.* **2007**, *33*, 28–39. [CrossRef]
45. Bult, M.; Verschuren, O.; Gorter, J.; Jongmans, M.; Piškur, B.; Ketelaar, M. Cross-cultural validation and psychometric evaluation of the Dutch language version of the Children's Assessment of Participation and Enjoyment (CAPE) in children with and without physical disabilities. *Clin. Rehabil.* **2010**, *24*, 843–853. [CrossRef]
46. Nordtorp, H.L.; Nyquist, A.; Jahnsen, R.; Moser, T.; Strand, L.I. Reliability of the Norwegian Version of the Children's Assessment of Participation and Enjoyment (CAPE) and Preferences for Activities of Children (PAC). *Phys. Occup. Ther. Pediatr.* **2012**, *33*, 199–212. [CrossRef]
47. Longo, E.; Badía, M.; Orgaz, B.; Verdugo, M.A. Cross-cultural validation of the Children's Assessment of Participation and Enjoyment (CAPE) in Spain. *Child Care Health Dev.* **2012**, *40*, 231–241. [CrossRef]
48. Colón, W.I.; Rodríguez, C.; Ito, M.; Reed, C.N. Psychometric evaluation of the Spanish version of the Children's Assessment of Participation and Enjoyment and Preferences for Activities of Children. *Occup. Ther. Int.* **2008**, *15*, 100–113. [CrossRef] [PubMed]
49. Ullenhag, A.; Krumlinde-Sundholm, L.; Granlund, M.; Almqvist, L. Differences in patterns of participation in leisure activities in Swedish children with and without disabilities. *Disabil. Rehabil.* **2013**, *36*, 464–471. [CrossRef] [PubMed]
50. Huang, Y.-Y.; Li, C.-Y.; Huang, I.-C.; Bendixen, R.; Chen, K.-L.; Weng, W.-C. Poster 7 the cross-cultural adaptation and psychometric evaluation of the Children's Assessment of Participation and Enjoyment-Chinese version. *Arch. Phys. Med. Rehabil.* **2013**, *94*, e13–e14. [CrossRef]
51. Fink, A.; Gebhard, B.; Erdwiens, S.; Haddenhorst, L.; Nowak, S. Reliability of the German version of the Children's Assessment of Participation and Enjoyment (CAPE) and Preferences for Activities of Children (PAC). *Child Care Health Dev.* **2016**, *42*, 683–691. [CrossRef] [PubMed]
52. Ullenhag, A.; Bult, M.; Nyquist, A.; Ketelaar, M.; Jahnsen, R.; Krumlinde-Sundholm, L.; Almqvist, L.; Granlund, M. An international comparison of patterns of participation in leisure activities for children with and without disabilities in Sweden, Norway and the Netherlands. *Dev. Neurorehabil.* **2012**, *15*, 369–385. [CrossRef] [PubMed]
53. Peña, E.D. Lost in translation: Methodological considerations in cross-cultural research. *Child Dev.* **2007**, *78*, 1255–1264. [CrossRef]
54. *IBM SPSS Statistics for Windows*; Version 26.0.; IBM Corp: Armonk, NY, USA, 2019.
55. George, D.; Mallery, M. *Using SPSS for Windows Step by Step: A Simple Guide and Reference, 11.0 Update*; Allyn & Bacon: Boston, MA, USA, 2003.
56. Hammel, J.; Magasi, S.; Heinemann, A.W.; Whiteneck, G.; Bogner, J.; Rodríguez, E. What does participation mean? An insider perspective from people with disabilities. *Disabil. Rehabil.* **2008**, *30*, 1445–1460. [CrossRef]
57. Mkabile, S.; Swartz, L. Caregivers' and parents' explanatory models of intellectual disability in Khayelitsha, Cape Town, South Africa. *J. Appl. Res. Intellect. Disabil.* **2020**, *33*, 1026–1037. [CrossRef]
58. Allison, L.; Strydom, A. Intellectual disability across cultures. *Psychiatry* **2009**, *8*, 355–357. [CrossRef]
59. Erhart, M.; Ellert, U.; Kurth, T.; Ravens-Sieberer, U. Measuring adolescents' HRQoL via self reports and parent proxy reports: An evaluation of the psychometric properties of both versions of the KINDL-R instrument. *Health Qual. Life Outcomes* **2009**, *7*, 77. [CrossRef]
60. Eiser, C.; Morse, R. Can parents rate their child's health-related quality of life? Results of a systematic review. *Qual. Life Res.* **2001**, *10*, 347–357. [CrossRef] [PubMed]
61. Barbosa, T.D.S.; Gavião, M.B.D. Oral health-related quality of life in children: Part III. Is there agreement between parents in rating their children's oral health-related quality of life? A systematic review. *Int. J. Dent. Hyg.* **2008**, *6*, 108–113. [CrossRef] [PubMed]
62. Sherifali, D.; Pinelli, J. Parent as proxy reporting. *J. Fam. Nurs.* **2007**, *13*, 83–98. [CrossRef] [PubMed]

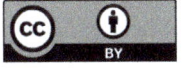 © 2020 by the authors. Licensee MDPI, Basel, Switzerland. This article is an open access article distributed under the terms and conditions of the Creative Commons Attribution (CC BY) license (http://creativecommons.org/licenses/by/4.0/).

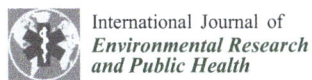

Article

Children in South Africa with and without Intellectual Disabilities' Rating of Their Frequency of Participation in Everyday Activities

Alecia Samuels [1,*], Shakila Dada [1], Karin Van Niekerk [1], Patrik Arvidsson [2,3] and Karina Huus [2]

1. Centre for Augmentative and Alternative Communication, University of Pretoria, Pretoria 0028, South Africa; shakila.dada@up.ac.za (S.D.); karin.vanniekerk@up.ac.za (K.V.N.)
2. CHILD Research Group, Swedish Institute for Disability Research, Jönköping University, 55111 Jönköping, Sweden; patrik.arvidsson@regiongavleborg.se (P.A.); karina.huus@ju.se (K.H.)
3. Centre for Research & Development, Uppsala University, Region Gävleborg, 801 88 Gävle, Sweden
* Correspondence: alecia.samuels@up.ac.za

Received: 16 August 2020; Accepted: 8 September 2020; Published: 15 September 2020

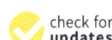

Abstract: In a low-and middle-income country (LMIC) such as South Africa, not much is known about how children with intellectual disabilities (ID) participate in everyday activities, as no studies to date have compared their participation to peers without ID from the same background. Using a newly developed, contextually valid measure of participation, Picture my Participation (PmP), 106 children with (73) and without ID (33), rated their frequency of participation in activities of daily living. Previous international research has established that children with ID tend to participate less frequently than children without ID in everyday activities outside of the school setting. However, much of this research is based on proxy ratings from caregivers rather than children with ID themselves. There is a growing body of evidence that suggests children with disabilities have uniquely different views of their own participation than their caregivers. The existing research evidence is also delimited to studies conducted predominantly in high income contexts (HICSs). Since it is universally acknowledged that participation patterns are affected by the environment, it is important to evaluate the generalizability of the current evidence to LMICs. The current study found that there were many similar patterns of participation between the two groups although significant differences were noted in social, community, leisure and self-care activities. We compare these results to findings from studies conducted in HICs and find that there are similarities but also differences across contexts. This study highlights the importance of gaining a child's perspective of participation and understanding how intellectual disability can affect participation relative to peers without ID in LMICS.

Keywords: participation; attendance; children with intellectual disabilities; low- and middle-income country; self-report; Picture my Participation; activities of daily living

1. Introduction

The WHOs International Classification of Functioning, Disability and Health (ICF) [1], more specifically its version for children and youth (ICF-CY) [2] is a framework that seeks to provide an understanding of children's functioning. It has brought about a change in the way we view outcomes for children with intellectual disability (ID) with the concept of participation increasingly seen as an important goal for this population. Participation is defined in the ICF-CY as a child's "involvement in a life situatio" which can be influenced by factors such as child characteristics (health conditions, body functions, and structures) and context (facilitators or barriers of the physical or social environment) [2].

King and colleagues [3] view participation in everyday activities as the context in which children develop competencies, where they gain an understanding of their strengths and abilities, form friendships and relationships, and ultimately make a contribution to their worlds. Participation is therefore both the ultimate goal of intervention and the context in which children develop [4].

The participation construct is especially important for children with ID since behavioral problems and social skills deficits tend to restrict their participation in most of their everyday environments such as home, school and community [5]. Some studies have suggested that many children with disabilities participate in less diverse activities as well as less frequently in activities than their typical peers [3]. Participation can contribute amongst others, to children with ID's health, self-esteem and psychological well-being [5]. Specifically, they may be at risk for increased sedentary lifestyles and social isolation [3].

While the ICF defines participation as "involvement in a life situation", this definition has been criticized by various authors as being difficult to operationalize and measure [6,7]. This difficulty stems from the failure of the ICF as a classification system to adequately differentiate the activity competence domain (measured as capacity, capability or performed skill in being able to execute an activity) from that of participation [8,9]. Consequently, many studies which claim to measure participation in childhood disability research tend to measure a broad range of constructs related to participation such as activity competence, preference, or aspects related to sense of self [9–11], rather than the social aspects of participation.

Granlund [6] and colleagues [12], based on a critical review of the language of participation used in the literature, recommend that participation be differentiated into the dimensions of "being there" (measured as time spent in or frequency of attendance in a life situation) and involvement (the experience of participation while attending in a life situation also referred to as engagement). Apart from a few exceptions, a systematic review of the literature on the participation of children with disabilities [5] revealed a tendency for the "being there" dimension of participation to be measured more often (i.e., frequency of access and inclusion in various activities of daily living) than involvement or engagement in these activities [13].

With specific reference to children and youth with ID, Shields and colleagues' [5] systematic review found that that when socio economic status is controlled, there are more similarities than differences in participation patterns pertaining to outside school activities between children with ID than peers without ID. Of the four studies that met the inclusion criteria for their review, children with ID were found to participate in a similar number of activities and to the same extent in terms of frequency for leisure activities (reading, watching television, computer games, listening to music) and physical community activities (e.g., sporting activities, biking, taking music or dance lessons). Both groups also participated with the same frequency in more informal, outdoor and accessible activities. Notable differences were reported in relation to the decreased number of social community activities and recreational activities participated in by children with ID, as well community activities, family enrichment activities and formal activities. Frequency of participation was different in relation to organized physical activities, playground activities with siblings, errands, dining out, as well as community activities such as visiting the library, or going to the movies. In contrast, children with ID tended to participate in a higher percentage—although less frequently—in community based social activities with their parents and other adults than with similar aged peers. According to Shields and colleagues [5] if the usual patterns of participation of children with ID are known in comparison to their peers without ID, it could potentially help us to understand whether or not they have opportunities to pursue activities that they enjoy which would contribute to their health and development.

The current systematic synthesis of literature on participation of children with ID, however, suffers from two biases found when measuring children with disabilities' participation. Firstly, much of the findings of the existing literature are based on proxy ratings from caregivers [10,14] Caregiver perspectives of participation may be very different to children's own self-reported experiences [3] as attested to in a recent study by Huus and colleagues [15] on perceptions of children with ID's human rights. Larger differences were found when children as self-raters were asked about whether they had things or friends to play with at home compared to their parent's proxy rating of this same question. This study also revealed that child-parent agreement can be affected by socio economic variables.

Secondly, the evidence base is currently delimited to studies conducted in high income contexts [16]. The ICF, based as it is on an ecological model of childhood development and a biopsychosocial perspective, acknowledges the situational nature of participation with the environment viewed as a key influencing factor [17]. In LMICs where resource limitations and negative attitudes towards people with disabilities are more acute [18], children with ID may be more restricted in their participation than their peers in high income contexts. It has been established that environmental factors such as cultural context [9] and socio-economic status [5] are related to children with disabilities' frequency of participation in different everyday activities. Both of these limitations on the current research evidence accentuate the importance of including children's own voices in perceptions of their participation in LMICs.

A recent systematic review focused on examining the participation construct in LMICs [16] revealed no studies to date in LMIC's where children with ID have evaluated their frequency of participation in various out of school environments. The current study thus sought to evaluate children with ID's ratings of their frequency of participation in various every-day contexts compared to their peers without intellectual disability in South Africa. Furthermore, since current self-report instruments of children's participation may not be contextually valid for use in LMICs, a new self-report measure for children with disabilities, Picture my Participation (PmP) [19], that takes into account culturally relevant activities that may be more relevant in LMICs, was used. More detail about the development and preliminary validation of the PmP in LMICs has been published elsewhere [19] and more detail about how it was used in this study is provided in the methodology of this paper. However, as one of the few self-report measures of participation that provides a child's perspective [20] it may provide a more valid understanding of the participation patterns of children with ID as well as the everyday activities they deem important [20]. While children as young as 4 to 5 years of age are able to reliably complete self-report measures if items and rating scales are suitably adapted [10]. Special consideration should be given to adapting measures for children with disabilities especially those with cognitive and communication impairments [20,21]. Measures for example that are cognitively accessible [21], i.e., that take a range of cognitive abilities into account and provide supports to reduce cognitive demands, increase the chances that respondents can interpret and respond to items as they were intended. The PmP provides visual supports using visual symbols for activity items and participation rating scales and takes the form of an interview with children with disabilities. These accessibility features thus contribute to more valid and reliable self-reporting [21].

2. Materials and Methods

2.1. Ethics

Ethical approval for the study was obtained from the University of Pretoria's Faculty of Humanities Research Ethics Committee (GW20180301HS) on the 10th of April 2018 and permission to conduct interviews was obtained from the local Department of Education and school principals. Informed consent was obtained from every child's primary caregiver, and assent was also sought from each participating child.

2.2. Recruitment

Dyads of caregivers and children were purposefully selected to participate in the study. All caregivers were required to be English literate, as they were required to complete the survey in English. Furthermore, the caregivers were required to be the primary caregiver of the child (that had to meet the criteria set for the children).

Children with ID were recruited from two special schools in Pretoria, South Africa that had English as the medium of instruction for teaching and learning. Up to 70% of children with disabilities in South Africa are not in school and when they do attend, most are still in separate schools for children with disabilities, termed special schools [22]. This situation continues despite progressive policies that are required to promote inclusive education. Children in these special schools come from diverse cultural and socioeconomic backgrounds.

In order to participate in the study, the children were required to (i) be older than 10 years and younger than 16 years. They were (ii) required to have attended a school with English as language of teaching and learning for a minimum of 2 years, in order ensure their ability to comprehend the instructions of the Picture my Participation tool. The participants were required to be (iii) diagnosed as having mild to moderate intellectual disability in order to be included in the group of children with disabilities. Furthermore, the children with ID were required to (iv) not have any functional hearing, visual or motor impairments.

The children without ID were recruited from mainstream schools in Pretoria, Gauteng, that all had English as the medium of teaching and learning. While in principle a mainstream school in South Africa refers to a neighborhood school that all children regardless of ability should be able to attend; in reality, however, it tends to cater to children who do not have special education needs [22]. All the children without ID were (i) between 10 years and 15 years and 11 months; (ii) had attended their current school for a minimum of 2 years and (iii) had never failed a grade at school. All recruited children were from an urban environment. Descriptive statistics regarding the participants can be viewed in Table 1.

Table 1. Descriptive information on the participants.

Demographic Variables	Children without ID	Children with ID
	n = 33	n = 79
Gender		
Male	11 (33.3%)	38 (48.1%)
Female	22 (66.7%)	36 (45.6%)
Missing	0	5 (6.3%)
Age		
9 years	3 (9.1%)	2 (2.5%)
10 years	16 (48.5%)	5 (6.3%)
11 years		13 (16.5%)
12 years	1 (3.0%)	16 (20.3%)
13 years	12 (36.4%)	14 (17.7%)
14 years	1 (3%)	11 (13.9%)
15 years	0	11 (13.9%)
16 years	0	2 (2.5%)
Missing	0	5 (6.3%)
Total family income		
Below R6000 per month	23 (69.7%)	55 (69.6%)
Above R6000 per month	7 (21.2%)	9 (11.4%)
Missing	3 (9.1%)	15 (19.0%)
Relationship of caregiver to child		
Father	7 (21.2%)	10 (12.7%)
Mother	25 (75.8%)	52 (65.8%)
Grandmother	0	1 (1.3%)
Other	1 (3.0%)	6 (7.6%)
Missing	0	10 (12.7%)
Employment status of caregiver		
Employed full-time	21 (63.6%)	35 (44.3%)
Part time	3 (9.1%)	12 (15.2%)
Unemployed	9 (27.3%)	22 (27.8%)
Missing	0	10 (12.7%)
Receiving social grant		
Yes	1 (3.0%)	26 (32.9%)
No	32 (97.05)	44 (55.7%)
Missing	0	9 (11.4%)
Highest education level of caregiver		
Grade 10 or less	1 (3.0%)	19 (24.1%)
Grade 12	9 (27.3%)	17 (21.5%)
Diploma	12 (36.4%)	10 (12.7%)
Degree	4 (12.1%)	5 (6.3%)
Postgraduate degree	1 (3.0%)	7 (8.9%)
Missing	6 (18.2%)	21 (26.6%)

2.3. Instruments

In order to determine children's eligibility for inclusion into the study, the following measures were completed with each child before the onset of conducting PmP interview. The Kaufman Brief Intelligence Test Second Edition (KBIT-2) [23] is a test of intelligence that is often used in research as a screening tool that can be administered by non-psychologists. Clinical researchers and specially trained postgraduate students with knowledge of the target group, completed this measure with children.

The Ten Questions Questionnaire (TQQ) [24] was completed by children's primary caregivers to rule out any hearing, vision or motor impairments. This is a screening tool that assesses the level and nature of a child's disability and includes 10 closed (yes/no) questions about whether the child has a problem or not in certain developmental areas.

In addition, the Learner Screening Tool by Educators (LeSTE) [25] was completed by teachers and the Line Drawings Test [26] was completed by a member of the research team with the participants. These tests provided additional information about the sensory and motor abilities of each child.

The PmP instrument was developed as a self-reported measure of participation of children in home, social and community activities within LMICs [19]. The PmP has two sections—Section 1 is completed by parents and Section 2 is a self-reported measure completed by an interviewer according to responses received from a child [19]. Section 1 starts with a consent form for the parent and is followed by demographic questions as well as the Ten Questions Questionnaire [24]. If the child meets the inclusion criteria, the parent will also complete the rest of the survey that contains the same questions pertaining to the frequency of the child's attendance and their perceived involvement in 20 activities as those included in the questions to the children.

Section 2 includes an assent form that is completed with a child before the commencement of the interview. Thereafter, children are asked to rate the frequency of their attendance in 20 different activities (developed from the ICF) according to a four-point symbol-based, visual Likert scale using Picture Communication Symbols (PCS). All 20 activities were also represented by a PCS symbol of the activity. The scale was also presented to the children visually by four PCS symbols that were displayed on a mat and kept in front of the child during the interview.

The symbols on the mat depicting the scale were of baskets with apples, filled to various degrees. "Always" on the scale was represented by a basket completely filled with apples, "sometimes" by a basket with three apples in it, "not really" by a basket with one apple and "never" by an empty basket. The Talking Mats methodology as described by Cameron and Murphy [27] was used and enabled the children to place the symbol of the activity that they were being asked about, under the appropriate visual Likert scale symbol displayed on the mat. The children were asked three trial questions to ensure that they understood the scale.

The children were also asked about their level of involvement in the 20 activities which they had to rate on a scale with "very", "somewhat" and "minimally" also represented in symbols on the mat. Thereafter, the children were required to state three activities that were most important to them. Following this, they were asked to indicate their perceived barriers and facilitators to participation for these three activities. In this paper, only the data on the frequency of attendance obtained from the children themselves will be analyzed and discussed. An interview with a child took approximately 30 min to complete.

2.4. Data Analysis

Statistical analysis was performed using SPSS software (version 25) (IBM Corp, Armonk, NY, USA). Since the data were not normally distributed, differences in participation in terms of frequency of attendance for each activity item on the PmP between groups of children with and without ID were analyzed using the non-parametric Mann–Whitney U test. This statistical test compares mean rank data and not the means as is typically done when the data are normally distributed.

P-values < 0.05 were considered as significant. Spearman's rank-order correlation was used to explore the relationship between the total scores of participation (a summary of frequencies of attendance for all activity items) between children with and children without disabilities.

3. Results

The results of a Mann–Whitney U test indicated several significant differences between the children with and without intellectual disabilities for 9 out of 20 items of the PmP (Table 2).

Table 2. Differences in participation (frequency of attendance) of each activity item between children with ID ($n = 73$) and children with typical development (TD) ($n = 33$).

PmP Items		Mean Rank	Mann–Whitney U	Z	Exact Sig. (2-taile)]
Personal care: Daily routines at home for personal care (dressing, choosing clothing, hair care, brushing teeth)	TD child	60.35	978.500	−1.982	0.048 *
	Child with ID	50.40			
Family mealtime: (with usual family members)	TD child	66.05	790.500	−3.242	0.001 *
	Child with ID	47.83			
Looking after his/her own health	TD child	67.50	742.500	−3.263	0.001 *
	Child with ID	47.17			
Gathering daily necessities for the family (water, food, picking vegetables, fuel)	TD child	50.05	1090.500	−0.812	0.419
	Child with ID	55.06			
Meal preparation with or for the family	TD child	68.75	632.000	−3.822	0.000 *
	Child with ID	45.28			
Cleaning at home: Cleaning up at home [clothing, household objects, laundry, rubbish, yard work	TD child	60.47	974.500	−1.683	0.092
	Child with ID	50.35			
Caring for family: Taking care of other family members	TD child	56.27	1113.000	−0.659	0.510
	Child with ID	52.25			
Caring for animals/pets: Taking care of animals (pet, or domestic livestock)	TD child	55.58	1136.000	−0.489	0.633
	Child with ID	52.56			
Family time: Interact with the family	TD child	69.92	662.500	−4.129	0.000 *
	Child with ID	46.08			
Celebrations: Family/community celebrations (birthdays, Weddings, Holiday gatherings)	TD child	60.30	980.000	−1.632	0.108
	Child with ID	50.42			
Playing with others: Getting together with other children in the community	TD child	58.06	1054.000	−1.083	0.280
	Child with ID	51.44			
Organised leisure: sport, clubs, music, art, dance	TD child	57.23	1081.500	−0.875	0.381
	Child with ID	51.82			
Quiet leisure (listening to music, reading)	TD child	65.59	805.500	−2.921	0.003 *
	Child with ID	48.03			
Religious and spiritual gatherings and activities	TD child	69.56	674.500	−3.900	0.000 *
	Child with ID	46.24			
Shopping and errands (market)	TD child	58.77	1030.500	−1.254	0.210
	Child with ID	51.12			
Social activities: Taking part in social activities in the community (parties, play group, parades)	TD child	64.30	815.000	−2.738	0.006 *
	Child with ID	47.82			
Visit to health centre (e.g., Doctor, dentist, other health care service)	TD child	53.05	1189.500	−0.109	0.949
	Child with ID	53.71			
School: Formal learning at school	TD child	68.53	708.500	−4.161	0.000 *
	Child with ID	46.71			
Overnight visits and trips	TD child	60.35	978.500	−1.634	0.104
	Child with ID	50.40			
Paid and unpaid employment	TD child	47.12	994.000	−1.520	0.125
	Child with ID	55.69			

* $p < 0.05$.

Firstly, children with ID indicated that they participated significantly less than TD children in several social activities and taking care of others. These activities included meal preparation: with or for the family ($p < 0.001$ *), spiritual activities: religious and spiritual gatherings and activities ($p < 0.001$*) as well as social activities: taking part in social activities in the community ($p = 0.006$ *). Furthermore, children with ID participated significantly less than TD children in several family life activities. These include family time: interact with the family ($p < 0.001$ *); family mealtime: (with usual family members) ($p = 0.001$ *); as well as quiet leisure (listening to music, reading) ($p = 0.003$ *).

Finally, several significant differences were observed between children with ID and children with typical development as the children with ID participated significantly less in personal care and development activities. These include school: formal learning at school ($p < 0.001$ *), personal care: daily routines at home for personal care ($p = 0.048$ *) as well as looking after their own health ($p = 0.001$ *).

A Spearman's rank-order correlation determined the relationship between the total scores, i.e., the summary of frequencies for every item, between children with and children without disabilities. There was a strong, positive correlation between children with and without disabilities, which was statistically significant (rs = 0.868, $p < 0.001$).

4. Discussion

Since it has been well established that factors within and outside of the child can act as barriers or facilitators of participation [2], we compare the findings of the current study to comparable studies undertaken in HICs on children with and without IDs frequency of attending various everyday activities. Where unexpected findings are noted, we cautiously infer from contextually relevant literature as to possible reasons that could account for differences. However, we are mindful that apart from obtaining demographic data such as economic status, we did not specifically measure how child characteristics or environmental factors could have accounted for the results.

In this study, the finding that children with and without ID from comparable socioeconomic backgrounds, display more similarities than differences in their frequency of attending everyday activities appears to be a consistent trend across low- and high-income contexts [5]. In South Africa, children with ID participated to the same extent in terms of frequency of attendance as children without ID in the majority of activities measured by the PmP. However, while there may be more similarities than differences between children with and without ID in terms of frequency of attendance across economic contexts, the actual activities where children with ID appear to have similar frequencies of attendance to their peers, tend to be different across economic contexts. In South Africa, similar patterns of participation to peers without ID are for activities taking place within the home environment and within the context of family routines such as household chores, taking care of family members, caring for pets and assisting with gathering basic necessities for the family. This may be a function of receiving more support in the home environment from family members than in outside contexts where they may not be present [19]. This is supported by King and colleagues [3] who found that children with ID had a higher frequency of participation in social activities in the home. This may be indicative of more support being offered in these environments from family members due to reduced physical, cognitive and social skills associated with this population [3].

In HICs, similar patterns of participation in terms of frequency of attendance between children with and without ID was noted in mainly leisure and community activities such as attending play groups, childcare and church [5]. These differences in the type of activities that were reported to have similar frequencies of participation between children with and without ID may be as a result of using different measuring instruments and therefore a function of content validity of instruments. In developing the PmP for LMICs, Arvidsson and colleagues [19] note the importance of having everyday activity items that are culturally relevant, i.e., meaningful and important for the population in a specific context.

However, there were also quite a few significant differences between children with and without ID, and these will be discussed in more detail in relation to specific activity types.

4.1. Social (Iutside the Home) and Community Life Activties

As noted above, while the present study found that there were many social activities in the home where children with ID participated similarly to peers without ID, notable differences included social activities outside the home, such as attending parties, playgroups or parades as well as community activities such as attending religious or spiritual gatherings. Findings of decreased frequency of participation for children with ID relative to peers without ID in social activities outside the home are similar to studies conducted in Australia [28] although in Canada, King and colleagues [3] found no differences between the two groups. Further investigation is therefore warranted into some of the potential barriers which may be unique to children with ID in South Africa and which could potentially explain the differences noted. Although we did not specifically test for any predictive or causative factors that would influence frequency of participation in out of home social and community activities, the South African literature alludes to potential physical access barriers in the community faced by people with ID, such as a lack of reliable, affordable and accessible public transport infrastructure [29] that could potentially limit children with ID's ability to participate in activities outside of the home.

As noted, participation can also be influenced by child characteristics such as an impairment in body structures and functions [2]. Children with ID in South Africa tend to have associated communication impairments in terms of receptive and expressive deficits [30,31] which can potentially limit their ability to independently access understandable information in their social environments [29], e.g., transport timetables and schedules. This may also be compounded by the fact that the special school in system South Africa rarely prioritizes literacy outcomes [32]. Thus, many children with ID exit the education system as non-literate, which can influence their ability to access knowledge and some degree of independence in social situations [29]. Communication difficulties may also limit children with IDs communicative interactions [30] in social situations such as parties or celebrations but their poor participation in social activities could also be affected by their associated deficits in social skills [5].

The significant differences between children with and without ID in terms of attendance of community activities such as religious or spiritual festivities is not supported by data from HICs, where children with and without ID display little difference when participating in this community activity [5]. The differences noted in the South African context may be a feature of the environment, such as attitudinal barriers towards people with intellectual disability [33].

Ndlovu argues that in some (although not all) indigenous African religions of Southern Africa, individuals with psychological and neurological impairments are often depicted as victims of witchcraft who should be "ritually, morally and physically cleansed of their affliction before they can be reintegrated into human society" [33] (p.32). For children with ID who have a lifelong health condition, these attitudinal barriers that equate the origins of ID with misfortune from the spiritual world, mitigate against inclusive practices and can result in continued marginalization and exclusion in religious and community life [34]. Again, we can only infer from the literature as to potential influencing factors. This will need to be empirically tested using study designs which specifically explore the impact of child characteristics and environmental factors such as physical, social and attitudinal barriers [35] on out of home social and community participation of children with ID.

4.2. Participation in Family Life and Indoor Leisure Activities

Differences in participation in family life and leisure activities in the home were also noted between children with and without ID in the current study. Children with ID indicated that they participated less frequently than children without ID in spending time with usual family members or interacting with the family members during mealtimes. This finding is somewhat inconsistent with studies conducted in Australia [28] where children with ID participated to the same extent as peers without ID in recreational activities with family members such as parents or with another adult: It is believed that family members are important forms of support for children with ID in situations which place a load on their cognitive and linguistic abilities [5]. However, this finding may reflect a preference for activities that are easier to engage in and for which they may not need as much support having developed the skills to participate independently [36].

This study also indicated that children with ID participated less frequently in quiet leisure time activities—such as listening to music or reading—than peers without ID. This is similar to results reported by Axelsson and Wilder [37] within the Swedish context, albeit with a more profound ID population. Less frequent participation in quiet leisure activities such as reading is also consistent with previous research [5], but as previously mentioned, poor prioritization of literacy outcomes for children with ID in South Africa [32] may account for a lack of participation in this activity.

Children with ID also indicated that they participated less frequently in their own personal care routines (dressing, brushing teeth, etc.) looking after their own health and development enhancing activities such as formal learning at school in comparison to their peers without ID. Due to the physical and cognitive demands associated with these activities, it may be a reflection that they may not have developed the functional skills needed to participate independently in these activities [3]. There is a strong body of evidence to suggest that children with ID in the South African context, like children with ID elsewhere, are at increased risk for oral health disease such as gingivitis and dental caries relative to the general population of similar age [38]. It is argued that the ability to maintain optimum oral health independently is difficult for this population and that support from caregivers for daily self-care activities and health remains high [39]. On the other hand, it has also been suggested that in some cultures, mothers' strong commitment to their caregiving role may impact on children with ID's ability to do personal care tasks for themselves [40]. More specifically, it has been argued that parents in collectivist cultures' strong values of care and protection may limit the ability of their children with IDs to develop functional independence in activities such as personal care routines [40]. However, the evidence for this argument is limited and would need to be investigated in much more depth for it to be seen as a significant barrier limiting children with IDs participation in self-care and health related activities.

Despite this study's findings of some significant differences in the frequency of participation in everyday activities between children with and without ID in the South African context, there is a growing realization in the country of the importance of participation and independence for children with ID in leisure, family and community life [41]. Some useful community-based rehabilitation interventions [42] that target the empowerment of the caregivers of children with disabilities to be advocates for their children, are starting to break down environmental barriers to their community participation. This is important as the decreased participation of children with ID from social, community and leisure activities, may have considerable implications for their social skills development and network of friendships within their peer cohort which are important for their quality of life and well-being [5].

5. Conclusions

This study, which compared the frequency of participation in everyday activities between children with and without ID from their own perspective using a contextually valid, self-report measure, is one of the first studies in South Africa to evaluate the similarities and differences in participation patterns for this population. While many similarities to studies undertaken in HICs were found, there were also some significant differences reported. At this stage, we were only able to infer from the literature as to possible reasons for this, as we did not measure any environmental factors or child characteristics which could account for the similarities and differences noted. We acknowledge this as an important limitation of the study which would need to be addressed in future research.

While children with ID participated similarly to peers without ID in the majority of activities in terms of frequency of attendance, it does not necessarily mean that they were involved in the activities to the same extent. This is an aspect which future research would need to address as well, since there are still very few studies—particularly in LMICs—which focus on the involvement dimension of participation [16]. Ultimately the knowledge of how children with ID participate in everyday activities will allow clinicians and researchers to gain better insight of how and where to target interventions to improve children with IDs' participation in everyday activities and which will ultimately contribute to their health and development [5].

This study, however, is one of the first in LMICs to evaluate and compare the participation of children with ID to their peers without ID in terms of frequency of attendance in activities from the perspective of children themselves. New participation tools, such as the PmP—which are more cognitively accessible for children with disabilities and take contextually relevant activities into account—represent an important step for increasing research knowledge about how children with ID participate in LMICs. Ultimately, this broadens the knowledge base and the external validity of participation research.

Author Contributions: Conceptualization, S.D., P.A. and K.H.; Formal analysis, A.S. and K.V.N.; Methodology, K.V.N. and P.A.; Project administration, S.D.; Writing—original draft, A.S.; Writing—review and editing, S.D., K.V.N., P.A. and K.H. All authors have read and agreed to the published version of the manuscript.

Funding: This research was funded by the National Research Foundation (NRF), South Africa, grant number 101566 and the Swedish Foundation for International Cooperation in Research and Higher Education (STINT), grant number SA2015-6253.

Acknowledgments: The authors would like to thank all the children and families who participated in this project as well as the Masters students in the Centre for Augmentative and Alternative Communication at the University of Pretoria who assisted with data collection.

Conflicts of Interest: The authors declare no conflict of interest. The funders had no role in the design of the study; in the collection, analyses, or interpretation of data; in the writing of the manuscript, or in the decision to publish the results.

References

1. World Health Organization. *The International Classification of Functioning, Disability and Health: ICF*; World Health Organization: Geneva, Switzerland, 2001.
2. World Health Organization. *The International Classification of Functioning, Disability and Health-Child and Youth: ICF-CY*; World Health Organization: Geneva, Switzerland, 2007.
3. King, M.; Shields, N.; Imms, C.; Black, M.; Ardern, C. Participation of children with intellectual disability compared with typically developing children. *Res. Dev. Disabil.* **2013**, *34*, 1854–1862. [CrossRef]
4. Law, M.; King, G.; King, S.; Kertoy, M.; Hurley, P.; Rosenbaum, P.; Young, N.; Hanna, S. Patterns of participation in recreational and leisure activities among children with complex physical disabilities. *Dev. Med. Child Neurol.* **2006**, *48*, 337–342. [CrossRef] [PubMed]
5. Shields, N.; King, M.; Corbett, M.; Imms, C. Is participation among children with intellectual disabilities in outside school activities similar to their typically developing peers? A systematic review. *Dev. Neurorehabilit.* **2014**, *17*, 64–71. [CrossRef]
6. Granlund, M. Participation–challenges in conceptualization, measurement and intervention. *Child Care Health Dev.* **2013**, *39*, 470–473. [CrossRef] [PubMed]
7. Coster, W.; Khetani, M.A. Measuring participation of children with disabilities: Issues and challenges. *Disabil. Rehabil.* **2008**, *30*, 639–648. [CrossRef] [PubMed]
8. Dean, E.E.; Fisher, K.W.; Shogren, K.A.; Wehmeyer, M.L. Participation and intellectual disability: A review of the literature. *Intellect. Dev. Disabil.* **2016**, *54*, 427–439. [CrossRef]
9. Imms, C.; Granlund, M.; Wilson, P.H.; Steenbergen, B.; Rosenbaum, P.L.; Gordon, A.M. Participation, both a means and an end: A conceptual analysis of processes and outcomes in childhood disability. *Dev. Med. Child. Neurol.* **2017**, *59*, 16–25. [CrossRef]
10. Adair, B.; Ullenhag, A.; Rosenbaum, P.; Granlund, M.; Keen, D.; Imms, C. Measures used to quantify participation in childhood disability and their alignment with the family of participation-related constructs: A systematic review. *Dev. Med. Child Neurol.* **2018**, *60*, 1101–1116. [CrossRef]
11. Adair, B.; Ullenhag, A.; Keen, D.; Granlund, M.; Imms, C. The effect of interventions aimed at improving participation outcomes for children with disabilities: A systematic review. *Dev. Med. Child Neurol.* **2015**, *57*, 1093–1104. [CrossRef]
12. Imms, C.; Adair, B.; Keen, D.; Ullenhag, A.; Rosenbaum, P.; Granlund, M. 'Participation': A systematic review of language, definitions, and constructs used in intervention research with children with disabilities. *Dev. Med. Child Neurol.* **2016**, *58*, 29–38. [CrossRef]
13. Axelsson, A.K.; Granlund, M.; Wilder, J. Engagement in family activities: A quantitative, comparative study of children with profound intellectual and multiple disabilities and children with typical development. *Child Care Health Dev.* **2013**, *40*, 523–534. [CrossRef]

14. Dada, S.; Andersson, A.; May, A.; Elgmark Andersson, E.; Granlund, M.; Huus, K. Agreement between participation ratings of children with intellectual disabilities and their primary caregivers. *Res. Dev. Disabil.* **2020**, *104*, 103715. [CrossRef]
15. Huus, K.; Granlund, M.; Bornman, J.; Lygnegård, F. Human rights of children with intellectual disabilities: Comparing self-ratings and proxy ratings. *Child Care Health Dev.* **2015**, *41*, 1010–1017. [CrossRef]
16. Schlebusch, L.; Huus, K.; Samuels, A.; Granlund, M.; Dada, S. Participation of young people with disabilities and/or chronic conditions in low- and middle-income countries: A scoping review. *Dev. Med. Child Neurol.* **2020**, 1–7. [CrossRef]
17. Anaby, D.; Hand, C.; Bradley, L.; Direzze, B.; Forhan, M.; Digiacomo, A.; Law, M. The effect of the environment on participation of children and youth with disabilities: A scoping review. *Disabil. Rehabil.* **2013**, *35*, 1589–1598. [CrossRef]
18. Bantjes, J.; Swartz, L.; Conchar, L.; Derman, W. Developing programmes to promote participation in sport among adolescents with disabilities: Perceptions expressed by a group of South African adolescents with cerebral palsy. *Int. J. Dis. Dev. Educ.* **2015**, *62*, 288–302. [CrossRef]
19. Arvidsson, P.; Dada, S.; Granlund, M.; Imms, C.; Bornman, J.; Elliott, C.; Huus, K. Content validity and usefulness of Picture My Participation for measuring participation in children with and without intellectual disability in South Africa and Sweden. *Scand. J. Occup. Ther.* **2019**, *27*, 336–348. [CrossRef]
20. Nilsson, S.; Björkman, B.; Almqvist, A.L.; Almqvist, L.; Björk-Willén, P.; Donohue, D.; Enskär, K.; Granlund, M.; Huus, K.; Hvit, S. Children's voices—Differentiating a child perspective from a child's perspective. *Dev. Neurorehabil.* **2015**, *18*, 162–168. [CrossRef]
21. Kramer, J.M.; Schwartz, A. Reducing barriers to patient-reported outcome measures for people with cognitive impairments. *Arch. Phys. Med. Rehabil.* **2017**, *98*, 1705–1715. [CrossRef]
22. Donohue, D.; Bornman, J. The challenges of realising inclusive education in South Africa. *S. Afr. J. Educ.* **2014**, *34*, 1–14. [CrossRef]
23. Kaufman, A.S.; Kaufman, N.L. *Kaufman Brief Intelligence Test*, 2nd ed.; Pearson, Inc.: Bloomington, MN, USA, 2004.
24. Durkin, M.S.; Wang, W.; Shrout, P.E.; Zaman, S.S.; Hasan, Z.M.; Desai, P.; Davidson, L.L. Evaluation of the ten questions screen for childhood disability: Reliability and internal structure in different cultures. *J. Clin. Epidemiol.* **1995**, *48*, 657–666. [CrossRef]
25. Naudé, T.E. The Effect of a Mathematical Aided Language Stimulation Programme for Subtraction Word-Problem Solving for Children with Intellectual Disabilities. Ph.D. Thesis, University of Pretoria, Pretoria, South Africa, 2015.
26. Dada, S. The Impact of Aided Language Stimulation on the Receptive Language Abilities of Children with Little or No Functional Speech. Ph.D. Thesis, University of Pretoria, Pretoria, South Africa, 2005.
27. Cameron, L.; Murphy, J. Enabling young people with a learning disability to make choices at a time of transition. *Br. J. Learn. Disab.* **2002**, *30*, 105–112. [CrossRef]
28. Solish, A.; Perry, A.; Minnes, P. Participation of Children with and without Disabilities in Social, Recreational and Leisure Activities. *J. Appl. Res. Intellect. Disabil.* **2010**, *23*, 226–236. [CrossRef]
29. McKenzie, J.A.; McConkey, R.; Adnams, C. Intellectual disability in Africa: Implications for research and service development. *Dis. Rehab.* **2013**, *35*, 1750–1755. [CrossRef]
30. Dada, S.; Huguet, A.; Bornman, J. The iconicity of picture communication symbols for children with English additional language and mild intellectual disability. *Augment. Altern. Commun.* **2013**, *29*, 360–373. [CrossRef]
31. Donohue, D.K.; Bornman, J.; Granlund, M. Household size is associated with unintelligible speech in children who have intellectual disabilities: A South African study. *Dev. Neuro* **2015**, *18*, 402–406. [CrossRef]
32. Bornman, J. Developing Inclusive Literacy Practices in South African Schools. In *Inclusive Practices and Principles in Literacy Education*; Forlin, C., Milton, M., Eds.; Emerald Publishing: Bingley, UK, 2017; Volume 11, pp. 105–122.
33. Ndlovu, H.L. African beliefs concerning people with disabilities: Implications for theological education. *J. Dis. Relat.* **2016**, *20*, 29–39. [CrossRef]
34. Chataika, T. Cultural and Religious Explanations of Disability and Promoting Inclusive Communities in Southern Africa. In *Searching for Dignity: Conversations on Human Dignity, Theology and Disability*; Claasens, J., Swarts, L., Hansen, L., Eds.; African Sun Media: Stellenbosch, South Africa, 2013; pp. 117–128.

35. King, G.; Law, M.; Hanna, S.; King, S.; Hurley, P.; Rosenbaum, P.; Kertoy, M.; Petrenchik, T. Predictors of the leisure and recreation participation of children with physical disabilities: A structural equation modelling analysis. *Child Health Care* **2006**, *35*, 209–234. [CrossRef]
36. Shields, N.; Synnot, A.; Kearns, C. The extent, context and experience of participation in out-of-school activities among children with disabilities. *Res. Dev. Disabil.* **2015**, *47*, 165–174. [CrossRef]
37. Axelsson, A.K.; Wilder, J. Frequency of occurrence and child presence in family activities: A quantitative, comparative study of children with profound intellectual and multiple disabilities and children with typical development. *Int. J. Dev. Dis.* **2014**, *60*, 13–25. [CrossRef]
38. Roberts, T.; Chetty, M.; Kimmie-Dhansay, F.; Stephen, L.X.G.; Fieggen, K. Dental needs of intellectually disabled children attending six special educational facilities in Cape Town: The new millennium. *S. Afr. Med. J.* **2016**, *106* (Suppl. 1), 94–97. [CrossRef]
39. Liu, Z.; Yu, D.; Luo, W.; Yang, J. Impact of oral health behaviors on dental caries in children with intellectual disabilities in Guangzhou, China. *Int. J. Environ. Res. Public Health* **2014**, *11*, 11015–11027. [CrossRef]
40. Kingsley, F.; Wickenden, M. Balancing priorities: British Bangladeshi mothers' perspectives on functional independence for their disabled children. *Br. J. Occup. Ther.* **2014**, *77*, 366–372. [CrossRef]
41. Capri, C.; Abrahams, L.; McKenzie, J.; Coetzee, O.; Mkabile, S.; Saptouw, M.; Hooper, A.; Smith, P.; Adnams, C.; Swartz, L. Intellectual disability rights and inclusive citizenship in South Africa: What can a scoping review tell us? *Afr. J. Dis.* **2018**, *7*, 1–17. [CrossRef] [PubMed]
42. Elphick, J.; De SasKropiwnicki, Z.; Elphick, R. "Our children have the right to an education too": Strategies employed by Orange Farm caregivers of children with disabilities in pursuit of the right to a basic education. *Dis. CBR Incl. Dev.* **2015**, *26*, 101–116. [CrossRef]

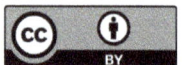

© 2020 by the authors. Licensee MDPI, Basel, Switzerland. This article is an open access article distributed under the terms and conditions of the Creative Commons Attribution (CC BY) license (http://creativecommons.org/licenses/by/4.0/).

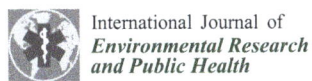

Article

The Role of Social Support in Participation Perspectives of Caregivers of Children with Intellectual Disabilities in India and South Africa

Shakila Dada [1,*], Kirsty Bastable [1] and Santoshi Halder [2]

1. Centre for Augmentative and Alternative Communication, Humanities Faculty, University of Pretoria, Pretoria 0002, South Africa; kgb0071978@gmail.com
2. Department of Education, University of Calcutta, Alipore Campus, 1 Reformatory St., Kolkata 700027, India; santoshi_halder@yahoo.com
* Correspondence: shakila.dada@up.ac.za

Received: 15 August 2020; Accepted: 3 September 2020; Published: 11 September 2020

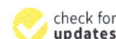

Abstract: Caregivers are an intrinsic component of the environment of children with intellectual disabilities. However, caregivers' capacity to support children's participation may be linked to the social support that they, as caregivers, receive. Social support may increase participation, educational, psychological, medical and financial opportunities. However, there is a lack of information on social support in middle-income countries. The current study described and compared the social support of caregivers of children with intellectual disabilities by using the Family Support Survey (FSS) in India and South Africa. The different types of social support were subsequently considered in relation to participation, using the Children's Assessment of Participation and Enjoyment (CAPE). One hundred caregiver–child dyads from India and 123 from South Africa participated in this study. The data were analysed using non-parametric measures. Indian caregivers reported greater availability of more helpful support than did the South African caregivers. Social support was associated with children's participation diversity (India) and intensity (South Africa). The child-/caregiver-reported participation data showed different associations with participation. Results from this study suggest that perceived social support of caregivers differs between countries and is associated with their child's participation. These factors need to be considered when generalising results from different countries.

Keywords: social support; family support survey; participation; intellectual disabilities; low- and middle-income country

1. Introduction

The introduction of the International Classification of Functioning, Disability and Health (ICF) [1] and the Child and Youth Version (ICF-CY) [2] highlighted participation as a critical health outcome [3]. Furthermore, participation has been highlighted as a human right for persons with disabilities at the United Nations Convention on the Rights of Persons with Disabilities [4]. Participation is described as an important means for achieving physical, social and academic development, cultural understanding, and community inclusion. It is argued that through participation, developmental skills are practiced until an outcome of learned skills is produced [5,6].

As the field of participation is growing, however, gaps in research have emerged. In spite of the fact that participation is reported to be influenced equally by personal and environmental factors [7–9], the bulk of research on participation has focused on personal factors. The current research has provided evidence of decreased participation for children with disabilities [9–14] and specific patterns of participation associated with the type and severity of a disability [15–19]. Studies considering the impact of environmental factors are more limited in number, but as highlighted by Anaby et al. in a scoping review on the effect of the environment on participation, family support and geographic location are facilitators of participation, while attitudes, the physical environment, policies and a lack of support serve as barriers to participation [20].

A paucity of research is also evident in relation to the effect of the income level of the country or culture on participation. Most children with disabilities in the world live in low- and middle-income countries [21], and environmental factors have been identified as an important participation-related concept. Hence, it would have been expected that research on participation in low- and middle-income countries would be common. However, the review by Anaby et al. [20], which identified 28 studies (and three reviews), all were conducted in high-income countries. A more recent scoping review by Schlebusch et al. [22] identified 78 studies on participation from low- and middle-income countries (55% conducted after the Anaby et al. [20] review). However, only 4% ($n = 6$) of these studies were from low-income countries, with 68% ($n = 53$) conducted in upper-middle-income countries. Furthermore, again only 4% ($n = 6$) of the studies in this review considered the effect of the environment on children's participation, while the remaining studies investigated participation as a process ($n = 7$), participation as an outcome ($n = 42$), child-related outcomes ($n = 14$), and the measurement of participation or related constructs ($n = 11$) [22]. All in all, there remains a lack of research on participation of children with disabilities from low- and middle-income countries, particularly in relation to environmental factors [22,23].

The importance of research on participation from low- and middle-income countries relates specifically to differences in the environment that may affect children with disabilities' participation. As indicated by Anaby et al. [20], environmental factors may function as facilitators of or barriers to the participation. Compared to their peers in high-income countries, children in low- and middle-income countries have been identified as being at greater risk from environmental influences such as poverty, reduced educational opportunities, violence and difficulty accessing healthcare [24–26]. In addition, the studies in the Anaby et al. review [20] were mostly from English-speaking countries embracing Eurocentric/western philosophies such as the U.S., the U.K., Canada, Australia and Europe [20], which see the individual as being independent from their community. This is in contrast to Afro-/Asia-centric philosophies that are founded on collectivism or see the self as inseparable from the community [27–29]. Differences in life philosophies may affect perceptions of self and disability, perceptions or availability of support, communication, and hence participation in these settings [27–29].

Within different cultural philosophies, the role of caregivers and the impact of factors such as caregiver support may affect participation. Unfortunately, limited research has been conducted in this area. Caregivers play a much greater role in finding [30,31] and facilitating [32] opportunities for participation for children with disabilities [20,33] than for children with typical development. In fact, the responsibility of ensuring that the rights of a child with intellectual disabilities are met, is reported to fall most often on caregivers [34–36]. Such responsibilities can create additional stress for caregivers and may limit their adaptability. Different forms of social support have been described as buffers for caregivers of children with disabilities to decrease stress and increase positive parenting [37,38]. When considering participation specifically, as expressed in the ICF-CY [2], "the role of the family environment and others in the immediate environment is integral to understanding participation, … ." [2], (p. xvi). Yet, little is known about the support experienced by caregivers of children [39], particularly in Afro-/Asia-centric countries [40]. Social support specifically is a process that "arises from formal support (medical or professional) and informal sources (extended family, friends, and neighbours) around the caregiver and family" [40], (p. 160). Social support is said to be a reciprocal interaction in which caregivers feel cared for, esteemed and valued, and in which they are engaged in a system of communication and mutual responsibility [41]. Social support enables caregivers of children with disabilities to mediate the stress that they face [38,42,43] by developing resilience [44] and increasing their situational appraisal [45] and coping strategies [46]. While reductions in stress are reported to increase well-being [47], the presence of social support for caregivers and the use of positive caregiving styles are reported to increase the quality of caregiving [48]. Nurturing the child's self-esteem can also result in better developmental outcomes for the child [40,48].

One distinct difference between Eurocentric and Afro-/Asia-centric households is the proportion of multi-generational households (both India and South Africa) [40,49]. Multigenerational households have been highlighted as able to provide resilience and growth where this might otherwise not have been possible [50–53]. The presence of older generations in the household can, however, also add to a caregiver's responsibilities. In Eurocentric cultures, help for an older generation is provided primarily when specific needs arise (for example injury or illness), and therefore multigenerational households are less common. In Afro-/Asia-centric cultures, simply "being old" is sufficient for the provision of additional support [51,52], and the provision of this support is culturally obligatory [52,53].

The influence of caregivers of children with disabilities on their child's participation is represented in the context- and environment-related constructs of the family of Participation-Related Constructs (fPRC) model [6]. In this model, caregivers constitute a key component of their child's context (part of the environment). They provide opportunities for participation, regulate the environment, and respond to their child [54]. In spite of this key role played by caregivers of children who have intellectual disabilities, only four studies [32] have made use of tools in which the caregivers reported on participation, and none of these considered factors specific to the caregiver which may affect participation [6]. From a systems perspective, the impact of caregiver factors on the participation of a child with intellectual disabilities can also be appreciated, as the influence of each level of the system on the other levels is highlighted. This perspective is supported by studies that identify the caregiver education level, income and social support structures [33,55] as factors that may have an effect on participation [33,56,57].

The final gap that has been noticed in the literature is the notion of diagnosis. The most commonly reported disability in terms of participation is cerebral palsy [20,58–63], and research on other conditions such as intellectual disabilities is sparse. Intellectual disability is a pervasive and lifelong condition in which children present significant limitations with regard to intellectual functioning and adaptive behaviour, prior to the age of 18 years [64]. In addition to the individual challenges experienced by children who have intellectual disabilities, environmental barriers may impede the achievement of human rights [34–36]. These may include a lack of opportunities for participation in education, recreation, leisure, sporting and community activities [10,65]. For children with intellectual disabilities, the combination of individual challenges and environmental barriers can result in decreased cognitive and linguistic skills, poor motor and social skills [66], social isolation and chronic health problems [32]. A systematic review of the participation of children with intellectual disabilities identified four studies that reported that children with intellectual disabilities participated to a similar extent in leisure activities, but less in social activities within the community, recreational activities, family enrichment activities and formal activities, than did their typically developing peers [32]. Other studies not included in the review indicated decreased participation in active-physical and skills-based activities [19,66,67] and a higher proportion of participation in social and recreational activities [19]. In addition, children with intellectual disabilities were noted to participate in a significantly greater number of activities at home [68], by themselves [19] or with adults, rather than with peers [10], in comparison to children with typical development. In addition, challenges in the participation of a child with an intellectual disability were found to affect not only the child, but also to place high levels of stress on the parents and family [30].

In conclusion, there is a need to describe the influence that the environmental component of caregiver support has on the participation of children with intellectual disabilities from low- and middle-income countries [33]. The current study aimed to measure, describe and compare the social support of caregivers of children with intellectual disabilities from India and South Africa, and to determine if there is an association between the social support reported by caregivers and the participation of their children as reported by caregivers and their children. India and South Africa were selected since both countries have been identified as having cultures in which households are more commonly multigenerational. However, India is a lower-middle-income country and has a very high reported prevalence of intellectual disability (≈6%), while South Africa is an upper-middle-income country and has a lower reported prevalence (≈2.25%) of intellectual disability [69,70].

2. Aims

This study had three key aims: firstly, to describe and compare the social support reported by caregivers of children with intellectual disabilities in India and South Africa; secondly, to determine if there was any association between the demographic factors and the social support reported by caregivers; thirdly, to determine if there was any association between the social support reported by caregivers and the participation of their children with intellectual disabilities.

The first hypothesis formulated for this study was that the social support available to caregivers in India and South Africa would be different. The second hypothesis suggested that demographic factors in India and South Africa would affect social support, and the third hypothesis stated that increased perceived social support would be associated with increased participation of the children with intellectual disabilities.

3. Materials and Methods

3.1. Study Design, Sampling and Participant Selection

A comparative group design was used for this study. Purposive sampling was used in schools for children with intellectual disabilities to identify participants. In both countries, education for children with disabilities is provided in special schools which can be either government funded or private. The support provided by these schools is dependent on a range of factors including context (rural/urban), funding and fees paid by parents. Both urban and rural schools were included in this study.

Inclusion criteria for caregiver–child dyads required children to be between the ages of 6 and 21, and to have a primary diagnosis of mild to moderate intellectual disability. Caregivers were required to be literate in Bengali, English, Afrikaans, isiZulu or isiXhosa, and children were required to speak Bengali, English, Afrikaans, isiZulu or isiXhosa. If a child's home language was not the same as the language in which the Children's Assessment of Participation and Enjoyment (CAPE) [71] was to be administered at their school, then the child needed to have been schooled in the language of the CAPE [71] for at least $1\frac{1}{2}$ years in order to be included in the study.

3.2. Ethics

Ethics approval for the study was obtained from the relevant ethics committees of the institutions of higher education in both countries. Permission was obtained from the appropriate departments and heads of schools or centres. In India, participants were identified in twelve schools and centres for children with disabilities. In South Africa, permission was obtained from the Department of Education in six provinces. Permission was also obtained from the principals and governing bodies of the schools identified. Eleven government schools and four private schools gave permission for their children to participate in the study.

3.3. Participants

A total of 223 caregiver–child dyads participated in the study, with 100 dyads from India and 123 from South Africa. The children had a mean age of 12:4 (years:months), and the sex composition of the sample was 61.3% male and 38.7% female. Although the reporting caregiver was primarily the child's mother (73.6%), fathers (15.6%) and other caregivers (10.8%) also reported on their children. More than half of the caregivers had at most a Grade 12 education (India 68%; South Africa 64%), and 64% of caregivers reported a household income of less than ZAR 30,000.00 (approximately EUR 1500.00) per month. Indian caregivers reported between one and six children residing in the household (M = 2), while the South African caregivers reported between one and 13 children (M = 3) in the household. Indian caregivers reported having grandparents living in the house in 67.4% of families, and other family members in 47.7% of families. South African caregivers reported having grandparents living in the house in 32.6% of families, and other family members in 52.3% of families. Statistically significant differences were evident in the demographic data of caregivers from India and South Africa.

The summarised demographic data of the participants are presented in Table 1.

Table 1. Demographic data of participants.

Demographic Factor	India (n = 100)	South Africa (n = 123)	Combined Data (n = 223)	Equivalence p-Value
Caregiver respondent (%) [1]				
Mother	33.8	39.8	73.6	
Father	6.1	9.5	15.6	0.129 [3]
Other	3.5	7.4	10.8	
Caregiver education (%) [1]				
Grade 11 or less	23.1	17.8	40.9	
Grade 12	7.1	17.8	24.9	0.000 *,[2]
Degree	12.0	8.9	20.9	
Other	2.2	11.1	13.3	
Household income per month (%) [1]				
<ZAR 4500 (≈EUR 220)	1.8	26.2	28.0	
ZAR 4501–ZAR 12,500 (≈EUR 600)	4.4	12.4	16.9	
ZAR 12,501–ZAR 30,000 (≈EUR 1500)	11.6	7.6	19.1	0.000 *,[2]
ZAR 30,001–ZAR 52,000 (≈EUR 2500)	5.8	3.6	9.3	
ZAR 52,001–ZAR 70,000 (≈EUR 3370)	6.2	3.1	9.3	
>ZAR 70,001 (≈EUR 3370)	14.7	2.7	17.3	
Number of children in the household (Median)	2.0	3.0	2.0	0.000 *,[2]
Grandparents in household (%) [1]	67.4	32.6	46.6	0.000 *,[2]
Additional family members in household (%) [1]	47.7	52.3	50.6	0.000 *,[2]
Employment (%) [1]				
Home executive/housewife	5.1%	20.8	14	
Not working currently	1.0	15.4	9.2	
Working part time	11.1	12.3	11.8	0.000 *,[2]
Working full time	82.8	43.1	60.3	
Other	0.0	8.5	4.8	
Child younger than 13 years (%) [1]	51.0	43.1	46.5	0.232 [2]
Child 13 years or older (%) [1]	49.0	56.9	53.5	
Sex (%) [1]				
Male	66.0	57.8	61.3	0.440 [3]
Female	34.0	42.2	38.7	

Note * the p value is significant. [1] Percentages may not add up to 100 due to rounding. [2] Pearson's chi-square $p < 0.05$. [3] Fisher's exact test–one-sided.

3.4. Materials

The availability of support to caregivers of children with intellectual disabilities in this study was determined using the Family Support Scale (FSS) [72]. The FSS [72] is a 19-component scale that asks caregivers to rate the helpfulness of support from various sources, for example, spouse, parents, friends, and parent groups. For each support source, the caregiver indicated on a Likert scale whether the support was not available (0), not at all helpful (1), sometimes helpful (2), generally helpful (3), very helpful (4) or extremely helpful (5). In the scoring of the FSS [72], the 19 sources were grouped into four factors—namely, family, spousal, social and professional support [73]. The FSS [72] was highlighted as a measure suitable for use with caregivers of children with disabilities in a scoping review on the subject [40], and was reported to have both internal consistency and stability across samples [73].

The participation of children was reported using the Children's Assessment of Participation and Enjoyment (CAPE) [71]. The CAPE [71] is a self-report questionnaire that has been developed for use with children/youth between the ages of 6 and 21 years, with and without disabilities. The CAPE [71] considers 55 activities grouped into domains (overall, informal and formal) or activity types (recreational, active-physical, social, skills-based and self-improvement). For each activity, five dimensions of participation are measured—namely, diversity, intensity, companionship, location and enjoyment [71]. A proxy report of the CAPE [71] was used to measure the caregivers' perceptions of their children's participation [74]. As reported in Dada, Bastable, Schlebusch and Halder [74] and available in this special edition of the Int. J. Eviron. Res. Public Health, the internal consistency of the CAPE [71] for this study was excellent ($0.923 < \alpha < 0.993$) [74,75].

All materials for this study were translated into Afrikaans, Bengali, Sepedi, isiXhosa, and isiZulu. Translation included forward and blind backward translation, as well as the consideration of linguistic, functional and cultural equivalence [76].

3.5. Data Collection

A total of 422 information packs were sent to caregivers via their child's school. The return rate in India was approximately 70% and South Africa approximately 55%.

The information pack included information on the study, a written consent form, the FSS [72], and the proxy version of the CAPE [71] in the language of teaching and learning at the child's school. The consenting caregivers completed these forms and returned them to the school in an envelope. The children whose caregivers consented were asked to provide assent and they completed the CAPE [71] in an interview at their school. All children in India assented and 98% of South African children assented. The CAPE [71] interview was conducted in close adherence to the instructions and using the visual supports provided in the manual. The interview was conducted in the language of teaching and learning at the school or the child's home language, with the researcher reading the questions to the child and recording their answers on the CAPE [71] forms. Children who assented, as well as those who did not, were provided with a token of appreciation (a ruler and an eraser).

3.6. Data Analysis

Data analysis for this study was conducted using SPSS version 26 (IBM, Armonk, NY, USA) [77]. Demographic data, data from the FSS [72] and from the CAPE [71] were analysed for normality first, and then using non-parametric tests including Pearson's chi-square, Fisher's exact test, Mann–Whitney U, Kruskal–Wallace, and the independent samples test. Internal consistency of the FSS [72] was evaluated using Cronbach's alpha [75]. Due to significant differences being evident in the demographic data of participants from India and South Africa, the analysis of the CAPE [71] and associations between the CAPE [71] and FSS [72] were conducted on each set of data independently, rather than as a single set.

The participation data from India and South Africa were compared to their respective FSS [72] data using Kendall's Tau$_b$ [78] to determine association. Although both Pearson's and Spearman's correlation coefficients are better known statistical coefficients, Kendall's Tau$_b$ has been shown to be less sensitive to outliers, thereby limiting the number of Type 1 errors and providing tighter confidence intervals and clearer interpretation [78,79]—specifically where sample sizes are smaller [80].

4. Results

The internal consistency of the FSS [72] is reported on first, followed by the social support perceived by caregivers. This is followed by the associations in demographic and FSS [72] data. The participation data are summarised (the full data are available in the paper titled: The participation of children with intellectual disabilities: Including the voices of children and their caregivers in India and South Africa, in this special edition), and associations between social support and participation are presented.

4.1. Internal Consistency of the FSS [72]

The internal consistency of the FSS [72] was determined using Cronbach's alpha. The FSS [72] presented with Cronbach's alpha coefficients between 0.748 and 0.780, which are considered acceptable [75,81].

4.2. Social Support Reported by Caregivers of Children with Intellectual Disabilities in India and South Africa

On average, caregivers in India and South Africa reported that family and spouse groups were generally helpful (family mean = 2.72, spouse mean = 2.70), and social and professional groups were sometimes helpful (social mean = 1.67, professional mean = 2.23). The caregiver's parents and spouse were most likely to be reported as extremely helpful. Parent groups, co-workers, social groups, church or spiritual support, early childhood intervention centres, and governmental and non-governmental agencies were most likely to be unavailable to caregivers. No significant differences were evident between social support factors for India and South Africa, except for spousal support ($p = 0.000$). For specific support sources, significant differences were evident between India and South Africa, both for the level of support reported and the sources available. Overall, the caregivers in India reported greater helpfulness from available support sources, but older children, co-workers or parent groups, social and religious groups, early childhood intervention and governmental/non-governmental services were not available to the majority of families. The South African caregivers, however, reported that social support groups were less helpful to them. Unavailable support in South Africa included relatives, spousal friends, friends, neighbours, other parents, parent and social groups, early childhood intervention and governmental/non-governmental services. The full social support results are indicated in Table 2.

Table 2. Caregiver-reported social support using the Family Support Survey (FSS) [72].

Family Support Scale [1]	India ($n = 100$)		South Africa ($n = 123$)		p-Value [2]/ Mann-Whitney U [2]
	Mode	% Not Available	Mode	% Not Available	
Family (Mean)	2.69	1.00	2.74	4.80	0.931 [3]
My parents	4.00	18.0	5.00	12.40	0.000 *
My relatives	4.00	5.00	0.00	33.90	0.000 *
My older children	0.00	70.00	0.00	19.30	0.000 *
Spousal (Mean)	3.23	3.00	2.23	6.50	0.000 *,[3]
My spouse's parents	4.00	25.00	0.00	30.60	0.000 *
My spouse's relatives	4.00	7.00	5.00	23.60	0.000 *
My spouse	5.00	7.00	0.00	24.50	0.000 *
My spouse's friends	4.00	13.00	0.00	42.50	0.000 *
Social (Mean)	1.54	2.00	1.78	14.60	0.230 [3]
My friends	4.00	13.00	0.00	35.10	0.000 *
My neighbours	4.00	8.00	0.00	36.00	0.000 *
Other parents	4.00	10.00	0.00	43.20	0.000 *
Co-workers	0.00	66.00	0.00	48.10	0.000 *
Parent group members	0.00	78.00	0.00	68.60	0.118
Social groups	0.00	89.00	0.00	59.40	0.000 *
Church/spiritual	0.00	96.00	0.00	40.40	0.000 *

Table 2. Cont.

Family Support Scale [1]	India (n = 100)		South Africa (n = 123)		p-Value [2]/ Mann-Whitney U [2]
	Mode	% Not Available	Mode	% Not Available	
Professional (Mean)	2.12	6.00	2.33	4.00	0.431 [3]
Family doctor	4.00	9.00	0.00	31.90	0.000 *
Early childhood intervention	0.00	91.00	0.00	52.30	0.000 *
School/day care	4.00	19.00	0.00	36.30	0.000 *
Professionals	4.00	16.00	5.00	27.50	0.000 *
Organisations Non-/Governmental	0.00	92.00	0.00	67.30	0.000 *

[1] Scores were measured on a Likert scale: 0 = not available; 1 = not at all helpful; 2 = sometimes helpful; 3 = generally helpful; 4 = very helpful; 5 = extremely helpful. [2] Pearson's chi-square, $p < 0.05$. [3] Mann–Whitney U, * P is significant when $p < 0.05$.

Associations between Demographic Factors and Social Support

In India, the association indicated increased family support when the caregiver was the mother ($Tau_b = 0.194$), whereas in South Africa, decreased family support was indicated when the caregiver was the mother ($Tau_b = -0.163$). Small positive associations between social support ($Tau_b = 0.201$) and employment ($Tau_b = 0.157$) were evident in India, while a small effect of home language on professional support was indicated for South Africa ($p = 0.262$). Associations between child sex and age were seen in India, with increased support for male ($Tau_b = -0.182$) and younger children ($Tau_b = 0.173$) [79]. The association data are presented in Table 3 below.

Table 3. Associations between demographic social support factors in India and South Africa.

Demographic Factors	Family		Spousal		Social		Professional	
	India	South Africa	India	South Africa	India	South Africa	India	South Africa
Relationship to child [1]	0.023 *	0.030 *	0.957	0.067	0.221	0.807	0.150	0.215
Education [1]	0.466	0.566	0.112	0.816	0.773	0.761	0.511	0.364
Employment [1]	0.940	0.112	00.577	0.205	0.016 *	0.139	0.547	0.249
Income [1]	0.716	0.315	0.041 *	0.946	0.858	0.013	0.540	0.262
Home language [2]	0.806	0.420	0.906	0.234	0.560	0.059	0.166	0.031 *
Number of children in the home [1]	0.218	0.246	0.711	0.311	0.290	0.814	0.290	0.287
Number of grandparents in the home [1]	0.693	0.214	0.136	0.350	0.335	0.824	0.587	0.419
Other relatives in the home [1]	0.637	0.545	0.712	0.649	0.913	0.602	0.090	0.309
Child's sex [1]	0.038 *	0.820	0.933	0.905	0.835	0.628	0.979	0.727
Child's age (<13/>13 years) [1]	0.443	0.507	0.224	0.169	0.042 *	0.070	0.859	0.826
Additional impairments [1]	0.724	0.296	0.723	0.597	0.396	0.175	0.091	0.129

* $p < 0.05$. [1] Tau_b. [2] Kruskal–Wallis.

4.3. Participation and Social Support for Children with Intellectual Disabilities in India and South Africa

4.3.1. Self-Reported Participation of Children with Intellectual Disabilities

Children in India and South Africa participated in a similar number of activities overall and with the same enjoyment. However, children from India were noted to participate more frequently at home with close family, while the children from South Africa participated less frequently at a relative's house with extended family (medium to large effects). The full participation data are available in Dada, Bastable, Schlebusch and Halder, in this special edition of the Int. J. Eviron. Res. Public Health.

4.3.2. Proxy-Reported Participation of Children with Intellectual Disabilities

Caregiver-reported participation differed from self-reported participation across both India and South Africa in terms of the number of social and skills-based activities participated in and to the level of enjoyment. No significant differences in the reporting of intensity, with whom, or where activities were conducted were evident. The full caregiver participation results are available in the Dada, Bastable, Schlebusch and Halder, in this special edition of the Int. J. Eviron. Res. Public Health.

4.4. Association between Social Support and Participation

4.4.1. Association between Social Support and Caregiver-Reported Participation of Children with Intellectual Disabilities in India and South Africa

Associations with the presence of family support sources were evident for the intensity of participation overall, in the informal domain and for self-improvement activities in South Africa. Family support was also associated with where formal and skills-based activities occurred in South Africa, but with caregiver-reported enjoyment in active-physical activities in India. Spousal factors were associated with the diversity of social activities in South Africa, with whom and where participation occurred overall, and with participation in the informal domain. In India, spousal support was associated with whom recreational activities occurred, and where informal and social activities took place. The social support factor was associated with the diversity of participation overall, in both the informal and formal domains in India. In South Africa, however, social support was associated with the intensity of participation overall, participation in the informal domain, and social activities. Intensity of participation in the formal domain as well as where participation in this domain occurred was associated with social support in India. Professional support was associated in India with the intensity of activities in the formal domain and social activities, but in South Africa, it was associated with participation with whom and participation in the informal domain. The association data are presented in Table 4.

Table 4. Association between social support factors and caregiver-reported participation.

Participation Domains or Activities	Family		Spousal		Social		Professional	
	India	South Africa	India	South Africa	India	South Africa	India	South Africa
Participation, as Reported by Caregivers								
Overall	0.248	0.850	0.923	0.343	0.05 *,1	0.735	0.504	0.625
Informal domain	0.165	0.846	0.902	0.549	0.123 *,3	0.462	0.681	0.960
Formal domain	0.244	0.365	0.776	0.181	0.017 *,1	0.882	0.852	0.301
Recreational activities	0.097	0.995	0.300	0.675	0.611	0.261	0.606	0.474
Active-physical activities	0.937	0.696	0.880	0.990	0.453	0.682	0.255	0.998
Social activities	0.335	0.221	0.542	0.044 *,1	0.062	0.863	0.378	0.496
Skills-based activities	0.322	0.214	0.369	0.107	0.207	0.963	0.252	0.265
Self-improvement activities	0.357	0.651	0.251	0.431	0.377	0.484	0.908	0.677
Participation Intensity, as Reported by Caregivers								
Overall	0.521	0.020 *,2	0.344	0.450	0.560	0.007 **,1	0.268	0.076
Informal domain	0.803	0.042 *,1	0.874	0.450	0.860	0.040 *,1	0.056	0.172
Formal domain	0.700	0.136	0.109	0.781	0.009 **,1	0.066	0.004 **,2	0.477
Recreational activities	0.793	0.744	0.430	0.831	0.790	0.187	0.821	0.421
Active-physical activities	0.913	0.174	0.849	0.690	0.238	0.545	0.723	0.083
Social activities	0.903	0.428	0.762	0.711	0.832	0.034 *,1	0.016 *,1	0.302
Skills-based activities	0.946	0.270	0.095	0.397	0.363	0.087	0.942	0.803
Self-improvement activities	0.458	0.029 *,1	0.754	0.366	0.842	0.075	0.098	0.705

Table 4. Cont.

Participation Domains or Activities	Family		Spousal		Social		Professional	
	India	South Africa	India	South Africa	India	South Africa	India	South Africa
Participation with Whom, as Reported by Caregivers								
Overall	0.688	0.300	0.250	0.048 *,1	0.379	0.055	0.878	0.046 *,1
Informal domain	0.766	0.261	0.256	0.042 *,1	0.544	0.035 *,1	0.513	0.018 *,1
Formal domain	0.665	0.407	0.429	0.278	0.131	0.654	0.311	0.887
Recreational activities	0.908	0.535	0.033 *,1	0.302	0.637	0.008 **,1	0.765	0.058
Active-physical activities	0.423	0.298	0.453	0.066	0.530	0.543	0.511	0.983
Social activities	0.700	0.212	0.193	0.081	0.465	0.134	0.053	0.348
Skills-based activities	0.276	0.114	0.451	0.250	0.784	0.232	0.134	0.716
Self-improvement activities	0.452	0.622	0.601	0.112	0.247	0.123	0.189	0.070
Participation Where, as Reported by Caregivers								
Overall	0.275	0.119	0.080	0.044 *,1	0.315	0.284	0.938	0.896
Informal domain	0.262	0.107	0.036 *,1	0.034 *,1	0.832	0.448	0.733	0.854
Formal domain	0.422	0.025 *,1	0.889	0.093	0.001 **,2	0.206	0.258	0.994
Recreational activities	0.797	0.651	0.739	0.751	0.243	0.056	0.439	0.338
Active-physical activities	0.275	0.044 *	0.233	0.045 *	0.130	0.781	0.589	0.539
Social activities	0.155	0.891	0.029 *,1	0.287	0.455	0.615	0.109	0.542
Skills-based activities	0.690	0.015 *,1	0.699	0.083	0.197	0.111	1.000	0.909
Self-improvement activities	0.241	0.251	0.992	0.122	0.671	0.123	0.135	0.459
Participation Enjoyment, as Reported by Caregivers								
Overall	0.121	00.761	0.305	0.424	0.145	0.694	0.036 *,2	0.283
Informal domain	0.079	0.801	0.273	0.800	0.993	0.817	0.046 *,1	0.205
Formal domain	0.444	0.603	0.425	0.036 *,1	0.045 *,1	0.968	0.647	0.848
Recreational activities	0.121	0.641	0.331	0.900	0.157	0.615	0.121	0.825
Active-physical activities	0.024 *,2	0.368	0.373	0.516	0.165	0.481	0.033 *,2	0.915
Social activities	0.089	0.533	0.100	0.795	0.256	0.230	0.590	0.199
Skills-based activities	0.137	0.123	0.763	0.685	0.575	0.518	0.267	0.546
Self-improvement activities	0.877	0.870	0.198	0.104	0.725	0.212	0.070	0.116

Tau$_b$ ** $p < 0.01$, * $p < 0.05$. Effect sizes: [1] Small effect: Tau$_b$ > 0.7, [2] Medium effect: Tau$_b$ > 0.21, [3] Large effect: Tau$_b$ > 0.50 [79].

4.4.2. Associations between Social Support and Child-Reported Participation of Children with Intellectual Disabilities in India and South Africa

Children in South Africa indicated associations between participation and family and social support, while children in India indicated connections between active physical activities and family. Intensity of participation in social (India) and recreational (South Africa) activities was associated with social support. An association between with whom recreational activities occurred and family support was evident in South Africa, while family support was associated with where participation occurred in India as well as South Africa. All effects identified were small [75]. Significant associations are reported in Table 5.

Table 5. Significant associations between social support factors and child-reported participation.

Participation Domains and Activities	Family		Spousal		Social		Professional	
	India	South Africa	India	South Africa	India	South Africa	India	South Africa
Participation, as Reported by Children								
Overall		0.009 **,1		0.243		0.048 *,1		0.525
Informal domain		0.010 *,1		0.228		0.040 *,1		0.363
Active-physical activities	0.048 *1	0.019 *,1	0.142	0.397	0.475	0.291	0.631	0.938
Social activities		0.010 *,1		0.062		0.007 *,1		0.191
Skills-based activities		0.022 *,1		0.098		0.053		0.756
Participation Intensity, as Reported by Children								
Social activities	0.701		0.438		0.041 *,1		0.571	
Recreational activities		0.068		0.336		0.012 *,1		0.053
Participation with Whom, as Reported by Children								
Recreational activities		0.033 *,1		0.539		0.758		0.066

Table 5. Cont.

Participation Domains and Activities	Family		Spousal		Social		Professional	
	India	South Africa	India	South Africa	India	South Africa	India	South Africa
Participation Where, as Reported by Children								
Formal domain	0.565		0.280		0.006 **,1	0.054		
Self-improvement activities	0.025 *,1		0.145		0.100	0.330		
Informal domain		0.014 *,1		0.416		0.202		0.928
Social activities		0.013 *,1		0.103		0.082		0.468
Participation Enjoyment, as Reported by Children								
Formal domain	0.049 *,1		0.216		0.301		0.072	
Active-physical activities		0.552		0.380		0.539		0.015 *,1
Self-improvement activities		0.013 *,1		0.112		0.629		0.527

Tau$_b$ ** $p < 0.01$, * $p < 0.05$. Effect sizes: [1] Small effect: Tau$_b$ > 0.7.

5. Discussion

Intellectual disability is one of the leading developmental disabilities in low- and middle-income countries [69,70]. For caregivers, a child with an intellectual disability can increase the stress and demands of parenting. Caregivers may find themselves solely responsible for ensuring that their child's rights are recognised and their needs are met [34–36]. Yet, in the face of increased demands, caregivers have reported a lack of support from outside of their immediate family [82,83]. Increased stress for caregivers can limit their ability to support their children and provide them with the required developmental opportunities [37,38] through participation in activities [6]. The relationship between the caregiver and the child's participation has been described as a related factor that may influence participation (the environment) [7–9,84]. For caregivers, however, social support has been described as a buffer to stress [37,38], which may increase their capacity to facilitate their child's participation. This study sought to describe the different types of social support experienced by caregivers of children with intellectual disabilities in India and South Africa (middle-income countries) and to identify whether there is an association between the social support reported by caregivers and the children's participation.

As discussed previously, the bulk of research on participation originated in high-income countries [22]. Hence, this study sought to provide information on participation of children with intellectual disabilities in two middle-income countries. In the initial analysis of demographic information from the participants it became clear that although both India and South Africa are middle-income countries, significant differences were evident in the demographics of the caregiver groups from these two countries. Education, income and employment differed significantly among the caregivers, with the South African caregivers reporting lower levels of education, income and employment. Such differences highlight the need for research across both low- and middle-income countries, as demographic differences alone make generalisation from one country to another challenging.

The presence of multigenerational households has been hypothesised to affect social support structures and to be widely prevalent in collectivist cultures. Nonetheless, only half of the families in this study came from multigenerational households, with Indian caregivers reporting significantly more multigenerational households than caregivers in South Africa—despite the fact that it has been suggested that multigenerational households may provide additional support for caregivers of children with disabilities [50–52]. Our study suggests that it cannot be assumed that households from traditionally collectivist countries will contain multiple generations, even if this has been a cultural norm in the past. Nowadays, industrialisation and globalisation have a clear impact on societal functioning [53].

In spite of the demographic differences identified between India and South Africa, social support from family, social and professional factors was reported as similar, but spousal support was significantly different. Caregivers from India reported more support from spousal sources—including their spouse, spouse's parents—and friends than did caregivers from South Africa, while approximately a quarter of South African caregivers reported that their spouse and relatives were not available. The lack of spousal availability in South Africa may result from the country's past, as the systematisation of migrant labour under apartheid split families by allowing only the working individual to stay in an urban area. As a result, families were divided, with mothers and children living in a different place from fathers. The forced separation of families under apartheid has had a significant effect on family structure in South Africa, which is still experienced today [85]. In Indian culture (in contrast), once married, some women would traditionally live with their husband's family, hence having a spouse available may also include the support of his family [53].

The demographic factors of relationship to child (family), employment (India, social), home language (South Africa, professional), child sex (India, family) and child age (India, social) were associated with social support reported by caregivers, although the associations showed small effects. The support experienced by caregivers may well be related to the social structure of the country, including how neighbours and friends support working parents, and cultural biases relating to sex and age [86–88]. For example, in India, male children are often revered while female children may be seen as a burden [89,90], while in South Africa professional support is most often available to caregivers in English or Afrikaans, which may not be their home language [91].

Overall participation of children with intellectual disabilities in India and South Africa was similar, but differences were evident in the formal domain, as well as in respect of active-physical and recreational activities. Weak positive associations with social support were evident across both the Indian and South African data in relation to the diversity of participation (mostly family support, but also spousal and social support). As participation in activities for children with intellectual disabilities requires (in many situations) the availability of the activities, as well as a partner to facilitate the child, the presence of additional family support may reduce the load on the caregiver and provide more opportunities for the child to participate. Similarly, spousal and social support may increase the number of opportunities for the child to participate.

The effect that social support given to caregivers of children with intellectual disabilities has on the participation of their child is evident in the associations identified between support sources and the caregiver-reported participation. In India, associations were seen most often between social and professional support and the formal domain, while in South Africa associations between spousal and social support were evident more often in the informal domain. These differences could be linked to the availability of resources. With lower income reported by caregivers in South Africa, it is possible that informal activities place less of a financial burden on caregivers. Importantly, however, the South African caregivers reported more households where the spouse was not available than did the Indian households. Thus, the association between both spousal and social support is logical, as when spousal support was not available, the South African caregivers relied on extended family and friends for support.

It is interesting to note the differences in associations evident between participation data as reported by the children and caregivers—this is in spite of the data not being significantly different [74]. The children's participation data were associated with family and social support, mostly in informal activities for South Africa, but primarily in formalised activities for India. Enjoyment was associated with professional support for active-physical activities in South Africa. This is a logical conclusion, in that children with special needs may require devices or support to participate in active-physical activities. Such support is often provided by professionals or professional organisations, for examples the special Olympics. Of interest, however, is that the enjoyment of formal (India) and self-improvement (South Africa) activities was associated with family support for children. In this regard it may be that self-improvement activities are participated in most frequently at home with family, or that these activities are most important to the family—hence all family members contribute towards the child's enjoyment in these areas.

Overall, the data from our study provide evidence that environmental factors play a role in the social support that caregivers of children with intellectual disabilities receive. Sequentially, social support plays a role in the participation of children with intellectual disabilities. Differences in the associations between social support and caregiver-reported participation point to demographic and cultural influences on the participation of children with intellectual disabilities. At the same time, differences in social support and participation associations between the child- and caregiver-reported participation data emphasise the subjective nature of social support and participation. Hence, results should not be generalised from one country to the next, even when aspects of their cultures appear similar at face value. When considering the participation of children with intellectual disabilities, the family environment should be examined as a whole, with reporting from multiple members in order to understand the factors that affect participation.

Considered in relation to current models of participation, the effects of social support were mostly weak, yet consistent across multiple areas of participation. Hence, they cannot be ignored in the consideration of participation of children with intellectual disabilities. Although current models of participation such as the fPRC [84] now include the child's context and environment, they have until recently focused more on the direct associations between the child and the environment.

5.1. Recommendations

Recommendations arising from this study include the exploration of the role of environmental factors in the participation of children with intellectual disabilities in other countries. Specifically, further research is recommended on the effects that social support interventions have on the participation of children who are typically developing and those with disabilities.

5.2. Limitations

The FSS [72] used in this study focuses on the perceived helpfulness of different types of social support but does not provide an opportunity for caregivers to report on the context of the support or to identify alternative supports that are needed [40]. Perhaps additional measures of the type of social support that is needed could have been included.

6. Conclusions

The social support provided to caregivers of children with intellectual disabilities in India and South Africa was similar in many respects. However, social support is sensitive to demographic factors such as employment and the relationship of the caregiver to the child. Caregivers of children with intellectual disabilities overwhelmingly reported a lack of social and professional support. In both India and South Africa, studies showed positive associations between participation and social support. For India, increased social support was associated with increased diversity of participation, while in South Africa it was associated with increased intensity of participation. Differences in results from different countries may preclude the generalisation of results relating to both social support and participation.

Author Contributions: The authors of this article contributed in the following areas: conceptualisation: S.D. and S.H.; methodology: S.D. and S.H.; validation: K.B. and S.D.; formal analysis: K.B.; investigation: S.D. and S.H.; resources: S.D. and S.H.; data curation: K.B., S.D. and S.H.; writing—original draft preparation: K.B. and S.D.; writing—review and editing: K.B., S.D. and S.H.; visualisation: K.B. and S.D.; supervision: K.B. and S.D.; project administration: S.D. and S.H.; funding acquisition: S.D. and S.H. All authors have read and agreed to the published version of the manuscript.

Funding: Funding from the National Institute of Humanities and Social Sciences/Indian Council of Social Science Research is hereby acknowledged. The content of this paper is solely the responsibility of the authors and does not necessarily represent the official views of the funders.

Acknowledgments: The authors would like to acknowledge the postgraduate students from the Master's in the Early Childhood Intervention programme who assisted with data collection.

Conflicts of Interest: The authors declare no conflict of interest. The funders had no role in the design of the study; in the collection, analysis or interpretation of data; in the writing of the manuscript, or in the decision to publish the results.

References

1. World Health Organisation. *The International Classification of Functioning, Disability and Health*; World Health Organisation: Geneva, Switzerland, 2001.
2. World Health Organisation. *International Classification of Functioning, Disability and Health—Child and Youth Version (ICF-CY)*; World Health Press: Geneva, Switzerland, 2007; ISBN 9789241547321.
3. Raghavendra, P.; Bornman, J.; Granlund, M.; Björck-Åkesson, E. The World Health Organization's International Classification of Functioning, Disability and Health: Implications for Clinical and Research Practice in the field of Augmentative and Alternative Communication. *Augment. Altern. Commun.* **2007**, *23*, 349–361. [CrossRef] [PubMed]
4. United Nations. *Convention on the Rights of Persons with Disabilities*; United Nations: Geneva Switzerland, 2006.
5. Murphy, N.; Carbone, P. Promoting the Participation of Children with Disabilities in Sports, Recreation, and Physical Activities. *Pediatrics* **2008**, *121*, 1057–1061. [CrossRef]
6. Imms, C.; Granlund, M.; Wilson, P.H.; Steenbergen, B.; Rosenbaum, P.L.; Gordon, A.M. Participation, both a means and an end: A conceptual analysis of processes and outcomes in childhood disability. *Dev. Med. Child Neurol.* **2017**, *59*, 16–25. [CrossRef] [PubMed]
7. Forsyth, R.J.; Colver, A.; Woolley, M.; Lowe, M. Participation of young severely disabled children is influenced by their intrinsic impairments and environment. *Dev. Med. Child Neurol.* **2007**, *49*, 345–349. [CrossRef] [PubMed]
8. Longo, E.; Badia, M. Research in Developmental Disabilities Patterns and predictors of participation in leisure activities outside of school in children and adolescents with Cerebral Palsy. *Res. Dev. Disabil.* **2013**, *34*, 266–275. [CrossRef]
9. Fauconnier, J.; Dickinson, H.O.; Beckung, E.; Marcelli, M.; McManus, V.; Michelsen, S.I.; Parkes, J.; Parkinson, K.N.; Thyen, U.; Arnaud, C.; et al. Participation in life situations of 8–12 year old children with cerebral palsy: Cross sectional European study. *BMJ* **2009**, *338*, b1458. [CrossRef]
10. Solish, A.; Perry, A.; Minnes, P. Participation of Children with and without Disabilities in Social, Recreational and Leisure Activities. *J. Appl. Res. Intellect. Disabil.* **2010**, *23*, 226–236. [CrossRef]
11. Eriksson, L.; Welander, J.; Granlund, M. Participation in everyday school activities for children with and without disabilities. *J. Dev. Phys. Disabil.* **2007**, *19*, 485–502. [CrossRef]
12. Law, M.; King, G.; King, S.; Kertoy, M.; Hurley, P.; Rosenbaum, P.; Young, N.; Hanna, S. Patterns of participation in recreational and leisure activities among children with complex physical disabilities. *Dev. Med. Child Neurol.* **2006**, *48*, 337–342. [CrossRef]
13. Raghavendra, P.; Olsson, C.; Sampson, J.; McInerney, R.; Connell, T. School participation and social networks of children with complex communication needs, physical disabilities, and typically developing peers. *Augment. Altern. Commun.* **2012**, *28*, 33–43. [CrossRef]
14. Hossein Memari, A.; Panahi, N.; Ranjbar, E.; Moshayedi, P.; Shafiei, M.; Kordi, R.; Ziaee, V. Children with Autism Spectrum Disorder and Patterns of Participation in Daily Physical and Play Activities. *Neurol. Res. Int.* **2015**, *2015*, 1–7. [CrossRef] [PubMed]
15. Shields, N.; Synnot, A.; Kearns, C. The extent, context and experience of participation in out-of-school activities among children with disability. *Res. Dev. Disabil.* **2015**, *47*, 165–174. [CrossRef] [PubMed]
16. Bult, M.K.; Verschuren, O.; Gorter, J.W.; Jongmans, M.J.; Piskur, B.; Ketelaar, M. Cross-cultural validation and psychometric evaluation of the Dutch language version of the Children's Assessment of Participation and Enjoyment (CAPE) in children with and without physical disabilities. *Clin. Rehabil.* **2010**, *24*, 843–853. [CrossRef]
17. Bedell, G.M.; Dumas, H.M. Social participation of children and youth with acquired brain injuries discharged from inpatient rehabilitation: A follow-up study. *Brain Inj.* **2004**, *18*, 65–82. [CrossRef]
18. Tint, A.; Maughan, A.L.; Weiss, J.A. Community participation of youth with intellectual disability and autism spectrum disorder. *J. Intellect. Disabil. Res.* **2017**, *61*, 168–180. [CrossRef] [PubMed]

19. King, M.; Shields, N.; Imms, C.; Black, M.; Ardern, C. Participation of children with intellectual disability compared with typically developing children. *Res. Dev. Disabil.* **2013**, *34*, 1854–1862. [CrossRef]
20. Anaby, D.; Hand, C.; Bradley, L.; Direzze, B.; Forhan, M.; Digiacomo, A.; Law, M. The effect of the environment on participation of children and youth with disabilities: A scoping review. *Disabil. Rehabil.* **2013**, *35*, 1589–1598. [CrossRef]
21. Olusanya, B.O.; Davis, A.C.; Wertlieb, D.; Boo, N.Y.; Nair, M.K.C.; Halpern, R.; Kuper, H.; Breinbauer, C.; de Vries, P.J.; Gladstone, M.; et al. Developmental disabilities among children younger than 5 years in 195 countries and territories, 1990–2016: A systematic analysis for the Global Burden of Disease Study 2016. *Lancet Glob. Health* **2018**, *6*, e1100–e1121. [CrossRef]
22. Schlebusch, L.; Huus, K.; Samuels, A.; Granlund, M.; Dada, S. Participation of young people with disabilities and/or chronic conditions in low- and middle-income countries: A scoping review. *Dev. Med. Child Neurol.* **2020**. [CrossRef]
23. Raghavendra, P. Participation of children with disabilities: Measuring subjective and objective outcomes. *Child Care Health Dev.* **2013**, *39*, 461–465. [CrossRef]
24. Grantham-mcgregor, S.; Cheung, Y.B.; Cueto, S.; Glewwe, P.; Richter, L.; Strupp, B. Child development in developing countries 1 Developmental potential in the first 5 years for children in. *Lancet* **2007**, *369*, 60–70. [CrossRef]
25. Walker, S.P.; Wachs, T.D.; Gardner, J.M.; Lozoff, B.; Wasserman, G.A.; Pollitt, E.; Carter, J.A. Child development in developing countries 2 Child development: Risk factors for adverse outcomes in developing countries. *Lancet* **2007**, *369*, 145–157. [CrossRef]
26. Lu, C.; Black, M.M.; Richter, L.M. Risk of poor development in young children in low-income and middle-income countries: An estimation and analysis at the global, regional, and country level. *Lancet Glob. Health* **2016**, *4*, e916–e922. [CrossRef]
27. Yin, J. Beyond postmodernism: A non-western perspective on identity. *J. Multicult. Discourses* **2018**, *13*, 193–219. [CrossRef]
28. Kubow, P.K. Exploring Western and non-Western epistemological influences in South Africa: Theorising a critical democratic citizenship education. *Compare* **2018**, *48*, 349–361. [CrossRef]
29. Ameka, F.K.; Terkourafi, M. What if . . . ? Imagining non-Western perspectives on pragmatic theory and practice. *J. Pragmat.* **2019**, *145*, 72–82. [CrossRef]
30. Douma, J.C.H.; Dekker, M.C.; Koot, H.M. Supporting parents of youths with intellectual disabilities and psychopathology. *J. Intellect. Disabil. Res.* **2006**, *50*, 570–581. [CrossRef]
31. Ruck, M.D.; Peterson-Badali, M.; Day, D.M. Adolescents' and Mothers' Understanding of Children's Rights in the Home. *J. Res. Adolesc.* **2002**, *12*, 373–398. [CrossRef]
32. Shields, N.; King, M.; Corbett, M.; Imms, C. Is participation among children with intellectual disabilities in outside school activities similar to their typically developing peers? A systematic review. *Dev. Neurorehabil.* **2014**, *17*, 64–71. [CrossRef]
33. Bedell, G.; Coster, W.; Law, M.; Liljenquist, K.; Kao, Y.C.; Teplicky, R.; Anaby, D.; Khetani, M.A. Community participation, supports, and barriers of school-age children with and without disabilities. *Arch. Phys. Med. Rehabil.* **2013**, *94*, 315–323. [CrossRef]
34. Gobrial, E. Mind the gap: The human rights of children with intellectual disabilities in Egypt. *J. Intellect. Disabil. Res.* **2012**, *56*, 1058–1064. [CrossRef] [PubMed]
35. United Nations General Assembly. Universal Declaration of Human Rights. *Int. J. Hum. Rights* **1998**, *2*, 84–88. [CrossRef]
36. Johnson, G.; Symonides, J. *Universal Declarattion of Human Right 1948*; The United Nations Educational, Scientific and Cultural Organization: Paris, France, 1948.
37. McConnell, D.; Savage, A.; Breitkreuz, R. Resilience in families raising children with disabilities and behavior problems. *Res. Dev. Disabil.* **2014**, *35*, 833–848. [CrossRef] [PubMed]
38. Sipal, R.F.; Sayin, U. Impact of Perceived Social Support and Depression on the Parental Attitudes of Mothers of Children Who are Deaf. *J. Child Fam. Stud.* **2013**, *22*, 1103–1111. [CrossRef]
39. Murphy, N.A.; Christian, B.; Caplin, D.A.; Young, P.C. The health of caregivers for children with disabilities: Caregiver perspectives. *Child. Care Health Dev.* **2007**, *33*, 180–187. [CrossRef]
40. Mantri-Langeveldt, A.; Dada, S.; Boshoff, K. Measures for social support in raising a child with a disability: A scoping review. *Child Care Health Dev.* **2019**, *45*, 159–174. [CrossRef]

41. Cobb, S. Social Support as a Moderator of Life Stress. *Psychosom. Med.* **1976**, *38*, 300–314. [CrossRef]
42. Migerode, F.; Maes, B.; Buysse, A.; Brondeel, R. Quality of Life in Adolescents with a Disability and Their Parents: The Mediating Role of Social Support and Resilience. *J. Dev. Phys. Disabil.* **2012**, *24*, 487–503. [CrossRef]
43. Ran Tak, Y.; McCubbin, M. Family stress, perceived social support and coping following the diagnosis of a child's congenital heart disease. *J. Adv. Nurs.* **2002**, *39*, 190–198. [CrossRef]
44. Benzies, K.; Mychasiuk, R. Fostering family resiliency: A review of the key protective factors. *Child Fam. Soc. Work* **2009**, *14*, 103–114. [CrossRef]
45. Mhaka-Mutepfa, M.; Cumming, R.; Mpofu, E. Grandparents Fostering Orphans: Influences of Protective Factors on Their Health and Well-Being. *Health Care Women Int.* **2014**, *35*, 1022–1039. [CrossRef] [PubMed]
46. Tang, F.; Jang, H.; Copeland, V.C. Challenges and resilience in African American grandparents raising grandchildren: A review of the literature with practice implications. *GrandFamilies Contemp. J. Res. Pract. Policy* **2015**, *2*, 1–31.
47. Casale, M.; Wild, L.; Cluver, L.; Kuo, C. Social support as a protective factor for depression among women caring for children in HIV-endemic South Africa. *J. Behav. Med.* **2015**, *38*, 17–27. [CrossRef]
48. Guralnick, M.J.; Hammond, M.A.; Neville, B.; Connor, R.T. The relationship between sources and functions of social support and dimensions of child- and parent-related stress. *J. Intellect. Disabil. Res.* **2008**, *52*, 1138–1154. [CrossRef] [PubMed]
49. Schlebusch, L.; Samuels, A.E.; Dada, S. South African families raising children with autism spectrum disorders: Relationship between family routines, cognitive appraisal and family quality of life. *J. Intellect. Disabil. Res.* **2016**, *60*, 412–423. [CrossRef] [PubMed]
50. Lee, Y.; Blitz, L.V.; Srnka, M. Trauma and resiliency in grandparent-headed multigenerational families. *Fam. Soc.* **2015**, *96*, 116–124. [CrossRef]
51. Samanta, T.; Chen, F.; Vanneman, R. Living Arrangements and Health of Older Adults in India. *J. Gerontol. Ser. B Psychol. Sci. Soc. Sci.* **2015**, *70*, 937–947. [CrossRef]
52. Burholt, V.; Dobbs, C. A support network typology for application in older populations with a preponderance of multigenerational households. *Aging Soc.* **2014**, *34*, 1142–1169. [CrossRef]
53. Breton, E. Modernization and Household Composition in India, 1983–2009. *Popul. Dev. Rev.* **2019**, *45*, 739–766. [CrossRef]
54. Raval, V.V.; Walker, B.L. Unpacking 'culture': Caregiver socialization of emotion and child functioning in diverse families. *Dev. Rev.* **2019**, *51*, 146–174. [CrossRef]
55. Piškur, B.; Beurskens, A.; Jongmans, M.J.; Ketelaar, M.; Norton, M.; Frings, C.; Hemmingsson, H.; Smeets, R. Parents' actions, challenges, and needs while enabling participation of children with a physical disability: A scoping review. *BMC Pediatr.* **2012**, *12*, 718. [CrossRef] [PubMed]
56. Hammal, D.; Jarvis, S.N.; Colver, A.F. Participation of children with cerebral palsy is influenced by where they live. *Dev. Med. Child Neurol.* **2004**, *46*, 292–298. [CrossRef] [PubMed]
57. Colver, A.F.; Dickinson, H.O. Study protocol: Determinants of participation and quality of life of adolescents with cerebral palsy: A longitudinal study (SPARCLE2). *BMC Public Health* **2010**, *10*, 280. [CrossRef] [PubMed]
58. Imms, C.; Reilly, S.; Carlin, J.; Dodd, K. Diversity of participation in children with cerebral palsy. *Dev. Med. Child Neurol.* **2008**, *50*, 363–369. [CrossRef]
59. Voorman, J.M.; Dallmeijer, A.J.; Schuengel, C.; Knol, D.L.; Lankhorst, G.J.; Becher, J.G. Activities and participation of 9- to 13-year-old children with cerebral palsy. *Clin. Rehabil.* **2006**, *20*, 937–948. [CrossRef]
60. Beckung, E.; Hagberg, G. Neuroimpairments, activity limitations, and participation restrictions in children with cerebral palsy. *Dev. Med. Child Neurol.* **2002**, *44*, 309–316. [CrossRef]
61. Chiarello, L.A.; Palisano, R.J.; Bartlett, D.J.; McCoy, S.W. A multivariate model of determinants of change in gross-motor abilities and engagement in self-care and play of young children with cerebral palsy. *Phys. Occup. Ther. Pediatr.* **2011**, *31*, 150–168. [CrossRef]
62. Bult, M.K.; Verschuren, O.; Jongmans, M.J.; Lindeman, E.; Ketelaar, M. What influences participation in leisure activities of children and youth with physical disabilities? A systematic review. *Res. Dev. Disabil.* **2011**, *32*, 1521–1529. [CrossRef]
63. Imms, C. Children with cerebral palsy participate: A review of the literature. *Disabil. Rehabil.* **2008**, *30*, 1867–1884. [CrossRef]

64. Schalock, R.L.; Luckasson, R.; Shogren, K. The Renaming of Mental Retardation: Understanding the Change to the Term Intellectual Disability. *Intellect. Dev. Disabil.* **2007**, *45*, 116–124. [CrossRef]
65. Tomlinson, M.; Yasamy, M.T.; Emerson, E.; Officer, A.; Richler, D.; Saxena, S. Setting global research priorities for developmental disabilities, including intellectual disabilities and autism. *J. Intellect. Disabil. Res.* **2014**, *58*, 1121–1130. [CrossRef] [PubMed]
66. Westendorp, M.; Houwen, S.; Hartman, E.; Visscher, C. Are gross motor skills and sports participation related in children with intellectual disabilities? *Res. Dev. Disabil.* **2011**, *32*, 1147–1153. [CrossRef] [PubMed]
67. Dahan-Oliel, N.; Mazer, B.; Riley, P.; Maltais, D.B.; Nadeau, L.; Majnemer, A. Participation and enjoyment of leisure activities in adolescents born at or less than 29 week gestation. *Early Hum. Dev.* **2014**, *90*, 307–314. [CrossRef] [PubMed]
68. Nelson, F.; Masulani-Mwale, C.; Richards, E.; Theobald, S.; Gladstone, M. The meaning of participation for children in Malawi: Insights from children and caregivers. *Child Care Health Dev.* **2017**, *43*, 133–143. [CrossRef] [PubMed]
69. The World Bank. IBA World Bank Open Data. Available online: https://data.worldbank.org/ (accessed on 23 October 2019).
70. Olusanya, B.O.; Wright, S.M.; Nair, M.K.C.; Boo, N.Y.; Halpern, R.; Kuper, H.; Abubakar, A.A.; Almasri, N.A.; Arabloo, J.; Arora, N.K.; et al. Global Burden of Childhood Epilepsy, Intellectual Disability, and Sensory Impairments. *Pediatrics* **2020**, *146*, e20192623. [CrossRef] [PubMed]
71. King, G.; Law, M.; King, S.; Hurley, P.; Rosenbaum, P.; Hanna, S.; Kertoy, M.; Young, N. *Children's Assessment of Participation and Enjoyment & Preferences for Activities of Children*; Pearson: San Antonio, TX, USA, 2004.
72. Dunst, C.J.; Trivette, C.M.; Jenkins, V. *Family Support Scale: Reliability and Validity*; Winterberry Press: Asheville, NC, USA, 1984.
73. Taylor, M.J.; Crowley, S.L.; White, K.R. Psychometric Investigation of the FSS and FRS. 1993. Available online: https://files.eric.ed.gov/fulltext/ED359249.pdf (accessed on 9 September 2020).
74. Dada, S.; Bastable, K.; Schlebusch, L.; Halder, S. The participation of children with intellectual disabilities: Including the voices of children and their caregivers in India and South Africa. *Int. J. Environ. Res. Public Health* **2020**, in press.
75. George, D.; Mallery, M. *Using SPSS for Windows Step by Step: A Simple Guide and Reference*; Allyn & Bacon: Boston, MA, USA, 2003.
76. Peña, E.D. Lost in translation: Methodological considerations in cross-cultural research. *Child Dev.* **2007**, *78*, 1255–1264. [CrossRef]
77. IBM Corporation. *IBM SPSS Statistics for Windows*; IBM Corporation: Armonk, NY, USA, 2017.
78. Miot, H.A. Correlation analysis in clinical and experimental studies. *J. Vasc. Bras.* **2018**, *17*, 275–279. [CrossRef]
79. Arndt, S.; Turvey, C.; Andreasen, N.C. Correlating and predicting psychiatric symptom ratings: Spearman's v versus Kendall's tau correlation. *J. Psychiatr. Res.* **1999**, *33*, 97–104. [CrossRef]
80. Bonett, D.G.; Wright, T.A. Sample size requirements for estimating Pearson, Kendall and Spearman correlations. *Psychometrika* **2000**, *65*, 23–28. [CrossRef]
81. Kimberlin, C.L.; Winterstein, A.G. Validity and reliability of measurement instruments used in research. *Am. J. Health Syst. Pharm.* **2008**, *65*, 2276–2284. [CrossRef] [PubMed]
82. Marquis, S.; Hayes, M.V.; McGrail, K. Factors Affecting the Health of Caregivers of Children Who Have an Intellectual/Developmental Disability. *J. Policy Pract. Intellect. Disabil.* **2019**. [CrossRef]
83. McConnell, D.; Savage, A. Stress and Resilience among Families Caring for Children with Intellectual Disability: Expanding the Research Agenda. *Curr. Dev. Disord. Rep.* **2015**, *2*, 100–109. [CrossRef]
84. Imms, C.; Adair, B.; Keen, D.; Ullenhag, A.; Rosenbaum, P.; Granlund, M. "Participation": A systematic review of language, definitions, and constructs used in intervention research with children with disabilities. *Dev. Med. Child Neurol.* **2016**, *58*, 29–38. [CrossRef]
85. Hall, K.; Richter, L.; Mokomane, Z.; Lake, L. (Eds.) *Children, Families and the State Collaboration and Contestation*; Children's Institute, University of Cape Town: Cape Town, South Africa, 2018; ISBN 9780620819343.
86. Chhichhia, B. Gender rights in post-colonial societies: A comparative study of Kenya and India. *Afr. J. Polit. Sci. Int. Relat.* **2020**, *5*, 1–13. [CrossRef]
87. Mitra, A.; Rao, N. Gender, water, and nutrition in India: An intersectional perspective. *Water Altern.* **2019**, *12*, 169–191.

88. Spary, C. *Gender, Development, and the State in India*; Taylor & Francis (Routledge): New York, NY, USA, 2019; ISBN 9780415610605.
89. Saraswat, D. Gender Composition of Children and Sanitation Behavior in India. 2018. Available online: https://papers.ssrn.com/sol3/papers.cfm?abstract_id=3020233 (accessed on 13 August 2020).
90. Singh, A.; Patel, S.K. Gender differentials in feeding practices, health care utilization and nutritional status of children in Northern India. *Int. J. Hum. Rights Healthc.* **2017**, *10*, 323–331. [CrossRef]
91. Pillay, M.; Tiwari, R.; Kathard, H.; Chikte, U. Sustainable workforce: South African Audiologists and Speech Therapists. *Hum. Resour. Health* **2020**, *18*, 1–13. [CrossRef]

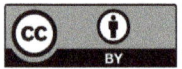

© 2020 by the authors. Licensee MDPI, Basel, Switzerland. This article is an open access article distributed under the terms and conditions of the Creative Commons Attribution (CC BY) license (http://creativecommons.org/licenses/by/4.0/).

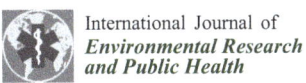

Article

Participation Restrictions among Children and Young Adults with Acquired Brain Injury in a Pediatric Outpatient Rehabilitation Cohort: The Patients' and Parents' Perspective

Florian Allonsius [1,*], Arend de Kloet [1], Gary Bedell [2], Frederike van Markus-Doornbosch [1], Stefanie Rosema [3], Jorit Meesters [1,4,5], Thea Vliet Vlieland [1,4] and Menno van der Holst [1,4,*]

[1] Basalt Rehabilitation Center, Department of Innovation, Quality and Research, 2543 SW The Hague, The Netherlands; A.deKloet@basaltrevalidatie.nl (A.d.K.); F.vanMarkus@basaltrevalidatie.nl (F.v.M.-D.); J.Meesters@basaltrevalidatie.nl (J.M.); t.p.m.vliet_vlieland@lumc.nl (T.V.V.)
[2] Department of Occupational Therapy, Tufts University, Medford, MA 02155, USA; gary.bedell@tufts.edu
[3] National Department Level, Specialists in Youth and Families, 1105 AZ Amsterdam, The Netherlands; stefanie.rosema@gmail.com
[4] Department of Orthopaedics, Rehabilitation and Physical Therapy, Leiden University Medical Center, 2333 ZA Leiden, The Netherlands
[5] Centre of Expertsie in Health Innovations, The Hague University of Applied Sciences, 2521 EN The Hague, The Netherlands
* Correspondence: f.allonsius@basaltrevalidatie.nl (F.A.); me.van.der.holst@basaltrevalidatie.nl (M.v.d.H.)

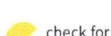

Abstract: Improving participation is an important aim in outpatient rehabilitation treatment. Knowledge regarding participation restrictions in children and young adults with acquired brain injury (ABI) is scarce and little is known regarding the differences in perspectives between patients and parents in the outpatient rehabilitation setting. The aims are to describe participation restrictions among children/young adults (5–24 years) with ABI and investigating differences between patients' and parents' perspectives. At admission in 10 rehabilitation centers, patients and parents were asked to complete the Child and Adolescent Scale of Participation (CASP; score 0–100; lower score = more restrictions) and injury/patient/family-related questions. CASP scores were categorized (full/somewhat-limited/limited/very-limited participation). Patient/parent-reported outcomes were compared using the Wilcoxon signed-rank test. 223 patients and 245 parents participated (209 paired-samples). Median patients' age was 14 years (IQR; 11–16), 135 were female (52%), 195 had traumatic brain injury (75%). The median CASP score reported by patients was 82.5 (IQR: 67.5–90) and by parents 91.3 (IQR: 80.0–97.5) (difference = $p < 0.05$). The score of 58 patients (26%) and 25 parents (10%) was classified as 'very-limited'. Twenty-six percent of children and young adults referred for rehabilitation after ABI had "very-limited" participation. Overall, parents rated their child's participation better than patients themselves. Quantifying participation restrictions after ABI and considering both perspectives is important for outpatient rehabilitation treatment.

Keywords: participation; rehabilitation; acquired brain injury; pediatric; patient-report; parent-report

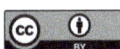

1. Introduction

Acquired brain injury (ABI) refers to irreversible damage to the brain which either has a traumatic cause; i.e., caused by external trauma (TBI) or a non-traumatic cause (nTBI); i.e., by internal causes [1]. It is a common diagnosis in children and young adults. The estimated yearly incidence rates in the Netherlands per 100,000 children and young adults are 288.9 (0–14 years) and 296.6 (15–24 years) for TBI and 108.8 (0–14 years) and 81.5 (15–24 years) for nTBI, respectively [2]. Due to natural brain adaptation, the majority of children and young adults with ABI will recover within the first year after brain injury [3]. However, on average, approximately 30% have persisting problems, and this group may benefit from rehabilitation treatment [1–5]. One of the ultimate goals of (outpatient) rehabilitation treatment is optimizing a patient's daily life participation [2,6–10]. However, despite its relevance, knowledge on participation restrictions of children and young adults with ABI referred for rehabilitation treatment is scarce. The currently available literature focuses on children (<14 years) with TBI in hospital-based cohorts [10–18].

Only a few studies focus on both patients' and parents' perspectives, and knowledge regarding outcomes on participation measuring both perspectives is even more scarce [9,12,14,19,20]. Moreover, for the pediatric rehabilitation-based population, and in the context of family-centered care, the question is whether the severity and nature of participation restrictions can best be rated by patients, parents or both, which is still an under-researched area [20–24].

Two relevant studies (a study in the United States (US) and a Dutch study) found strong internal structure validity and internal consistency between the patient and parent reported versions of the outcome measures i.e., the Child and Adolescent Scale of Participation (CASP) [9,20]. Yet, discrepancies between patients' and parents' perspectives were found, where parents reported lower scores than the patients [9,20]. However, the study conducted in the US only focused on youth aged 11–17 years and with chronic conditions/disabilities, and making comparison to patients with ABI difficult [20]. The Dutch study focused on patients with ABI a small age range (14–25 years), and used a relatively small sample size (n = 49) from only one rehabilitation center [9]. This rehabilitation-based study in which the primary focus was on fatigue outcomes, investigated participation as well and found multidirectional relationships between participation and fatigue as well as considerable participation restrictions among patients with ABI as measured with the CASP (median 82.5, IQR 68.8, 92.3) [9].

Other studies based on hospital-based cohorts, report that 25–80% of children and young adults with either TBI (mild/moderate/severe) or nTBI (i.e., stroke, tumor) experience participation restrictions after ABI [2,6,7,9,10,14,16,17,25–36]. This wide range is due to differences in definition of participation, outcome measures, inclusion criteria (i.e., age, type and severity, hospital based) and time points (i.e., time since onset of ABI) used in these studies [36]. In both children and young adults, participation restrictions after ABI tend to persist for a long time which negatively influences life development [37]. Negative consequences could affect the development of physical, psychological and social emotional skills and competencies, as well as the shaping of identity, health and wellbeing in adulthood [2,7,9,16,17,25,30–36,38–40].

Regarding the factors associated with participation restrictions, several studies found that more participation restrictions after pediatric ABI were associated with (among others), diminished health-related quality of life (HRQoL), and negative patient and environmental influences i.e., more patient's motor, cognitive, behavioral and emotional consequences [7,12,16,22,23,36,41,42]. To date, these influences were not investigated among children and young adults with ABI who were referred for outpatient rehabilitation treatment.

The present study aims to investigate among children and young adults with ABI (5–24 years with TBI or nTBI) who were referred for outpatient rehabilitation treatment (not having received any prior rehabilitation treatment):

1. the nature and severity) of participation restrictions;
2. differences regarding patients' and parents' perspectives on patients' participation restrictions;
3. the association between HRQoL and patient- and environmental factors on the one side and participation restrictions on the other side.

2. Materials and Methods

2.1. Design

Data from patients with ABI (and/or their parents) that were referred for outpatient rehabilitation treatment on the basis of continuing and/or expected problems, related to their brain injury were analyzed. These patients had not received any outpatient rehabilitation treatment yet. This study was part of a larger multi-center study on family impact, fatigue, participation and quality of life and associated factors in the Dutch ABI population (children and young adults). The study was started in 2015 in 10 Dutch rehabilitation centers, using a consensus-based set of patient/parent-reported outcome measures (PROMs) at admission as part of routine care. The reports of these PROMs were used for clinical goal setting in rehabilitation practice. The protocol for this study was reviewed by the medical ethics committee of the Leiden University Medical Center (P15.165), and an exempt from full medical ethical review was provided. For the current article the 'Strengthening the Reporting of Observational studies in Epidemiology' (STROBE) guidelines were used [43].

2.2. Patients

All children and young adults aged 5–24 years with a diagnosis of ABI, who were referred for outpatient rehabilitation treatment to a participating rehabilitation center and their parent(s) were eligible to participate. If patients and/or parents were unable/limited to write and/or understand the Dutch language, they were not invited by the center's health care professionals to complete the questionnaires. Patients over the age of 16 years had to give their parents' permission for completing the questionnaires according to the Dutch law of healthcare decision making.

2.3. Data Collection

Demographic and injury characteristics were extracted from the medical records by health professionals employed by the rehabilitation centers where patients had their appointment. For the outcomes related to participation, quality of life and child and environmental outcomes a (digital) questionnaire was administered to patients and/or their parents. Patients and parents were given the opportunity to complete this questionnaire prior to the first appointment during their visit at the outpatient rehabilitation clinic. If a patient (in case of a young adult) came without parents to the appointment, parents were asked to complete the questionnaires either on paper or digitally within one week after the first appointment. Unique links to the digital questionnaires were sent to the participants by e-mail by the medical health professionals working at the rehabilitation centers. Data were recoded, and thereafter anonymously stored in a central database at Basalt rehabilitation center in The Hague (The Netherlands). Finally, after analyzing the data, the centers received the results to use for clinical practice.

2.4. Assessments

2.4.1. Demographic and Injury Characteristics

Information regarding demographics and injury-related characteristics included: date of birth, date of injury, date of referral to rehabilitation, age at the start of the first appointment i.e., the difference between date of birth and date of referral to rehabilitation and gender i.e., male/female. Time between onset of ABI and referral to rehabilitation was calculated and thereafter divided into 2 groups: referred for rehabilitation within 6 months, and after 6 months after ABI onset. The categorization of ABI was divided in: TBI/nTBI. If known, the TBI severity levels were divided into either mild, or moderate/severe (based on the Glasgow Coma Scale at hospital admission [44]). NTBI causes were divided into stroke/cerebrovascular accidents, brain tumors, meningitis/encephalitis, hypoxia/intoxication, and other.

2.4.2. Participation Outcome Measure

The Child and Adolescent Scale of Participation (CASP) was administered to patients and parents to measure participation restrictions of the patient. The CASP is part of the "Child and Family Follow-up Survey" (CFFS) [45]. The CFFS, including CASP was validated for children, young adults and youth with ABI, was translated in the Dutch language, and is considered feasible and reliable tools to assess participation restrictions [2,17,20,25,45–48]. Patient-report (both children and young adults) and parent-report versions of the CASP were available and used both in the present study [17,20,47]. The CASP is a 20-item questionnaire, yielding a total score, and 4 domain scores including: home & community living activities; 5 items, home participation; 6 items, community participation; 4 items, and school/work participation; 5 items. Activities regarding participation are rated on a 4-point scale: 4 = age expected (full participation), 3 = somewhat limited, 2 = very limited, and 1 = unable. Items marked as" not applicable" do not receive a score. Scores for each item are summed and divided by the maximum possible score based on the number of items rated. The results, multiplied by 100, give a final score between 0–100, which counts for both the total score and the domain scores. The higher the scores, the closer a patient is participating to age-expected participation levels in daily life.

2.4.3. Four-Level Categorization

For the present study, a 4-level categorization system was developed to distinguish between levels of participation restrictions of patients for use in clinical practice. First, a draft version of a 4-level categorization was created by five of the authors based on preliminary analysis of the CASP data gathered for the present study and consensus discussions (F.A., A.d.K., M.H., G.B. and T.V.V.). We thereafter presented the categorization to a group of physicians and psychologists in the field, and to the remaining authors who are all experts in the field. Together, consensus was reached on the categorization and it was agreed to use it for further analyses in the present study. The 4-level categorization was made as follows:

- Category 1, CASP score 100–97.5: Full participation; participating in activities the same as or greater than peers, with or without assistive devices or equipment.
- Category 2, CASP score 97.5–81.0: Somewhat limited participation; participating in activities a bit less than peers. The patient may also need occasional supervision or assistance.
- Category 3, CASP score 81.0–68.5: Limited participation; participating in activities less than peers. The patient may also need supervision or assistance.
- Category 4, CASP score 68.5 or less: Very limited participation; participating in activities much less than peers, the patient may also need a lot of supervision or assistance.

2.4.4. Secondary Outcome Measures

When assessing participation restrictions, patient (i.e., children and young adults) factors, environmental factors as well as health related quality of life were described using the following outcome measures:

- Child/young adults' factors: The Child and Adolescent Factors Inventory (CAFI). The 15-item CAFI is a parent-report outcome measure consists of a list of problems or impairments related to the patients' health, cognitive, physical and psychological functioning. The CAFI is also part of the CFFS. Each item is rated on a 3-point scale: 1 = No problem; 2 = Little problem; 3 = Big problem. The final score is the sum of all item ratings divided by the maximum possible score of 54 (e.g., 36/54 = 0.67). This score then was multiplied by 100 to create an outcome on a 0–100-point scale. Higher scores indicate a greater extent of problems [45].
- Environmental factors: Child and Adolescent Scale of Environment (CASE): The 18-item CASE is a parent-reported outcome measure and is designed to assess the frequency and impact of environmental barriers experienced by children and young adults with disabilities. The CASE is also part of the CFFS. Similar to the CAFI, each item is rated on a 3-point scale: 1 = No problem; 2 = Little problem; 3 = Big problem and the final score is calculated in the same way. Again, higher scores indicate a greater extent of problems [45].
- Health-related Quality of Life (HRQoL): The 23-item Pediatric Quality of Life InventoryTM Generic Core Scales 4.0 (PedsQL™ GCS 4.0) is a patient-report and parent-report outcome measure and is used to determine the patients' HRQoL [49] It is available in a Dutch language version and is validated for different age ranges and diagnoses (also

for the for the pediatric TBI population) [50] It yields a total-score and 4 dimension-scores i.e., physical functioning (8 items), emotional functioning (5 items), social functioning (5 items), school/work functioning (5 items) [49] Items are answered on a Likert-scale (0 = never to 4 = almost always) and thereafter linearly transformed to a 0–100 scale (0 = 100, 1 = 75, 2 = 50, 3 = 25, 4 = 0). The results, items summed and divide by the number of items answered gives a final score between 0–100, with lower scores indicating diminished HRQoL [49,51].

2.5. Statistical Analysis

2.5.1. Characteristics

Patients' injury, demographic and family related characteristics were described using descriptive statistics. All continuous variables were expressed as medians with interquartile ranges (IQR) and means with standard deviations (SD), based on their distributions (Kolmogorov-Smirnoff (K-S) test). Characteristics were presented for the total group and for the group of children (5–17 years) and the group of young adults (18–24 years) separately. The age categorization for children and young adults is in line with the Committee on Improving the Health, Safety, and Well-Being of Young Adults (Washington DC, 2015) and previous Dutch studies in patients with ABI [50,52–54].

2.5.2. Primary/Secondary Outcome Measures

Regarding the primary (CASP) and secondary outcome measures (CAFI, CASE, PedsQL™ GCS-4.0), descriptive statistics were used to describe both the patient-report and the parent-report total scores of the CASP and the PedsQL™ GCS-4.0 and, if applicable, the domain scores. The CAFI and CASE were described similar as the CASP and the PedsQL™ GCS-4.0 but were only parent-report outcome measures. All outcomes were expressed as medians with IQRs (K-S test). To assess the potential correlation between the total scores of the CASP, PedsQL™ GCS 4.0 for HRQoL (patient/parent-report) and the CAFI/CASE (parent-report), Spearman correlations were calculated (Rho; ρ) and were considered: very strong, if >0.70; strong, if 0.40–0.69; moderate, if 0.30–0.39; weak, if 0.2–0.29; and negligible, if <0.19 [55].

2.5.3. Four-Level Group Categorization (CASP)

To interpret how limited the patients' participation restrictions were (patient-report and parent-report), the 4-level group categorization was used i.e., "full participation"/ "somewhat limited"/"limited"/"very limited" participation. The CASP median (IQR) total scores are presented for all 4 group category levels. Per group (1 to 4), patient characteristics i.e., age, gender, time between administration to rehabilitation and ABI onset (<6 months or ≥6 months between onset and referral), cause; TBI/nTBI; and severity levels TBI; mild/moderate-severe, were reported (using descriptive statistics). Finally, within-group median (IQR) total scores of the CAFI/CASE/PedsQL™ GCS-4.0 were reported.

2.5.4. Comparing Patients' and Parents' Perspectives

To compare outcomes, data from the patient-report and parent-report CASP versions, Wilcoxon signed-rank tests were used, for children and young adults separately. To test agreement between patients and parents additionally the Intraclass Correlation Coefficients (absolute agreement, single measures; ICC's) were calculated both for the CASP total and CASP domain scores. ICC scores were considered: poor, if <0.40; moderate, if 0.41–0.60; good, if 0.61–0.80; excellent, if >0.81 [56]. Regarding the results obtained by using the 4-level categorization system, Weighted kappa (K_w) with linear weights was used to assess agreement between patients' and parents' scores [57,58]. The Strength of agreement is considered: poor, if < 0.20; fair, if 0.21–0.40; moderate, if 0.41–0.60; good, if 0.61–0.80; very good, if 0.81–1.00 [57–59]. A Bonferroni correction was performed to account for multiple testing (the α-value divided by the number of analyses on the dependent variable did not exceed 0.05). Outcomes were described for the total group, for children (5–17 years), and for young adults (18–24 years) separately. Descriptive statistics were used to describe the CASP median (IQR) total scores, domain scores and categorization (counts, percentages). Differences/similarities in participation restriction categorization were described as follows: patients scoring in the same category as their parents, patients scoring themselves 1 to 3 categories lower than their parents, and patients scoring themselves 1 to 2 categories higher than their parents.

All analyses were performed using SPSS 24.0 for Windows (IBM, SPSS Statistics for Windows, Version 24.0. IBM Corp, Armonk, NY, USA). The level of significance was set at $p < 0.05$ for the Spearman Rho correlation, Wilcoxon signed rank and ICC tests.

3. Results

3.1. Characteristics

Patient, family and injury related characteristics are described in Table 1. The flow of all eligible participants for the current analyses can be found in Figure 1. The data of two-hundred-sixty patients, (217 children (83%) and 43 young adults (17%)) and/or their parents was analysed. In total, there were 223 patient- and 245 parent-reported questionnaires completed and there were 209 patient-parent pairs (see Table 1 and Figure 1). One hundred and ninety-five (75%) patients had TBI of which 151 were mild TBI (77%). One hundred and thirty-five patients were female (52%). Ninety-six patients (39%) were referred to the rehabilitation center more than six months after brain injury onset. The median age of the patients in the group of children (5–17 years) was 14 years (IQR 11–16), and 18 (IQR 18–19) in the ≥18-year-old age group.

Table 1. Patient, family and injury characteristics of children and young adults with acquired brain injury (ABI) referred to an outpatient rehabilitation center.

Patient Injury and Demographic Related Characteristics	Children 5–17 y, n = 217	Young Adults ≥18 y, n = 43	Total Cohort 5–24 y, n = 260
Gender: Female n (%)	112 (52%)	23 (54%)	135 (52%)
Age (years) at admission median (IQR)	14 (11–16)	18 (18–20)	14 (11–16)
Time (months) between ABI onset and referral to rehabilitation median (IQR)	4.0 (1–18)	4 (2–19)	4 (1–18)
>6 months n (%)	87 (40%)	17 (40%)	104 (40%)
Traumatic brain injury (TBI) n (%)	160 (74%)	35 (81%)	195 (75%)
Severity levels TBI * n (%)			
Mild	124 (78%)	27 (77%)	151 (77%)
Moderate-severe	15 (9%)	5 (14%)	20 (10%)
Unknown	21 (13%)	3 (9%)	24 (13%)
Non-traumatic brain injury (nTBI) n (%)	57 (26%)	8 (19%)	65 (25%)
Causes nTBI n (%)			
Tumor	25 (44%)	2 (25%)	27 (41%)
Stroke	11 (19%)	5 (63%)	16 (25%)
Encephalitis/meningitis	10 (17%)	1 (12%)	11 (17%)
Hypoxia/intoxication	2 (4%)	0 (0%)	2 (3%)
Other/unknown	9 (16%)	0 (0%)	9 (14%)
Family Related Characteristics	Children 5–17 y, n = 209	Young adults ≥18 y, n = 36	Total Cohort 5–24 y, n = 245
Living in a single-parent household n (%)	34 (16%)	8 (22%)	42 (17%)
Cultural background parents: non-Dutch n (%)	16 (8%)	2 (6%)	18 (7%)
Educational level parent** number (%)			
Low	7 (3%)	3 (8%)	10 (4%)
Intermediate	41 (20%)	6 17%)	47 (19%)
High	162 (77%)	27 (75%)	188 (77%)

* Based on Glasgow Coma Scale at hospital admission: "mild"—13–15, "moderate"—9–12, "severe" < 8 ** Educational level parent: low—prevocational practical education or less, intermediate—prevocational theoretical education and upper secondary vocational education, high—secondary education, higher education and/or university level education.

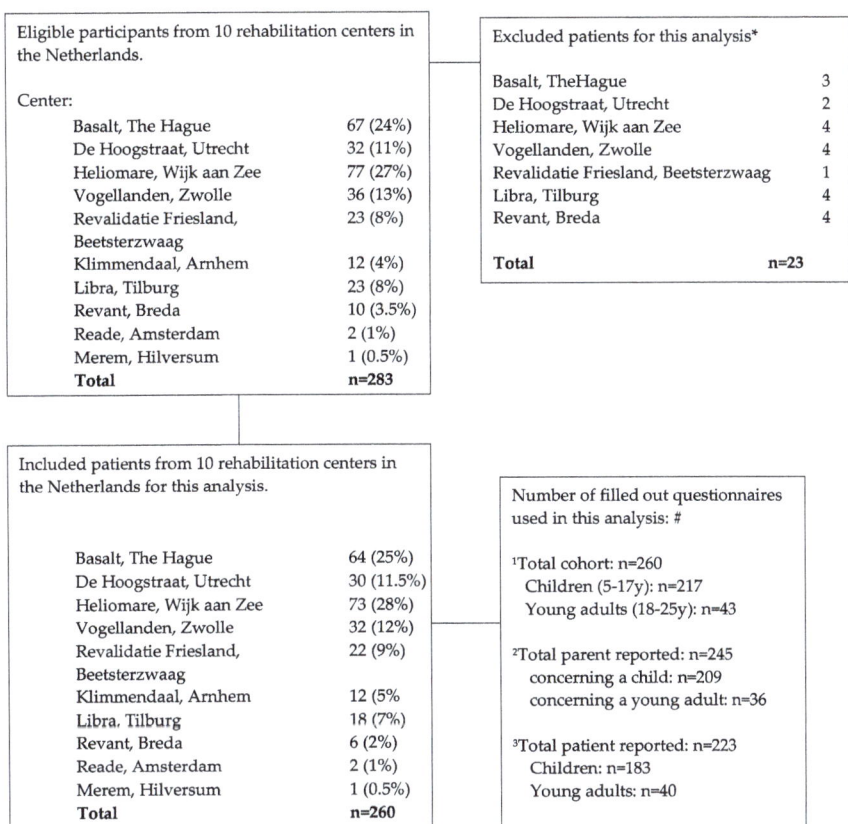

Figure 1. Flow of children and young adults with ABI admitted for rehabilitation and eligible for the present analysis. * Missing participants: $n = 11$ no official ABI diagnosis, $n = 12$ incomplete questionnaires. # Number of filled out questionnaires used in this analysis (total/patient-reported/parent-reported): [1]; number of questionnaires filled out by the patient, the parents or both in total and per age group (children, adolescents and young adults). [2]; number of questionnaires filled out by parents only in total and per age group (children, adolescents and young adults). [3]; number of questionnaires filled out by patients only (self-reported) in total and per age group (children, adolescents and young adults).

3.2. Participation Outcomes

Regarding participation outcomes in our population, as seen in Table 2, the median CASP total score reported by patients ($n = 223$) was 82.5 (IQR: 67.5–90.0), and by parents ($n = 245$) was 91.3 (IQR: 80.0–97.5). As seen in Table 2, Figure 2a,b, the lowest scores were found in the domain score "community participation" i.e., median patient-report score 75.0 (IQR: 56–92), median parent-report score 87.5 (IQR: 75–100). The highest median scores were found in the 'home participation' domain score for patients (87.5, IQR: 75–96), and in the "school/work participation" domain score for parents (95.0, IQR: 83–100).

Table 2. Total and domain scores on the CASP, CAFI, CASE and PedsQL™ GCS-4.0 (HRQoL) of children and young adults with acquired brain injury (ABI) and mutual correlations.

Outcome Measure	Domain Scores/Total Scores	Patient Report n = 223 Median (IQR)	Parent Report n = 245 Median (IQR)
CASP [1]	Total Score	82.5 (68–90)	91.3 (80–98)
	Home/community living activities	80.0 (63–90)	90.0 (75–100)
	Home participation	87.5 (75–96)	91.7 (83–100)
	Community participation	75.0 (56–92)	87.5 (75–100)
	School/work participation	85.0 (67–95)	95.0 (83–100)
PedsQL™ GCS-4.0 (HRQoL) [2]	Total score	65.2 (53–78)	60.9 (48–75)
	Physical health	68.8 (50–86)	68.8 (47–81)
	Emotional functioning	65.0 (45–85)	60.0 (40–75)
	Social functioning	80.0 (65–90)	75.0 (60–95)
	School/work functioning	50.0 (35–65)	50.0 (30–60)
CAFI [3]	Total Score	NA	56.9 (49–65)
CASE [3]	Total Score	NA	39.0 (33–51)
Correlations [$]		Patient Report n = 223 Rho	Parent Report n = 245 Rho
CASP total score	HRQoL total score	ρ 0.67 **	ρ 0.62 **
CASP total score	CAFI total score	NA	ρ 0.60 **
CASP total score	CASE total score	NA	ρ 0.53 **

[1] CASP: Child and Adolescent Scale of Participation, 0–100 with lower scores indicating more participation restrictions. [2] PedsQL™ Generic Core Scales 4.0 for Health-related quality of life (HRQoL): 0–100 with lower scores indicating lower HRQoL. [3] CAFI: Child and Adolescent Factors Inventory (CAFI), and CASE: Child and Adolescent Scale of Environment, 0–100 with higher scores indicating more problems. [$] ρ = Spearman's rho (ρ) correlation. ** $p < 0.001$.

Secondary outcome measures are also presented in Table 2. Regarding HRQoL, the median PedsQL™ GCS-4.0 patient-report total score was 65.2, (IQR: 53–78), and the median parent-report score was 60.9 (IQR: 48–75). The parent-report median scores in the CAFI (child/young adult factors) and CASE (environmental factors) were: 56.9 (IQR: 49–65) and 39.0 (IQR: 33–51), respectively. Spearman's rho correlations between the CASP scores and the CAFI/CASE and HRQoL were significant ($p < 0.01$) and strong ranging between: ρ 0.53–0.67.

3.3. Four-Level CASP Categorization

Table 3 shows within-group (patient/injury-related) characteristics, and CASP/CAFI/CASE/HRQoL scores of participation restrictions (patient-report and parent-report where applicable) in our cohort, organized by the 4-level CASP participation restrictions categorization. Eighty-nine percent of the patients, and 73% of the parents reported patients' participation restrictions in more than one CASP domain. Forty-three percent (patient-reported) and 45% (parent-reported) reported CASP total scores that fell in the "somewhat limited" category. Twenty six percent (patient-report) and 10% (parent-report) reported CASP total scores that fell in the "very limited" category. In this "very limited" category, median CASP scores were 57.9 (IQR: 50–64) for patient-report data, and 61.4 (IQR: 49–65) for parent-report data. Patients who fell in this 'very limited' category, had a median age of 15 years (both in the patient and parent-reported category), 45–52% were female, 64–78% had a TBI and 33–40% were referred for rehabilitation more than 6 months after ABI onset. Lower participation CASP scores, i.e., category levels up to category 4, also showed lower (diminished) patient and parent report HRQoL scores, and higher (more problems) parent report CAFI/CASE scores.

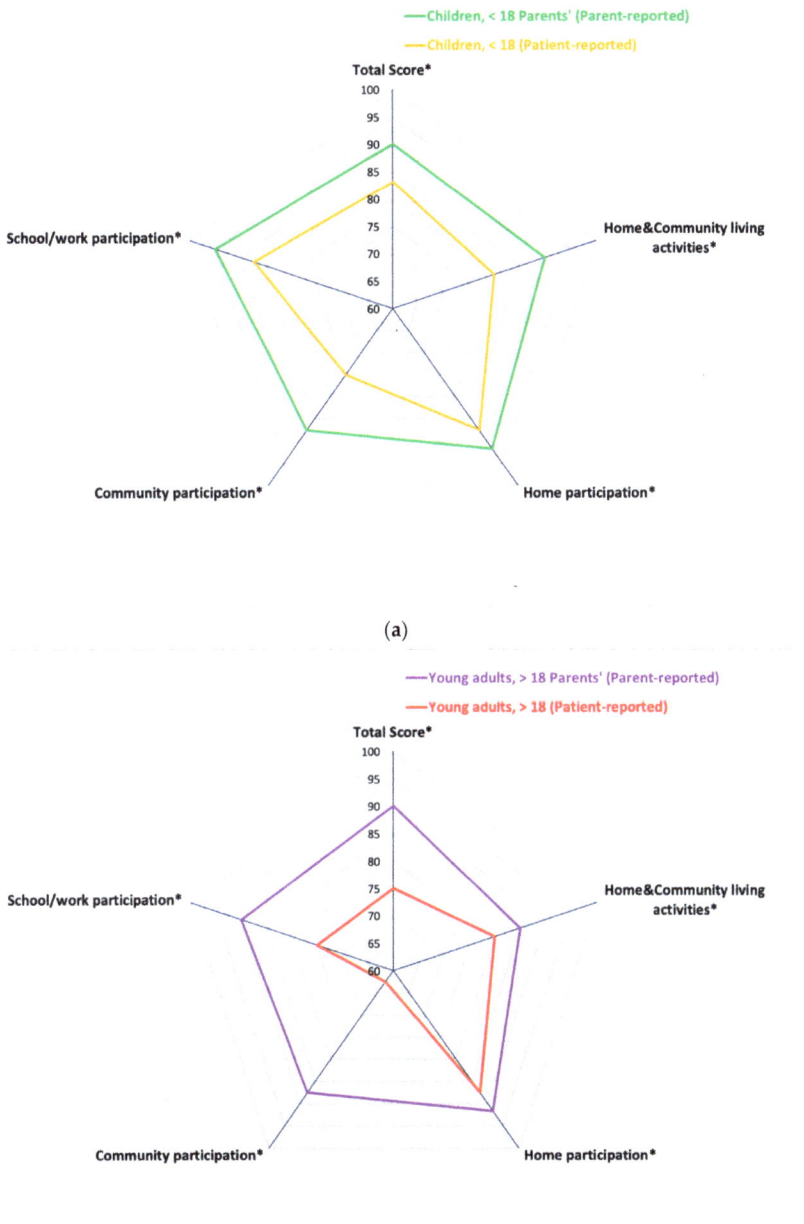

Figure 2. (a) Differences in CASP scores between Patients and Parents in children (5–17 years) with ABI. * CASP: Child and Adolescent Scale of Participation, 0–100 with lower scores indicating more participation restrictions. (b) Differences in CASP scores between Patients and Parents in young adults (18–24 years) with ABI. * CASP: Child and Adolescent Scale of Participation, 0–100 with lower scores indicating more participation restrictions.

Table 3. Within group characteristics of children and young adults with acquired brain injury (ABI) based on CASP participation restriction categorization.

Patient-Report (CASP) n = 223 (100%)

Category	n (%)	CASP # Totalscore Median (IQR)	Age: Median (IQR)	Gender Female: n (%)	$ Admin to Rehab ≥6 m: n (%)	Cause TBI: n (%)	Severity TBI Mild: n (%)	a HRQoL Median (IQR)
1 Full participation	25 (11%)	98.7 (98–99)	15 (12–16)	12 (48%)	13 (52%)	18 (72%)	14 (88%)	80.4 (75–86)
2 Somewhat limited participation	95 (43%)	86.8 (84–91)	14 (12–16)	50 (53%)	35 (37%)	72 (76%)	55 (86%)	75 (63–82)
3 Limited participation	45 (20%)	75 (71–78)	15 (11–17)	29 (64%)	15 (33%)	32 (71%)	24 (83%)	62 (52–68)
4 Very limited participation	58 (26%)	57.9 (50–64)	15 (13–16)	26 (45%)	15 (33%)	45 (78%)	39 (97%)	47.3 (38–58)

Parent-Report (CASP) n = 245 (100%)

Category	n (%)	CASP # Totalscore Median (IQR)	Age: Median (IQR)	Gender: Female: n (%)	$ Admin to Rehab ≥6 m n (%)	Cause: TBI	Severity TBI: Mild	a HRQoL Median (IQR)	b CAFI Median (IQR)	b CASE Median (IQR)
1 Full participation	67 (27%)	100 (98–100)	15 (11–16)	33 (49%)	24 (36%)	58 (87%)	45 (92%)	75 (63–83)	47.1 (43–57)	34.4 (33–36)
2 Somewhat limited participation	111 (45%)	91.3 (88–94)	13 (10–15)	59 (53%)	43 (39%)	79 (71%)	62 (86%)	64.1 (54–77)	56.9 (51–63)	39.8 (33–50)
3 Limited participation	42 (17%)	76.3 (73–80)	14 (10–16)	23 (55%)	19 (45%)	28 (67%)	24 (89%)	47.8 (41–55)	63.7 (55–71)	48.8 (43–62)
4 Very limited participation	25 (10%)	61.4 (49–65)	15 (12–17)	13 (52%)	10 (40%)	16 (64%)	12 (92%)	42.4 (35–48)	64.7 (59–74)	53.2 (41–67)

CASP: Child and Adolescent Scale of Participation, 0–100 with lower scores indicating more participation restrictions. Categories: [1] Full participation: Group 1, Between 97.5–100: Participating in activities the same as or more than other peers, [2] Somewhat limited participation: Group 2, Between 97.5–81: Participating in activities somewhat less than other peers, [3] Limited participation: Group 3: Between 81–68.5: Participating in activities less than other peers, [4] Very limited participation: Group 4, Below (<) 68.5: Participating in activities much less than other peers. [45] $ Time (months) between administration to rehabilitation and ABI onset (more than 6 months). a Patient and parent-report PedsQL™ Generic Core Scales 4.0 for health-related quality of life (HRQoL), 0–100 with lower scores indicating lower HRQoL. b Parent-report CAFI: Child and Adolescent Factors Inventory, and Parent-report CASE: Child and Adolescent Scale of Environment, 0–100 with higher scores indicating more problems.

3.4. Differences in Patients' and Parents' Perspectives

In Table 4, the differences in participation outcomes between patients and parents (paired samples) is reported. Regarding the total paired-sample group (n = 209), there was moderate agreement in participation total CASP and domain outcomes between patients and their parents i.e., ICC = 0.42–0.57, all $p < 0.001$. In the group of children (5–17 years, n = 176) moderate agreement was found between patients' and their parents' total CASP and domain scores (ICC = 0.43–0.55, all $p < 0.001$). In the young adult ($\geq$ 18 years, n = 33) group, there was poor-moderate patient/parent agreement between patient- and parent report scores on all CASP domains (ICC = 0.37–0.59, all $p < 0.001$). Regarding the categorical data on the 4-level categorization system, a fair to moderate agreement was found between the patients and parents; "moderate" in children; K_w: 0.42 (95%CI 0.32–0.52, $p < 0.001$), and "fair" in young adults; K_w: 0.27 (95%CI 0.08–0.46, $p < 0.05$). Regarding the differences in categorization between patients and their parents, in the total paired-sample group, 38% of the patients scored themselves in a lower CASP level category than their parents. In the group of children, the same percentage was found (38%), while in the young adult group 51% scored themselves in a lower category than their parents.

Table 4. Differences and similarities between patient and parent CASP participation scores and categories.

	Paired Samples Total Group (5–24 Years) n = 209			
CASP	Patient Report Median (IQR)	Parent Report Median (IQR)	Wilcoxon Z [#]	ICC [$]
Total Score	82.5 (68–90)	90.0 (80–97)	−8.2 **	0.54
Home/community living activities	80.0 (63–90)	90.0 (75–100)	−5.9 **	0.51
Home participation	87.5 (75–96)	91.7 (83–100)	−5.9 **	0.42
Community participation	75.0 (56–92)	87.5 (75–100)	−8.5 **	0.51
School/work participation	85.0 (66–90)	95.0 (80–100)	−6.2 **	0.57

CASP Categorization	Patient report Number (%)	Parent Report Number (%)	Patient/Parent Categorization ^	Number (%)
			Same as parents	110 (53%)
- Full	23 (11%)	51 (24%)	Different from parents	99 (47%)
- Somewhat limited	92 (44%)	98 (47%)	a: 1 category worse	54 (26%)
- Limited	41 (20%)	37 (18%)	b: 2 categories worse	15 (7%)
- Very limited	53 (25%)	23 (11%)	c: 3 categories worse	10 (5%)
	K_w: 0.40 (95%CI 0.31–0.49), $p < 0.001$		d: 1 category better	18 (9%)
			e: 2 categories better	2 (1%)

	Paired Samples Children (5–17 Years) n = 176			
CASP	Patient Report Median (IQR)	Parent Report Median (IQR)	Wilcoxon Z [#]	ICC [$]
Total Score	83.1 (69–90)	90.0 (80–97)	−7.4 **	0.54
Home/community living activities	80.0 (63–90)	90.0 (75–100)	−5.2 **	0.51
Home participation	87.5 (75–96)	91.7 (83–100)	−5.4 **	0.43
Community participation	75.0 (56–92)	87.5 (75–100)	−7.4 **	0.52
School/work participation	87.5 (70–96)	95.0 (82–100)	−5.6 **	0.55

CASP Categorization	Patient Report Number (%)	Parent Report Number (%)	Patient/Parent Categorization ^	Number (%)
			Same as parents	99 (53%)
- Full	20 (11%)	41 (23%)	Different from parents	77 (47%)
- Somewhat limited	83 (47%)	86 (49%)	a: 1 category worse	42 (24%)
- Limited	30 (17%)	31 (18%)	b: 2 categories worse	11 (6%)
- Very limited	43 (24%)	18 (10%)	c: 3 categories worse	8 (5%)
	K_w: 0.42 (95%CI 0.32–0.52), $p < 0.001$		d: 1 category better	14 (8%)
			e: 2 categories better	2 (1%)

Table 4. Cont.

CASP	Paired Samples Young Adults (18–24 Years) n = 33			
	Patient report Median (IQR)	Parent report Median (IQR)	Wilcoxon Z [#]	ICC [$]
Total Score	75.0 (65–86)	90.0 (78–99)	−3.6 **	0.56
Home/community living activities	80.0 (66–90)	85.0 (75–100)	−2.8 *	0.52
Home participation	87.5 (75–90)	91.7 (79–100)	−2.3 *	0.37
Community participation	62.5 (50–84)	87.5 (75–100)	−4.0 *	0.48
School/work participation	75.0 (55–90)	90.0 (74–100)	−2.8 *	0.59

CASP Categorization	Patient report Number (%)	Parent Report Number (%)	Patient/Parent Categorization [^]	Number (%)
- Full	3 (9%)	10 (30%)	Same as parents	12 (37%)
- Somewhat limited	9 (27%)	12 (36%)	Different from parents	21 (63%)
- Limited	11 (33%)	6 (18%)	a: 1 category worse	11 (33%)
- Very limited	10 (30%)	5 (15%)	b: 2 categories worse	4 (12%)
			c: 3 categories worse	2 (6%)
	K$_w$: 0.27 (0.08–0.46), $p < 0.05$		d: 1 category better	4 (12%)
			e: 2 categories better	0 (0%)

[1] CASP: Child and Adolescent Scale of Participation, 0–100 with lower scores indicating more participation restrictions. [#] Z scores for Wilcoxon signed-rank test for nonparametric data outcomes * $p < 0.05$, ** $p < 0.001$; [$] ICC; Intraclass Correlation Coefficients rated: <0.40: poor; 0.41–0.60: moderate; 0.61–0.80 good; >0.81: excellent. K$_w$: Weighted Kappa interpretation (categorical CASP score): <0.20: poor, 0.21–0.40: fair, 0.41–0.60: moderate, 0.61–0.80: good, 0.81–1.00: very good—agreement. [^] Patient categorization compared to parents' categorization: The differences in categorized participation between patients and their parents, a: Patients that scored 1 category worse than their parents, b: Patients that scored 2 categories lower than their parents, c: Patients that scored 3 categories lower than their parents, d: Patients that scored 1 category better than their parents, e: Patients that scored 2 categories better than their parents.

4. Discussion

According to data gathered before/on the first appointment for routine outpatient rehabilitation for children and young adults with ABI and their parents in multiple rehabilitation centers, 88% (patient-reported) and 73% (parent-reported) of the patients have participation restrictions that can be classified as "somewhat limited" to "very limited", with a considerable number of patients (25, parent reported and 58, patient reported) that can be classified as "very limited". The large majority was classified in the "somewhat limited" category. Overall, patients consistently reported more severe participation restrictions than parents. There was a greater discrepancy in the levels of participation restrictions between patients and parents in the young adult group compared to the children group.

4.1. Participation Restrictions

These results confirm that experiencing participation restrictions is common in pediatric patients with brain injuries (TBI/nTBI) [2,6,7,9,12,16,17,25,30–36,41]. Furthermore, the results we found, pointed out that the rehabilitation referred group had more participation restrictions compared to a Dutch hospital-based cohort [2]. In the current analyses of data among patients referred to an outpatient rehabilitation center, the vast majority reported participation restrictions in one or more domains of the CASP. This proportion was relatively high as compared to the 25–80% reported in a systematic review of studies on participation restrictions in children and youth with ABI including in hospital-based cohorts [7]. The current analyses found that the majority of patients was classified as "somewhat limited". These patients could also be "at risk" regarding restricted participation. In clinical practice it could also be important to monitor the patients that score relatively better than patients with more limited participation. However, future research must confirm this hypothesis by further looking into the "somewhat limited" patients. Concerning the prevalence of participation restrictions in young adults, some differences with the literature were found. A previous rehabilitation-based study, with patient and parent-reported data that focused on patients with ABI in the age group of 14–25, reported similar participation restrictions when compared to the results of the total sample from the current analyses [9]. However, more participation restrictions were found in the young adult group in the current analyses [9]. Differences could possibly be explained by differences in age inclusion. Results suggest that young adults experience more participation restrictions than children. This could be explained by the greater appeal made on for example independence, planning and coping in this transitional age group.

4.2. Community Participation

For both patient-report and parent-report CASP outcomes and in all (age) groups (<18 years/>18 years/total), the lowest scores were found in the domain 'community participation' which includes participation related to e.g., social play/leisure activities with friends, events, sports, doing groceries, communicating with others in the neighborhood. [45,47]. Restrictions in community participation could also be related to the fact that children and young adults with ABI often have difficulties in social functioning, emotional functioning, and processing sensory stimuli (after ABI onset). These competences are needed when participating in the community [7,37]. However, other factors (e.g., environmental resources, stigma, family support, as well as time allocation), may also influence community participation [14,42].

4.3. Correlations with the CASP and CAFI/CASE/HRQoL

In comparison to a previous Dutch study in a hospital cohort with a higher CASP total score, the mutual correlations of the CASP with the CAFI, and CASE (parent-report), were higher in this rehabilitation-based population [2]. Regarding HRQoL, in line with previous literature participation was found to be highly correlated with HRQoL (patient-report and parent-report) [9,16,35]. These results underline the interdependence of limitations on the level of participation (CASP), child/young adult factors e.g., body functions and structures (CAFI), environmental factors (CASE) and HRQoL (PedsQL GCS-4.0). These findings also support the assumption that the CASP, PedsQL GCS-4.0, CAFI and CASE are more suitable among patients that were administered to outpatient rehabilitation (and filled out the questionnaires at admission) than in patients that were in a hospital (hospital-based).

4.4. Notable Results Found in the Current Rehabilitation-Based Population

Notable results were found in the current analyses among the outpatient rehabilitation-based population, which were not found in previous studies [36,41].

- Firstly, the majority of children and young adults with a mild TBI reported scores in the "very limited" category. These results suggest that the TBI population experience participation restrictions no matter the initial TBI severity. Therefore, targeting and monitoring these restrictions for all TBI severities is relevant at admission to rehabilitation treatment.
- Secondly, late referral (over 6 months) to outpatient rehabilitation was common across all participation category groups based on the CASP total scores, in example; "somewhat limited participation category"–"very limited participation category". "One-third up to 45% of the patients in the different participation categories were referred for rehabilitation more than 6 months after ABI onset. This was also common among more than one-third of the patients in the "very limited" category. Several explanations can be given for a delay in referral. Medical specialists and general practitioners could potentially underestimate (long-term) problems/restrictions of patients or simply do not recognize them and/or they may not be familiar with pediatric ABI care pathways. Parents and patients do not know what signals or problems to be alert of, may tend to choose a "wait and see" approach before seeking help and/or are not familiar with ABI support pathways [5].

These findings should be discussed with professionals in acute care to increase awareness of possible consequences of later rehabilitation referral and to ultimately improve referral policies and procedures.

4.5. Differences in Perspectives

Regarding patients' and parents' perspectives, moderate agreement between patient and parent reported CASP (total and domain) scores were found. Previous studies underlined the importance of measuring both patients' and parents' perspectives to assess outcomes [20,36]. One Dutch study regarding adolescents and young adults with ABI found a difference between the patients and the parents CASP total score outcomes, similar to what we found in the results of the analyses [9]. Parents tend to report less participation restrictions for their children than the patients themselves, which is in contrast to previous studies with other outcomes (e.g., HRQoL; where parents usually report lower scores than their children) [9,16,17,25,30–33,35,40]. This was also found in our analyses. A large part of the patients in our cohort scored themselves in another CASP level category than their parents did. These discrepancies in reporting outcomes may be explained due to the fact that most participation activities (of the children and young adults) occur outside of the home environment where parents are not present and also, young adults spend more time away from parents than children. Our results suggest that assessing both patients' and parents' perspectives is important in order to identify differences and similarities. By using both perspectives, a broader view on overall functioning is attained, providing health care professionals the opportunity to consider both patients' and parents' perspectives when collaborating on rehabilitation goals, and make sure parents play an active role in today's often proposed family-centered care [14].

4.6. Categorization of Severity of Participation Restrictions

In the currently analyzed data, a 4-level categorization was created that correspond to specific CASP score ranges to reflect the overall degree of participation restriction. This categorization was based on previously identified levels of participation suggested by one of the authors (G.B.). To date, CASP outcomes were described as just a score between 0 and 100 (lower score = more participation restrictions). To facilitate a better interpretation of the score in clinical practice, we proposed a categorization of the total score into four levels. This 4-level categorization can be used next to the original 0–100 score) to compare and report CASP outcomes. The use of cut-off values may help to contextualize and differentiate the scores for clinical practice (i.e., indication for rehabilitation, evaluation of intervention) and research. All statistical comparisons of patients' and parents' scores in the present study consistently demonstrated a considerable discrepancy. Poor agreement was also seen using the proposed 4-level categorization, substantiating the validity of that division. Regarding the 4 categories, the majority of the patients and their parents reported CASP scores in the 'somewhat limited', the 'limited' and 'very limited' categories. A quarter of the children and almost one-third of the young adults scored in the most restricted, i.e., "very limited" category. Parent and patient-report scores differed in participation restriction category in almost half of the of cases, with parent scores and categories demonstrating lower levels of participation restriction as previously described. Future longitudinal studies could use this new categorization to further evaluate its utilization, and/or to investigate recovery outcomes over time (e.g., moving to higher category level of participation) during rehabilitation treatment related to interventions.

4.7. Limitations

Describing analyses and results among rehabilitation referred patients resulted in a number of limitations. First, there was a relatively small sample of young adults compared to the sample of children (43 vs. 217). The explanation is merely organizational: most rehabilitation centers have a separate pediatric (<16 or <18 years) and adult ($\geq$18 years) department where only the pediatric department was involved. Only two centers had a separate department for young adults (18–25 years) and included young adults. However, the number of included young adults was large enough to analyze and report outcomes for separately. Since, due to age and life phase, in the young adult group is a different group of patients it is recommended to include this group of patients in transition fully in future pediatric studies. Secondly, not for all patients paired sample data was available, making the analysis for the differences/similarities between patients' and parents' perspectives only possible for a portion of our analyses (*n* = 209). However, since we had paired sample data available for the majority of patients, we believe that outcomes are generalizable. Third, the CASP is known to have a ceiling effect [17,47] Nonetheless, in contrast to other studies reporting ceiling effects in children and young adults with ABI, these were less evident in the present analyses making the CASP a more suitable instrument for use in rehabilitation cohorts (versus patients that are hospitalized) of patients with ABI [2,17,20,47]. Furthermore, an alternative instrument that also focusses on the ABI population is lacking [17]. Finally, results of patient/parent rated outcome measures could be biased, i.e., by limitations in motivation or patients' and/or parents' moment bound 'stress and mood'.

4.8. Directions for Future Research

Interesting follow up projects could be longitudinal studies monitoring participation over time and evaluative studies using the CASP to explore the effect of rehabilitation programs for children and young adults with ABI and their families, since optimizing participation is an important rehabilitation goal. In these studies, the newly developed categorization of participation outcomes could be used and further investigated on its usefulness and robustness. Future studies should include the search for the best available participation outcome measures particularly given the number of promising participation-focused, multi-setting interventions that recently have been developed to improve participation outcomes for individual children, youth, and families [21–24]. The next challenge is to drive implementation of participation-based interventions on a larger scale, and research should be focused on enabling strategies and on cost-effectiveness of these interventions. The CASP and our newly proposed categorization of participation restrictions could support this process.

5. Conclusions

A substantial portion of patients (ages 5–24 years) with acquired brain injury referred to an outpatient rehabilitation center in The Netherlands had "limited" to "very-limited" participation. Patients reported greater participation restrictions than their parents and disparities between patient reported and parent reported participation restrictions were greater in young adults than in children. Furthermore, a strong correlation was found between patient and environmental factors (CAFI and CASE), HRQoL (PedsQL GCS-4.0), and participation (CASP). Most restrictions were found in the 'community participation' domain. A large part of the patients with a late referral (>6 months) to rehabilitation after ABI onset reported "very limited" participation. Early referral is important as this may reduce participation restrictions. Taking into account both patients' as well as parents' perspectives is important in outpatient rehabilitation treatment in order to guide both patients and their parents appropriately during treatment. Furthermore, the categorization of CASP scores into 4 categories might be useful for clinical practice and research, but more study is needed to understand how this can be applied and inform participation focused clinical and practical decisions.

Author Contributions: All authors listed have contributed sufficiently to the project to be included as authors, and all those who are qualified to be authors are listed in the author byline. The authors that contributed in this research were: F.A., A.d.K., G.B., F.v.M.-D., S.R., J.M., T.V.V., M.v.d.H. and were responsible for: Conceptualization, F.A., A.d.K. and M.v.d.H.; methodology, F.A., M.v.d.H.; software, F.A., M.v.d.H.; validation, F.A., G.B., A.d.K., M.v.d.H.; formal analysis, F.A., M.v.d.H.; investigation, F.A., M.v.d.H., A.d.K.; resources, A.d.K.; data curation, F.A., A.d.K., M.v.d.H.; writing—original draft preparation, F.A.; writing—review and editing, A.d.K., G.B., F.v.M.-D., J.M., T.V.V., S.R., M.v.d.H.; visualization, F.A., M.v.d.H.; supervision, T.V.V., A.d.K., M.v.d.H.; project administration, A.d.K., T.V.V.; funding acquisition, A.d.K. All authors have read and agreed to the published version of the manuscript.

Funding: This research was funded by Hersenstichting (PZ2015.01.10) and the Revalidatiefonds (R2014.124).

Institutional Review Board Statement: The protocol for this study was reviewed by the medical ethics committee of the Leiden University Medical Center (P15.165), and an exempt from full medical ethical review was provided.

Data Availability Statement: Data used in this study is stored in a central database at Basalt Rehabilitation center, The Hague in the office of innovation, quality and research and can be available when requested.

Acknowledgments: We would like to thank all the patients and their families participating in this study. Further we would like to thank Cedric Kromme, and Åsa Mennema for contributing to this study by collecting and processing the data into the central database. Finally, we would like to thank all clinical health care professionals and medical secretaries of the participating rehabilitation centers contributing in this study i.e., Basalt in the Hague, De Hoogstraat in Utrecht, Heliomare in Wijk aan Zee, Vogellanden in Zwolle, Klimmendaal in Apeldoorn, Revalidatie Friesland in Beesterswaag, Libra Rehabilitation&Audiology in Tilburg, Revant Breda, Merem in Hilversum and Reade in Amsterdam.

Conflicts of Interest: The authors declare no conflict of interest.

References

1. Greenwald, B.D.; Burnett, D.M.; Miller, M.A. Congenital and acquired brain injury. 1. Brain injury: Epidemiology and pathophysiology. *Arch. Phys. Med. Rehabil.* **2003**, *84*, S3–S7. [CrossRef] [PubMed]
2. De Kloet, A.J.; Hilberink, S.R.; Roebroeck, M.E.; Catsman-Berrevoets, C.E.; Peeters, E.; Lambregts, S.A.; van Markus-Doornbosch, F.; Vlieland, T.P.M.V. Youth with acquired brain injury in The Netherlands: A multi-centre study. *Brain Inj.* **2013**, *27*, 843–849. [CrossRef]
3. Barlow, K.M.; Crawford, S.; Stevenson, A.; Sandhu, S.S.; Belanger, F.; Dewey, D. Epidemiology of postconcussion syndrome in pediatric mild traumatic brain injury. *Pediatrics* **2010**, *126*, e374–e381. [CrossRef]
4. Micklewright, J.L.; King, T.Z.; O'Toole, K.; Henrich, C.; Floyd, F.J. Parental distress, parenting practices, and child adaptive outcomes following traumatic brain injury. *J. Int. Neuropsychol. Soc.* **2012**, *18*, 343–350. [CrossRef] [PubMed]
5. Feary, N.; McKinlay, A. Impact of mild traumatic brain injury understanding on intended help-seeking behaviour. *J. Child Health Care* **2020**, *24*, 78–91. [CrossRef]
6. Ezekiel, L.; Collett, J.; Mayo, N.E.; Pang, L.; Field, L.; Dawes, H. Factors Associated With Participation in Life Situations for Adults With Stroke: A Systematic Review. *Arch. Phys. Med. Rehabil.* **2019**, *100*, 945–955. [CrossRef]
7. De Kloet, A.J.; Gijzen, R.; Braga, L.W.; Meesters, J.J.L.; Schoones, J.W.; Vliet Vlieland, T.P.M. Determinants of participation of youth with acquired brain injury: A systematic review. *Brain Inj.* **2015**, *29*, 1135–1145. [CrossRef] [PubMed]
8. Ilmer, E.C.; Lambregts, S.A.; Berger, M.A.; de Kloet, A.J.; Hilberink, S.R.; Roebroeck, M.E. Health-related quality of life in children and youth with acquired brain injury: Two years after injury. *Eur. J. Paediatr Neurol.* **2016**, *20*, 131–139. [CrossRef] [PubMed]
9. Van Markus-Doornbosch, F.; van der Holst, M.; de Kloet, A.J.; Vliet Vlieland, T.P.M.; Meesters, J.J.L. Fatigue, Participation and Quality of Life in Adolescents and Young Adults with Acquired Brain Injury in an Outpatient Rehabilitation Cohort. *Dev. Neurorehabil.* **2019**, *23*, 328–335. [CrossRef]
10. Imms, C.; Adair, B.; Keen, D.; Ullenhag, A.; Rosenbaum, P.; Granlund, M. 'Participation': A systematic review of language, definitions, and constructs used in intervention research with children with disabilities. *Dev. Med. Child Neurol.* **2016**, *58*, 29–38. [CrossRef]
11. Galvin, J.; Froude, E.H.; McAleer, J. Children's participation in home, school and community life after acquired brain injury. *Aust. Occup. Ther. J.* **2010**, *57*, 118–126. [CrossRef]
12. Van Tol, E.; Gorter, J.W.; DeMatteo, C.; Meester-Delver, A. Participation outcomes for children with acquired brain injury: A narrative review. *Brain Inj.* **2011**, *25*, 1279–1287. [CrossRef] [PubMed]
13. Law, M.; Anaby, D.; DeMatteo, C.; Hanna, S. Participation patterns of children with acquired brain injury. *Brain Inj.* **2011**, *25*, 587–595. [CrossRef] [PubMed]
14. Bedell, G.; Coster, W.; Law, M.; Liljenquist, K.; Kao, Y.C.; Teplicky, R.; Anaby, D.; Khetani, M.A. Community participation, supports, and barriers of school-age children with and without disabilities. *Arch. Phys. Med. Rehabil.* **2013**, *94*, 315–323. [CrossRef]
15. Renaud, M.I.; Lambregts, S.A.; de Kloet, A.J.; Catsman-Berrevoets, C.E.; van de Port, I.G.; van Heugten, C.M. Activities and participation of children and adolescents after mild traumatic brain injury and the effectiveness of an early intervention (Brains Ahead!): Study protocol for a cohort study with a nested randomised controlled trial. *Trials* **2016**, *17*, 236. [CrossRef] [PubMed]
16. Lambregts, S.A.M.; Smetsers, J.E.M.; Verhoeven, I.; de Kloet, A.J.; van de Port, I.G.L.; Ribbers, G.M.; Catsman-Berrevoets, C. Cognitive function and participation in children and youth with mild traumatic brain injury two years after injury. *Brain Inj.* **2018**, *32*, 230–241. [CrossRef]

17. Resch, C.; Van Kruijsbergen, M.; Ketelaar, M.; Hurks, P.; Adair, B.; Imms, C.; De Kloet, A.; Piskur, B.; Van Heugten, C.M. Assessing participation of children with acquired brain injury and cerebral palsy: A systematic review of measurement properties. *Dev. Med. Child Neurol.* **2020**, *62*, 434–444. [CrossRef] [PubMed]
18. Keetley, R.; Westwater-Wood, S.; Manning, J.C. Exploring participation after paediatric acquired brain injury. *J. Child Health Care* **2020**. [CrossRef]
19. Catroppa, C.; Crossley, L.; Hearps, S.J.; Yeates, K.O.; Beauchamp, M.; Rogers, K.; Andetrson, V. Social and behavioral outcomes: Pre-injury to six months following childhood traumatic brain injury. *J. Neurotrauma* **2015**, *32*, 109–115. [CrossRef]
20. McDougall, J.; Bedell, G.; Wright, V. The youth report version of the Child and Adolescent Scale of Participation (CASP): Assessment of psychometric properties and comparison with parent report. *Child Care Health Dev.* **2013**, *39*, 512–522. [CrossRef]
21. Moore, M.; Robinson, G.; Mink, R.; Hudson, K.; Dotolo, D.; Gooding, T.; Ramirez, A.; Zatzick, D.; Giordano, J.; Crawley, D.; et al. Developing a Family-Centered Care Model for Critical Care After Pediatric Traumatic Brain Injury. *Pediatr. Crit. Care Med.* **2015**, *16*, 758–765. [CrossRef]
22. Imms, C.; Mathews, S.; Richmond, K.N.; Law, M.; Ullenhag, A. Optimising leisure participation: A pilot intervention study for adolescents with physical impairments. *Disabil. Rehabil.* **2016**, *38*, 963–971. [CrossRef]
23. Anaby, D.; Pozniak, K. Participation-based intervention in childhood disability: A family-centred approach. *Dev. Med. Child Neurol.* **2019**, *61*, 502. [CrossRef]
24. Karpa, J.; Chernomas, W.; Roger, K.; Heinonen, T. Families' Experiences Living with Acquired Brain Injury: "Thinking Family"-A Nursing Pathway for Family-Centered Care. *Nurs. Res. Pract.* **2020**, *2020*, 8866534. [CrossRef]
25. Renaud, M.I.; Lambregts, S.A.M.; van de Port, I.G.L.; Catsman-Berrevoets, C.E.; van Heugten, C.M. Predictors of activities and participation six months after mild traumatic brain injury in children and adolescents. *Eur. J. Paediatr. Neurol.* **2020**, *25*, 145–156. [CrossRef]
26. Kersey, J.; McCue, M.; Skidmore, E. Domains and dimensions of community participation following traumatic brain injury. *Brain Inj.* **2020**, *34*, 708–712. [CrossRef] [PubMed]
27. Erler, K.S.; Whiteneck, G.G.; Juengst, S.B.; Locascio, J.J.; Bogner, J.A.; Kaminski, J.; Giacino, J.T. Predicting the Trajectory of Participation After Traumatic Brain Injury: A Longitudinal Analysis. *J. Head Trauma Rehabil.* **2018**, *33*, 257–265. [CrossRef]
28. Vos, L.; Poritz, J.M.P.; Ngan, E.; Leon-Novelo, L.; Sherer, M. The relationship between resilience, emotional distress, and community participation outcomes following traumatic brain injury. *Brain Inj.* **2019**, *33*, 1615–1623. [CrossRef] [PubMed]
29. Wrightson, J.G.; Zewdie, E.; Kuo, H.C.; Millet, G.Y.; Kirton, A. Fatigue in children with perinatal stroke: Clinical and neurophysiological associations. *Dev. Med. Child Neurol.* **2020**, *62*, 234–240. [CrossRef] [PubMed]
30. Di Battista, A.; Soo, C.; Catroppa, C.; Anderson, V. Quality of life in children and adolescents post-TBI: A systematic review and meta-analysis. *J. Neurotrauma* **2012**, *29*, 1717–1727. [CrossRef] [PubMed]
31. Anderson, V.; Brown, S.; Newitt, H.; Hoile, H. Educational, vocational, psychosocial, and quality-of-life outcomes for adult survivors of childhood traumatic brain injury. *J. Head Trauma Rehabil.* **2009**, *24*, 303–312. [CrossRef] [PubMed]
32. Green, L.; Godfrey, C.; Soo, C.; Anderson, V.; Catroppa, C. A preliminary investigation into psychosocial outcome and quality-of-life in adolescents following childhood traumatic brain injury. *Brain Inj.* **2013**, *27*, 872–877. [CrossRef]
33. Neuner, B.; von Mackensen, S.; Krumpel, A.; Manner, D.; Friefeld, S.; Nixdorf, S.; Frühwald, M.; DeVeber, G.; Nowak-Göttl, U. Health-related quality of life in children and adolescents with stroke, self-reports, and parent/proxies reports: Cross-sectional investigation. *Ann. Neurol.* **2011**, *70*, 70–78. [CrossRef] [PubMed]
34. Kristiansen, I.; Strinnholm, M.; Stromberg, B.; Frisk, P. Clinical characteristics, long-term complications and health-related quality of life (HRQoL) in children and young adults treated for low-grade astrocytoma in the posterior fossa in childhood. *J. Neurooncol.* **2019**, *142*, 203–210. [CrossRef]
35. Boosman, H.; Winkens, I.; van Heugten, C.M.; Rasquin, S.M.; Heijnen, V.A.; Visser-Meily, J.M. Predictors of health-related quality of life and participation after brain injury rehabilitation: The role of neuropsychological factors. *Neuropsychol. Rehabil.* **2017**, *27*, 581–598. [CrossRef] [PubMed]
36. Anaby, D.; Law, M.; Hanna, S.; Dematteo, C. Predictors of change in participation rates following acquired brain injury: Results of a longitudinal study. *Dev. Med. Child Neurol.* **2012**, *54*, 339–346. [CrossRef] [PubMed]
37. Camara-Costa, H.; Francillette, L.; Opatowski, M.; Toure, H.; Brugel, D.; Laurent-Vannier, A.; Meyer, P.; Dellatolas, G.; Watier, L.; Chevignard, M. Participation seven years after severe childhood traumatic brain injury. *Disabil. Rehabil.* **2019**, *42*, 2402–2411. [CrossRef] [PubMed]
38. Huebner, R.A.; Johnson, K.; Bennett, C.M.; Schneck, C. Community participation and quality of life outcomes after adult traumatic brain injury. *Am. J. Occup. Ther.* **2003**, *57*, 177–185. [CrossRef]
39. McLean, A.M.; Jarus, T.; Hubley, A.M.; Jongbloed, L. Associations between social participation and subjective quality of life for adults with moderate to severe traumatic brain injury. *Disabil. Rehabil.* **2014**, *36*, 1409–1418. [CrossRef]
40. Petersen, C.; Scherwath, A.; Fink, J.; Koch, U. Health-related quality of life and psychosocial consequences after mild traumatic brain injury in children and adolescents. *Brain Inj.* **2008**, *22*, 215–221. [CrossRef]
41. Iverson, G.L.; Gardner, A.J.; Terry, D.P.; Ponsford, J.L.; Sills, A.K.; Broshek, D.K.; Solomon, G.S. Predictors of clinical recovery from concussion: A systematic review. *Br. J. Sports Med.* **2017**, *51*, 941–948. [CrossRef]
42. Van Baalen, B.; Ribbers, G.M.; Medema-Meulepas, D.; Pas, M.S.; Odding, E.; Stam, H.J. Being restricted in participation after a traumatic brain injury is negatively associated by passive coping style of the caregiver. *Brain Inj.* **2007**, *21*, 925–931. [CrossRef]

43. Cuschieri, S. The STROBE guidelines. *Saudi J. Anaesth.* **2019**, *13*, S31–S34. [CrossRef]
44. Jain, S.; Iverson, L.M. *Glasgow Coma Scale*; StatPearls: Treasure Island, FL, USA, 2020.
45. Bedell, G.M. Developing a follow-up survey focused on participation of children and youth with acquired brain injuries after discharge from inpatient rehabilitation. *NeuroRehabilitation* **2004**, *19*, 191–205. [CrossRef] [PubMed]
46. Golos, A.; Bedell, G. Responsiveness and discriminant validity of the Child and Adolescent Scale of Participation across three years for children and youth with traumatic brain injury. *Dev. Neurorehabil.* **2018**, *21*, 431–438. [CrossRef]
47. Bedell, G. Further validation of the Child and Adolescent Scale of Participation (CASP). *Dev. Neurorehabil.* **2009**, *12*, 342–351. [CrossRef] [PubMed]
48. De Bock, F.; Bosle, C.; Graef, C.; Oepen, J.; Philippi, H.; Urschitz, M.S. Measuring social participation in children with chronic health conditions: Validation and reference values of the child and adolescent scale of participation (CASP) in the German context. *BMC Pediatr.* **2019**, *19*, 125. [CrossRef]
49. Varni, J.W.; Limbers, C.A.; Burwinkle, T.M. Parent proxy-report of their children's health-related quality of life: An analysis of 13,878 parents' reliability and validity across age subgroups using the PedsQL 4.0 Generic Core Scales. *Health Qual. Life Outcomes* **2007**, *5*, 2. [CrossRef]
50. Limperg, P.F.; Haverman, L.; van Oers, H.A.; van Rossum, M.A.; Maurice-Stam, H.; Grootenhuis, M.A. Health related quality of life in Dutch young adults: Psychometric properties of the PedsQL generic core scales young adult version. *Health Qual. Life Outcomes* **2014**, *12*, 9. [CrossRef] [PubMed]
51. McCarthy, M.L.; MacKenzie, E.J.; Durbin, D.R.; Aitken, M.E.; Jaffe, K.M.; Paidas, C.N.; Slomine, B.S.; Dorsch, A.M.; Berk, R.A.; Christensen, J.R.; et al. The Pediatric Quality of Life Inventory: An evaluation of its reliability and validity for children with traumatic brain injury. *Arch. Phys. Med. Rehabil.* **2005**, *86*, 1901–1909. [CrossRef]
52. Haverman, L.; Limperg, P.F.; van Oers, H.A.; van Rossum, M.A.; Maurice-Stam, H.; Grootenhuis, M.A. Psychometric properties and Dutch norm data of the PedsQL Multidimensional Fatigue Scale for Young Adults. *Qual. Life Res.* **2014**, *23*, 2841–2847. [CrossRef]
53. Gordijn, M.; Cremers, E.M.; Kaspers, G.J.; Gemke, R.J. Fatigue in children: Reliability and validity of the Dutch PedsQL Multidimensional Fatigue Scale. *Qual. Life Res.* **2011**, *20*, 1103–1108. [CrossRef] [PubMed]
54. Engelen, V.; Haentjens, M.M.; Detmar, S.B.; Koopman, H.M.; Grootenhuis, M.A. Health related quality of life of Dutch children: Psychometric properties of the PedsQL in the Netherlands. *BMC Pediatr.* **2009**, *9*, 68. [CrossRef]
55. Mutch, C.; Tisak, J. Measurement error and the correlation between positive and negative affect: Spearman (1904, 1907) revisited. *Psychol. Rep.* **2005**, *96*, 43–46. [CrossRef]
56. Bartko, J.J. The intraclass correlation coefficient as a measure of reliability. *Psychol. Rep.* **1966**, *19*, 3–11. [CrossRef] [PubMed]
57. Cohen, J. Weighted kappa: Nominal scale agreement with provision for scaled disagreement or partial credit. *Psychol. Bull.* **1968**, *70*, 213–220. [CrossRef] [PubMed]
58. Fleiss, J.L.; Levin, B.; Paik, M.C. *Statistical Methods for Rates and Proportions*, 3rd ed.; John & Wiley & Sons, Inc.: Hoboken, NJ, USA, 2003.
59. Altman, D.G. *Practical Statistics for Medical Research*; Chapman & Hall/CRC Press: New York, NY, USA, 1999.

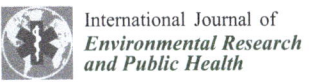

Article

Participation Profile of Children and Youth, Aged 6–14, with and without ADHD, and the Impact of Environmental Factors

Tair Shabat [1], Haya Fogel-Grinvald [1], Dana Anaby [2] and Anat Golos [1,*]

1 School of Occupational Therapy, Faculty of Medicine, Hebrew University, Jerusalem 91240, Israel; tair.shitiat@mail.huji.ac.il (T.S.); hayagrin@gmail.com (H.F.-G.)
2 School of Physical and Occupational Therapy, McGill University, Montreal, QC H3G 1Y5, Canada; dana.anaby@mcgill.ca
* Correspondence: anat.golos@mail.huji.ac.il; Tel.: +972-50-4935636

Abstract: Background: Children and youth with attention deficit hyperactivity disorder (ADHD) may experience difficulties in participation, but few studies examine their participation and the environmental factors affecting participation. This study explored the participation and the environmental factors of children and youth, with and without attention deficit hyperactivity disorder (ADHD), in the following three settings: home, school, and community. Materials and Methods: Parents of 65 participants aged 6–14 (M = 9.91, SD = 1.87) with and without ADHD completed the Participation and Environment Measure for Children and Youth (PEM-CY) questionnaire, which evaluates participation and environmental factors, along with demographic and screening questionnaires. Results: The ADHD group ($n = 31$) scored significantly lower than the non-ADHD group ($n = 34$) in "frequency" at home, "involvement", and overall environmental support in all settings, with parents expressing a greater desire to change their child's home and community participation. For the ADHD group, a relationship was found between environmental support and involvement in all three settings. Conclusions: The findings demonstrated differences in the participation of children and youth with ADHD across different settings, compared to those without ADHD, and confirmed the effect of environmental factors on participation, especially involvement. It is essential to consider participation measures and environmental factors when designing interventions for children and youth with ADHD.

Keywords: children and youth; ADHD; participation; frequency; involvement; environment; well-being

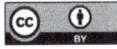

1. Introduction

The International Classification of Functioning, Disability and Health (ICF) of the World Health Organization (WHO) defines participation as "involvement in a life situation" [1], which is considered an important outcome measure for rehabilitation and intervention [1,2], as well as the focus and goal of many health and rehabilitation disciplines [3]. Participation in meaningful activities has a positive influence on health and well-being and is essential for the development of a person's abilities and self-efficacy [4,5], as well as for skill acquisition and learning among children and youth [6]. Participation is a multidimensional concept that includes various dimensions such as frequency and involvement. Participation frequency is considered as an objective aspect, referring, for example, to the number of times a person participates in an activity [7], while involvement refers to the feelings and personal experience of participation and includes various elements such as motivation, adherence, satisfaction, and emotional engagement [7–10].

The participation of children and youth with different health conditions (such as attention deficit hyperactivity disorder (ADHD) and autism spectrum disorder (ASD) and/or disabilities was found to be limited, compared to that of children with typical development [11–13]. For example, it was found that children with disabilities participate less frequently and/or are less involved in activities in the home, school, and community settings, compared to their peers with typical development [14–16].

One of the health conditions that may affect the participation of children and youth in different settings is attention deficit hyperactivity disorder (ADHD). This is a neurodevelopmental disorder characterized by attention deficit and/or impulsivity and hyperactivity, whose prevalence among children and youth is estimated at about 5%. Symptoms of ADHD persist in adulthood, with prevalence among adults estimated at about 2.5% [17,18]. A diagnosis of ADHD is based on the appearance of six or more criteria (such as lack of attention to details, difficulty organizing tasks, etc.), related to inattention, hyperactivity, and/or impulsivity, some of which appear prior to age 12; and these symptoms must occur in at least two life environments in a way that impairs functioning and quality of life [17].

ADHD has far-reaching and long-term consequences in all functioning areas, as it affects various aspects of a person's life, including daily functioning, employment, social participation, and family stability [17,18]. Studies among ADHD populations have often focused on specific impairments and/or functioning areas in which the implications of ADHD arise. For example, Shimoni et al. [19] and Engel-Yeger and Ziv-On [20] reported that children with ADHD participate less frequently in most leisure activities, receive less enjoyment from formal leisure activities, and show a lower preference for participation in some leisure activities, such as physical and social leisure activities, compared to children without ADHD. Additional studies indicated difficulties in social functioning of children and youth with ADHD compared to their peers [21,22], affecting their participation in various social activities [19,20].

Social difficulties of children and youth with ADHD may include peer rejection, inappropriate behavior, and/or difficulties with social skills such as collaboration, taking turns, reciprocity, and focus on conversation and play [21,22]. In addition, this population may experience difficulties in academic functioning [23,24], putting them at greater risk for low academic achievement, suspensions and expulsion from school, more absences, and even dropping out permanently, compared to populations without ADHD [25,26]. While these studies focus on one area of functioning, Harpin [27] described difficulties in the participation of a population with ADHD in multiple settings, and Lavi et al. [28] also reported significantly lower participation of adolescents with ADHD in daily activities and in school and home participation, compared to their peers without ADHD.

In summary, most studies examining the functioning of children and youth with ADHD are often focused on their specific difficulties and disabilities rather than their overall participation. In addition, there are few studies describing the participation profile of children and youth with ADHD compared to their peers without ADHD, particularly with respect to different settings (home, school, and community). Thus, a need exists to expand professional knowledge of the effects of ADHD on the participation of children and youth with this diagnosis, as it impacts their daily life in various settings [19].

In addition to health conditions, various environmental factors, such as physical and sociocultural factors, may also affect a person's development and participation [1,3,29,30]. Environmental factors can either support or hinder (erect barriers to) participation [3]. It is therefore important to examine the environmental factors and their impact on participation [31]. Not surprisingly, people with disabilities often identify relationships between environmental factors, participation, and quality of life. This highlights the need to assess the environmental impact on their participation at the community and social levels [29]. Research has found that the environmental domains noted in the ICF influence the participation of children with disabilities [32]. For example, the study by Bedell et al. [14], which examined community participation of children with and without disabilities, indicated that parents of children with disabilities more often rated environmental factors as barriers to participation and more rarely as supports, compared to parents of children without disabilities. Furthermore, it appears that the environment plays a unique role in influencing participation in different settings (home, school, and community). Specifically, environmental barriers were found to directly affect the frequency of participation and involvement in all settings, whereas environmental supports only influenced involvement in home and community settings, and participation frequency in the community setting [11].

However, despite increasing research on the contribution of environmental factors in explaining the participation of children and youth with disabilities, the majority of these studies have focused on children with physical disabilities [32], autism [33], or developmental coordination disorder (DCD) [34]. A number of studies conducted among children and youth with ADHD have addressed the relationship between environment and functioning. They have identified factors such as attitudes and social–family environment as relevant in conducting a functional assessment of this population [35,36]. One qualitative study showed that over half of the participants described a particular aspect of ADHD as context-dependent, which may indicate an association between environment and ADHD symptoms [37]. In a review article, Dvorsky and Langberg [38] reported that social and family support, particularly social acceptance and positive parenting, has a positive effect and can even prevent the negative effects of ADHD. They also noted that research examining such supportive and protective factors is still in its infancy, suggesting further exploration.

All this points to the need for an in-depth examination of how environmental factors impact the participation of children and youth with disabilities [32]. Specifically needed is a comparison of those with ADHD to their peers without ADHD, in a range of settings, with attention given to the relationship between environmental supports and participation patterns. Our study addressed this need by examining the participation profile of children and youth with ADHD, and the environmental factors that may influence their participation. The results may contribute to a deeper understanding of the participation of children and youth with ADHD, thereby assisting in assessment and contributing to the development and implementation of appropriate intervention programs for this population.

The present study focuses on examining the participation of children and youth (aged 6–14) with and without ADHD, in home, school, and community settings, identifying the environmental supports for and barriers against participation, and examining the availability of supporting resources. Our specific objectives were to examine the following: (a) the differences between children and youth with and without ADHD with respect to participation patterns (in terms of frequency, involvement), desire for change, and the overall environmental support in each of the settings (home, school, and community); (b) the relationship between the overall environmental support and the participation patterns (frequency and involvement) in the different settings in each group (with and without ADHD); and (c) the differences in the participation patterns between the different settings (home, school, and community), and to describe the environmental factors (support and barriers) that influence participation of children and youth with ADHD.

2. Materials and Methods

2.1. Study Design

A descriptive quantitative and comparison cross-sectional design was used.

2.2. Participants

The study population included 65 parents of children and youth, aged 6–14, most of them (about 60%) from urban areas in the central district of Israel, who were recruited by voluntary response sampling. Most parents were married (89.5%), were aged 45 and under (mothers: 73.4%; fathers: 65.1%), and had an academic education (mothers: 83.6%; fathers: 74.6%). The participants were divided into the following two groups: (a) an ADHD group (31 participants) and (b) a non-ADHD group (34 participants) matched in age range and adjusted for gender and socioeconomic status (according to the level of family income). The inclusion criteria for each group were children and youth whose parents reported that they did (ADHD group) or did not (non-ADHD group) receive a diagnosis of ADHD from a qualified professional, with all reports confirmed by the ADHD Questionnaire (see

Instruments, Section 2.3). The exclusion criteria for both groups were as follows: (a) the parents' lack of fluency in the Hebrew language; (b) attendance of the child/adolescent in a special education environment; and (c) one or more of the following diagnoses for the child/adolescent: cerebral palsy, autism, epilepsy, Tourette syndrome, intellectual disability, psychiatric disorder, and/or brain injury, according to their parents' report in the demographic questionnaire (see Instruments, Section 2.3). In the ADHD group, at least half of the parents reported learning, sensory, and emotional–behavioral difficulties of their children. As seen in Table 1, both groups included participants with an average age of 9–10 years, most were boys (over 64%), and were from average or high socioeconomic strata. No significant differences were found in the characteristics between the two groups with respect to age, gender, or family socioeconomic status.

Table 1. Demographic characteristics of the participants.

		Children and Youth with ADHD		Children and Youth without ADHD			
		n	Mean (SD)	n	Mean (SD)		
Age		31	10.37 (1.83)	34	9.48 (1.83)	$t_{(63)} = -1.95$ [a]	$p = 0.056$
		n	%	n	%		
Gender	male	20	64.52	22	64.71	$\chi^2_{(1)} = 0.0$ [b]	$p = 0.987$
	female	11	35.48	12	35.29		
Socioeconomic status	below average	3	9.68	0	-	$\chi^2_{(2)} = 3.50$ [b]	$p = 0.174$
	average	14	45.16	16	47.06		
	above average	14	45.16	18	52.94		

Attention deficit hyperactivity disorder (ADHD); a—Independent-samples *t*-test; b—Chi-squared test for independence.

2.3. Instruments

2.3.1. A demographic Questionnaire

A demographic questionnaire was developed for this study as a parental reporting tool. Its purpose was to characterize the study population, as well as to provide information about the child/adolescent and his/her family. The personal details in the questionnaire included items such as age, gender, country of birth, educational framework, health condition, and family income.

2.3.2. The Attention Deficit and Hyperactivity Screening Questionnaire

The Attention Deficit and Hyperactivity Screening Questionnaire [17] is a parent-report questionnaire that identifies symptoms of ADHD according to the criteria found in the Diagnostic and Statistical Manual of Mental Disorders, Fifth Version (DSM-5) [17]. It includes 18 criteria rated by the parent on a scale of 4 grades (3 = "very much", 0 = "not at all"). The questions are divided into criteria related to attention and hyperactivity, with suspected ADHD indicated by a score of 2 or higher in at least 6 of the 9 criteria for attention, and/or in at least 6 of 9 criteria related to hyperactivity and/or impulsivity. This questionnaire was used as an exclusion criterion for the non-ADHD group.

2.3.3. The Participation and Environment Measure for Children and Youth (PEM-CY)

The Participation and Environment Measure for Children and Youth (PEM-CY) [8] is a parent-report instrument that examines participation and environmental factors affecting the participation of school-age children (5–17 years of age) across the following three settings: home, school, and community. The PEM-CY participation items represent broad types of activities typically performed in each setting, i.e., home (10 activities), school (5 activities), and community (10 activities). For each activity type, parents are asked to note the following: (a) how frequently their child participates ("never" = 0 to "daily" = 7); (b) how involved their child is while participating ("minimally" = 1 to "very" = 5); and (c) whether they desire change in their child's participation ("no" or "yes"; if "yes", parents identify the type of change desired: "frequency", "involvement", and/or "variety"). Parents are then asked whether certain features of the environment help or hinder their child's participation in activities in each setting ("not an issue", "usually helps", "sometimes helps/makes harder", "usually makes harder"). They are also asked about perceived adequacy/availability of supporting resources ("not needed", "usually yes", "sometimes yes/no", "usually no"). The PEM-CY has been found to have moderate-to-good internal consistency (Cronbach's α = 0.59–0.83) in the participation scales. Its test–retest reliability was found to be moderate at school ($r = 0.58$), and high at home ($r = 0.84$) and in the community ($r = 0.79$). Additionally, high reliability was found in the environment scale ($r > 0.76$). This measure identifies significant differences in participation patterns and environmental factors between children with and without disabilities [12], supporting its construct validity. It also has been effectively used in the Israeli context.

2.4. Procedure

This study was approved by the Ethics Committee of the Hebrew University, Jerusalem, Israel (No. 27032018). Ads for recruiting subjects were posted on social networks and relevant forums; for the ADHD group, therapists working with children and youth with ADHD were also contacted. Parents who showed interest and agreed to participate in the study received an explanatory letter and filled out the questionnaires electronically, via email, or manually, according to their preference. The data were collected without identifying personal and/or computer information. Screening of the returned questionnaires was performed according to the exclusion and inclusion criteria (see Participants, Section 2.2).

2.5. Data Analysis

Statistical analysis was performed using the SPSS version 25.0 (Statistical Package for the Social Sciences, Armonk, NY, USA) [39], with a significance level of 0.05. Descriptive statistics were used to describe the study population, including participants' background data distribution, and the environmental factors (supports and barriers) impacting the ADHD group. Differences between the two groups in gender and socioeconomic status were examined using the chi-squared test for independence, and an independent-samples t-test was used for the age variable. For each setting (home, school, community), the participation patterns (frequency and involvement) were measured using mean variables. The desire for change in their child's participation was measured as the percent of activities in which the parents indicated that desire. In addition, according to the PEM-CY manual's guidelines, a variable was calculated for the overall environmental factors supporting participation ("overall environmental support" (in each setting separately). All environment questions were recoded into 3-point scale by merging "Not an issue/Not needed" with "Usually helps/Usually yes". The sum of all the environment ratings was divided by the maximum possible score within a setting, and multiplied by 100 (higher scores indicated more support of children's participation or more availability of the supporting resource). In order to compare the participation patterns, the desire for change, and the overall environmental support between the two groups (with and without ADHD), one-way MANOVA analysis was used. Effect-size calculation was conducted using partial eta squared, with $\eta^2 > 0.14$ defined as high effect, $0.06 < \eta^2 < 0.13$ as medium, and $0.01 < \eta^2 < 0.05$ as low [40]. In order to examine the relationship between the overall environmental support and the participation patterns (frequency and involvement) within each group, Pearson's correlations were calculated. In order to examine the differences among the three settings in the participation patterns (frequency and involvement) of the ADHD group, a one-way repeated measures ANOVA was used with Bonferroni correction.

3. Results

3.1. Comparison of Participation and the Overall Environmental Support between Groups in the Different Settings

Differences in participation patterns between the two groups were examined using a one-way MANOVA analysis. The differences between the groups on the combined dependent variables were statistically significant for frequency ($F_{(3, 61)} = 3.91$, $p = 0.013$; partial $\eta^2 = 0.16$) and for involvement ($F_{(3, 61)} = 14.16$, $p < 0.001$; partial $\eta^2 = 0.41$). As seen in Table 2, follow-up univariate ANOVAs showed significant differences with medium-to-high effect sizes in the frequency aspect in the home setting, and in the involvement aspect in all three settings. That is, the ADHD group was found to participate less frequently at home and was less involved in the three settings, compared to the non-ADHD group. It should be noted that no significant differences were found between the groups in the frequency aspect in the school setting.

Table 2. Comparison of participation patterns (frequency and involvement), desire for change, and the overall environmental support in the different settings between the two groups.

Measure	Setting	With ADHD (n = 31) mean (SD)	Without ADHD (n = 34) mean (SD)	$F_{(1, 63)}$	η^2
Frequency (8-point scale)	Home	5.77 (0.66)	6.08 (0.45)	5.10 *	0.08
	School	4.60 (1.28)	4.35 (0.93)	0.85	0.01
	Community	3.17 (1.06)	3.61 (0.80)	3.60	0.05
Involvement (5-point scale)	Home	3.50 (0.60)	4.30 (0.39)	41.55 ***	0.40
	School	3.89 (0.86)	4.35 (0.59)	6.40 **	0.09
	Community	3.74 (0.91)	4.30 (0.54)	9.12 **	0.13
		mean in percent (SD)	mean in percent (SD)		
Desire for change	Home	68.92 (24.21)	47.35 (23.23)	13.43 ***	0.18
	School	47.58 (33.59)	32.45 (30.45)	3.63	0.05
	Community	42.90 (24.56)	27.64 (22.47)	6.85 **	0.10
Overall environmental support	Home	83.78 (8.58)	94.11 (6.38)	27.52 ***	0.31
	School	82.54 (10.67)	94.89 (6.76)	30.98 ***	0.33
	Community	96.42 (12.66)	94.82 (7.67)	10.45 **	0.14

Notes: * $p < 0.05$, ** $p < 0.01$, *** $p < 0.001$.

The combined dependent variable of the desire for change significantly differs between the two groups ($F_{(3, 61)} = 4.83$, $p = 0.004$, partial $\eta^2 = 0.19$). In follow-up univariate ANOVAs, significant differences were found between the groups with medium-to-high effect sizes in the home and community settings, meaning that parents in the ADHD group were more interested in change than parents in the non-ADHD group at home and in the community, but not at school.

Examining the differences between the groups with respect to the overall environmental support, a significant difference between groups was found for the three combined settings ($F_{(3, 60)} = 13.39$, $p < 0.001$, partial $\eta^2 = 0.40$), along with significant differences with high effect sizes that were found between the two groups in each setting. Thus, the ADHD group reported the overall environmental support to be lower than the non-ADHD group, indicating that, among the ADHD group, the environmental factors are less supportive of children's participation or are less available to lend support.

3.2. Correlation between Overall Environmental Support and Participation Patterns in all Settings and for Each of the Groups

Pearson's correlations were calculated to explore the relationships between environmental support and the participation patterns for each of the groups. As seen in Table 3, no significant correlation was found between the overall environmental support and frequency of participation. However, significant positive correlations were found between overall environmental support and involvement of both groups in the home settings (Figure 1). In the school and community settings, significant positive correlations were found for the ADHD group, but not for the non-ADHD group (Figures 2 and 3). In conclusion, the ADHD group showed a positive and significant relationship between overall environmental support and involvement in each of the settings, whereas with the non-ADHD group a similar relationship was found only in the home setting.

Table 3. Pearson's correlations between environmental support and participation patterns (frequency and involvement) among children with and without attention deficit hyperactivity disorder (ADHD).

	Overall Environmental Support	
	Children with ADHD (n = 31)	Children without ADHD (n = 34)
Frequency		
Home	0.06	0.23
School	0.27	0.3
Community	0.03	0.24
Involvement		
Home	0.38 *	0.37 *
School	0.49 **	0.2
Community	0.47 **	−0.02

Notes: * $p < 0.05$, ** $p < 0.01$; Pearson's correlations (r).

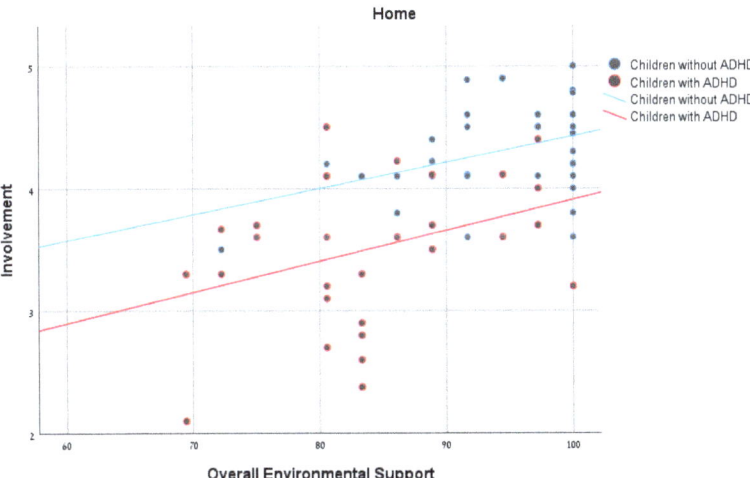

Figure 1. Correlations between overall environmental support and involvement among children with and without attention deficit hyperactivity disorder (ADHD) in the home environment.

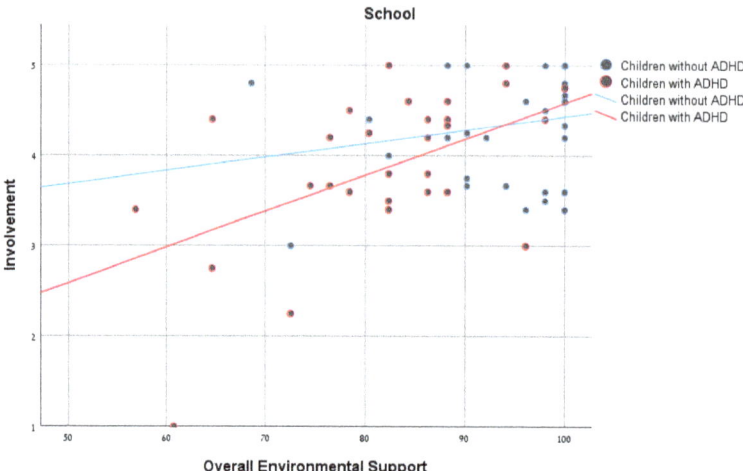

Figure 2. Correlations between overall environmental support and involvement among children with and without ADHD in the school environment.

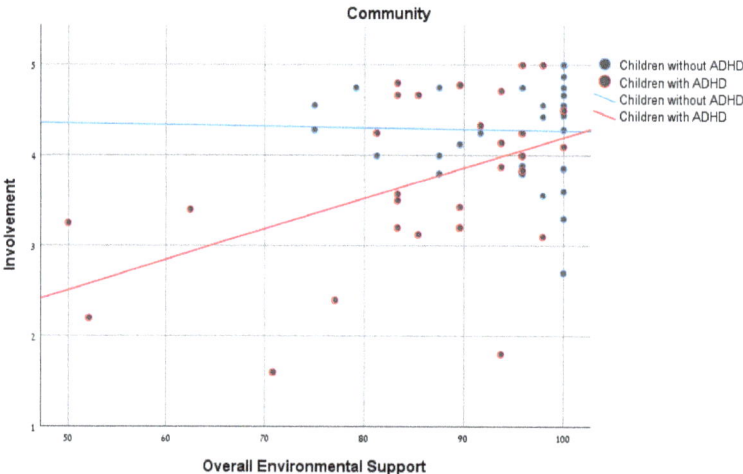

Figure 3. Correlations between overall environmental support and involvement among children with and without ADHD in the community environment.

3.3. Differences in Participation Patterns and Prevalence of Environmental Factors Impacting the ADHD Group

One-way repeated measures ANOVAs were conducted to determine whether there was a statistically significant difference in the ADHD group's participation among the different settings. Frequency of participation significantly changed with the settings as follows: $F_{(2, 60)} = 79.738$, $p < 0.001$, partial $\eta^2 = 0.73$. Pairwise comparisons with Bonferroni correction showed all three settings significantly differed from one another ($p < 0.001$). The frequency of participation at home was found to be higher than in the school and the community environments, and the frequency of participation in the school was found to be higher than in the community (Figure 4).

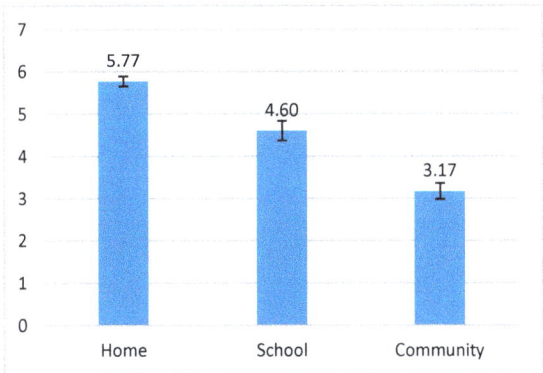

Figure 4. Frequency of participation of the ADHD group in the three settings.

Involvement in participation also significantly changed with the settings as follows: $F_{(2, 60)} = 3.943$, $p = 0.025$, partial $\eta^2 = 0.12$. In pairwise comparisons with Bonferroni correction, the mean of involvement at home was significantly lower than in school ($p < 0.05$), but no significant differences were found when comparing the involvement at home and school to the involvement in the community (Figure 5).

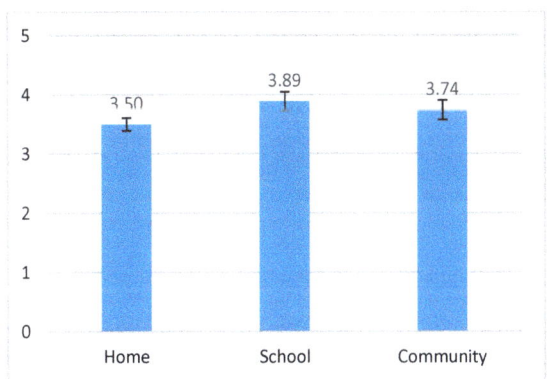

Figure 5. Involvement in participation of the ADHD group in the three settings.

The ADHD group's description of supports and barriers affecting participation in the different settings was evaluated by calculating the percentage of participants' consensus. Examining the supports, it appears that, in the home environment, "the attitudes and actions of therapists and other professionals" were reported as the most supportive factor (27.60%). In the school environment, the most supportive factor reported was "relationships with peers" (32.30%), followed by "the attitudes and actions of teachers, coaches, or staff" (25.80%). The result was similar for the community environment, where the most supportive factor for the ADHD group was "attitudes and actions of other members of the community" (29%).

Examining the barriers of the ADHD group, it was found that, in the home environment, "the cognitive demands" were reported as the most common inhibitors (38.70%). In the school environment, "the cognitive demands" and "the sensory stimulation" were the most frequently reported inhibitory factors (45.20% for each of them). Similar inhibitory factors were reported in the community environment, leading with sensory stimulation (19.40%) and cognitive demands (16.10%).

4. Discussion

This study was designed to examine the participation profile as affected by environmental factors (supports and barriers) among children and youth with ADHD, compared to their peers without ADHD. Additionally, the study set out to examine the relationship between overall environmental support and participation patterns (frequency and involvement) in each group, in the following three settings: home, school, and community.

4.1. Comparison of Participation Patterns, Desire for Change, and Overall Environmental Supports

Regarding the comparison of the participation patterns and the desire for change, it was found that, in the home environment, children and youth with ADHD participated less frequently and were less involved than their peers without ADHD. These findings are consistent with previous research suggesting that children with disabilities participate less frequently and are less involved at home, compared with typically developing children [16]. They also support the findings of Lavi et al. [28], showing that adolescents with ADHD participate less in the home environment than their peers without ADHD. In addition, as expected, our study found that parents of children and youth with ADHD reported a greater desire for change in their children's participation in the home environment, compared to the non-ADHD group. This suggests that the parents of children with ADHD were less satisfied with their child's participation patterns. A possible explanation for this is the difficulty in balancing the stability of the family with the need to assist a child/adolescent with ADHD [27,41], which is made even more challenging by parents' exposure to their child's ever-present difficulties in this environment.

Regarding the school setting, our findings indicated that children and youth with ADHD were less involved than children and youth without this diagnosis. This may be due to the difficulties in the social functioning of children and youth with ADHD, which comprise four of the five school-related activities in the PEM-CY questionnaire. Indeed, other studies of children with ADHD indicate high rates of peer rejection, low teacher ratings of their social skills in the classroom, difficulty in social involvement, along with difficulty in cooperation and in reciprocal conversation while playing with others [21,22]. Additionally, this finding was consistent with a previous study indicating that children and youth with disabilities (including ADHD) are less involved in the school environment than their typically developing peers [15].

However, in our study, no significant difference was found between the groups in frequency of participation in the school environment. A possible explanation for this is that participation frequency is influenced by school policy and routine [15], which may possibly obscure the differences between the groups. In addition, no significant differences were found between the groups in the desire for change in school environment participation. This may be related to the fact that the school environment is less accessible or familiar to parents.

Regarding the community environment, our findings indicated that the ADHD group was less involved than the non-ADHD group. This is similar to the study by Engel-Yeger and Ziv-On [20], which found that children with ADHD preferred to participate less in most leisure activities, and also received less enjoyment from formal leisure activities, compared to children without ADHD. Since involvement typically includes elements such as motivation and personal preference, which can be considered participation-related constructs [10], it may be assumed that the lower preference among children with ADHD to participate in the leisure activities that most often occur in the community environment would affect their involvement here. However, our study found no significant difference in frequency of participation between groups in the community environment. This finding is not consistent with the study of Bedell et al. [14], according to which children and youth with disabilities participate less frequently and are less involved in community activities than typically developing peers. A possible explanation is the difference in group characteristics, that is, the study described above included diagnoses in addition to ADHD, such as orthopedic defects, developmental delay, and autism, which may affect both the frequency and the ability to participate in activities. In addition, our study showed that parents of children and youth with ADHD reported a greater desire for change in their children's participation in the community, compared to those without ADHD. A possible explanation is that parents perceive themselves as influencing their children's participation in community activities, given their role in registering their children for such activities and encouraging them to participate.

Overall, our findings indicated lower involvement in the ADHD group compared to the non-ADHD group in all three settings. Since the construct of involvement refers to the level of concentration, emotional involvement, satisfaction, and attention when performing an activity [8], it is not unlikely that children and youth with ADHD will experience difficulty in maintaining attention and active partnership throughout a particular activity. In accordance with the lower involvement of children and youth with ADHD in all settings, the implementation of training programs for parents and teachers, as well as outreach programs in the community setting, can be beneficial for promoting their participation, personal involvement, and well-being. Regarding overall environmental support, this study found a significant difference between the groups in each of the three settings, meaning that environmental factors were less supportive of, or were less available to lend support to, the participation of children and youth with ADHD, compared to the non-ADHD group. These findings support the literature, which documents differences in the environmental support given to children with and without disabilities in different settings, and highlights the fact that there are more environmental barriers that affect the participation of children with disabilities, compared to children without disabilities [12,13]. A specific example of this is reflected in the study by Coster et al. [15], who found that parents of students with disabilities were significantly more likely to report patterns of the school environment that hindered participation, and that the resources needed to support their child's participation were not adequate, compared to students without disabilities.

4.2. Relationship between Overall Environmental Support and Participation Patterns

The results of the study found no significant association between environmental supports and participation frequency, for either of the groups (with and without ADHD). A similar finding was reported in the study of Rosenberg et al. [30], which examined the effect of environmental barriers on participation among children with mild developmental disabilities and found no significant correlation between environmental barriers and the number of activities in which the child participated (diversity) or the child's participation frequency (intensity). These results may be explained by the fact that the ADHD group can easily attend an activity, since they do not necessarily need major accessibility. However, our study did find a significant association between environmental support and involvement in all three settings among children and youth with ADHD, and in the home setting among children and youth without ADHD. It seems that, for the ADHD group, being involved (which means to be fully immersed in the activity) can be more challenging. This reinforces the understanding that participation is a multidimensional concept whose assessment requires addressing various aspects [7,9,31], including frequency and subjective measures such as involvement.

Our findings demonstrated a positive connection between environmental support and involvement among children and youth with ADHD in all the settings, confirming the need for environmental support to promote participation. In light of the importance of participation and its contribution to development, health, and well-being of children and youth, further examination is advisable to better understand the effects of increased participation on the well-being of this population.

It should be noted that, in the ADHD group, a significant correlation was found in all three settings, whereas in the non-ADHD group the correlation was found to be significant only in the home environment. These differences between groups indicate that, for children and youth with ADHD, the environmental supports are more significant influences on their involvement in activities in different settings.

4.3. Comparison of Frequency and Involvement between the Different Settings and a Description of the Environmental Factors

In comparing the different settings for frequency and involvement patterns, the home was found to be the environment in which children and youth with ADHD participated most frequently, yet they were less involved. A possible explanation for this is that the home environment is the main place where most daily tasks are performed [42]. As such, it contains activities that may take place in the family routine at a high frequency, such as household chores (e.g., setting the table and cleaning the room) and personal care management (e.g., maintaining hygiene and brushing teeth), as well as other unstructured informal activities, such as play, arts and crafts, and getting together with other people, that often require a child's initiative. At the same time, the child/adolescent may be dependent on another person, particularly his or her parents, when performing activities in this environment [34], which may result in lower involvement. An example of this was given in the study of Dunn et al. [43], who examined participation among children and youth with ADHD in various household tasks, and highlighted their need for support from family members while performing them; this tendency may also affect other activities reflected in the present study.

In contrast, school was found to be an environment where children and youth with ADHD are mostly involved in school activities, which may be related to the school activities themselves that are more structured. Our results, however, were limited to activities included in the PEM-CY questionnaire, which do not necessarily highlight the difficulties of this population in executive functions [44,45] and academic functioning [24,26]. These difficulties are underrepresented in the questionnaire items related to school activities, but are more prominent in home activities such as homework preparation, school preparation, and household chores.

According to our results, the community showed the lowest frequency of participation among children and youth with ADHD. This may result from the nature of community activities, such as group events or traveling, which may occur less frequently than home and school activities. Significantly, this low frequency was also reported by the non-ADHD group, an outcome supported by various studies that used the PEM-CY and similarly indicated highest participation frequency at home and lowest in the community [12,13,34]. However, it is important to note that these studies did not examine the frequency differences among the three settings, but rather compared groups with and without disabilities in different participation patterns.

Examining the environmental supports and barriers influencing children and youth with ADHD indicated that the factors which stood out most frequently as inhibitors, in all three settings, were the activity demands, and in particular the cognitive demands (e.g., concentration, attention, and problem-solving). This finding is consistent with the cognitive difficulties of the ADHD population related to attention, concentration [17], and executive functions, all of which impair their participation in various occupations throughout the day [28]. In addition to these, social demands (at home and school) and physical demands (in the community) were also reported as inhibiting participation among this population. The findings relate to activity demands, given the confirmed interactions between the person, the environment, and the activity [14]; therefore, changing the activity demands in the environment may promote participation. Interventions that include this adaptation of activity demands may promote the participation of children and youth with ADHD in the various settings. Adaptations in the activity demands, and in particular in the cognitive demands, can be applied by professional training and guidelines to parents, teachers, and community members who are involved in the participation of this population.

Another major barrier for children and youth with ADHD in school and the community is the sensory stimulation (e.g., amount and/or type of sound, noise, light, temperature, textures of objects, and crowds). This refers to distractions due to unrelated stimuli, and it may therefore reflect the high prevalence of comorbidity associated with sensory modulation dysfunction [46]. Reports of sensory interference highlight the need to assess environmental sensory conditions (for example, by using the Sensory Processing Measure and/or the Sensory Profile Questionnaire) and to consider them when designing interventions, in order to promote participation. Reducing sensory stimuli such as classroom decorations, and/or performing community activities in a relatively quiet environment, may be examples of such sensory adjustments.

Regarding the supports, other people's attitudes and actions were found to promote the participation of children and youth with ADHD in the three settings (e.g., babysitters and other professionals at home; teachers and staff at school; and members of the community, such as shopkeepers and instructors). Indeed, according to the literature, positive attitudes in the community and culture can promote participation [32], with the strongest evidence for social protective factors being found in social acceptance having a positive effect on the symptoms of the disorder [38]. In addition, relationships with peers emerged as one of the strongest supports for children and youth with ADHD. The fact that this factor was found to be helpful in school was interesting, given that it is adult support through their presence and supervision that is sometimes perceived as providing confidence among children with ADHD in the school environment [47].

Given that the environment is a potentially modifiable factor, there is considerable value in identifying which features of the home, school, and community environments are barriers to participation, so that interventions can be directed appropriately [7]. Therefore, these findings that indicate specific environmental factors constituting supports (people's attitudes and actions, and relationships with peers) or barriers (activity demands and sensory stimulation) to participation of children and youth with ADHD may greatly contribute to the well-being of that population.

4.4. Research Limitations and Recommendations for Further Research

The present study has a number of limitations, for which further research is recommended. First, the study focused on a convenience sample of 65 children and youth with and without ADHD aged 6–14 years, which is a wide age range. Moreover, most of them have average or above-average socioeconomic status, live in the central district of Israel, and have parents with an academic education. Further studies need to include a larger and more representative sample of the two groups, including smaller age ranges, various socioeconomic strata and areas of residence, with varying levels of parents' education, in order to enable better generalization of the findings. In addition, further studies should include children and youth with various health conditions, following the literature related to the range of health-related characteristics among representative study samples. Second, the information was based on parents' reports regarding their children's diagnosis of ADHD and the study criteria. Further research could include additional information from a professional regarding the ADHD type and comorbidity, such as sensory modulation dysfunction, learning disabilities, and/or DCD, which is common in this population [27,46,48]. Additionally, it is recommended to include other perspectives, such as the child/youth themselves and/or others (teachers and caregivers), especially regarding settings outside the home. It should also be noted that parents with ADHD are more likely to have children with ADHD [27]; this may affect parents while answering a long questionnaire like the PEM-CY, as well as their responsiveness to participating in the study. Therefore, it is recommended to substitute or add tools, including semi-structured interviews with parents, in order to facilitate questionnaire completion and deepen their understanding of the participation patterns. Moreover, this study included one measure for evaluating participation, which is a multidimensional and complex concept that no single dimension of measurement is likely to fully capture [7]. In following up the study results, further research should use additional measures related to the more subjective patterns inherent in this concept. Finally, further examination of the environmental supports and barriers, as well as the impact of environmental supports on the involvement and well-being of children and youth with ADHD, may also contribute to the expansion of professional knowledge.

5. Conclusions

This study described the participation profile, environmental factors (supports and barriers), and the relationship between overall environmental support and the participation patterns of frequency and involvement, among children and youth with and without ADHD, aged 6–14, based on parental reports. The findings indicated that, compared to their peers without ADHD, children and youth with ADHD participate less frequently in the home setting, they are less involved in all three settings, and their parents are more interested in changing their participation at home and in the community. Information about the specific activities to which parents want to see change is clinically important, as it can guide goal setting and targeted intervention. At the same time, children and youth with ADHD reported lower overall environmental support. Our findings showed a relationship between environmental support and involvement of children and youth with ADHD in all three settings, in contrast to children and youth without ADHD. These differences between groups reflect the interactional nature of participation, while confirming the need for environmental support to promote participation mainly among children and youth with ADHD.

In addition, differences in their participation patterns were found in various settings. These findings highlight the need for a broad examination of participation in different settings. As mentioned above, since participation is a multidimensional concept, its assessment requires addressing multiple aspects, including subjective measures such as involvement.

Different environmental factors were found to support or inhibit the participation of children and youth with ADHD, such as other people's attitudes and actions, relationships with peers, activity requirements (particularly cognitive), and sensory stimuli. This knowledge can lead to a greater effort to evaluate environmental support for children and youth with ADHD and improve their participation patterns (particularly their involvement) in various activities in different settings. The resulting development of intervention programs will benefit this population and contribute to their well-being.

Author Contributions: Investigation and Writing, T.S.; Statistical consulting, Writing—Data analysis and Results, H.F.-G.; Professional advisor, D.A.; Primary Investigation, Writing, and Corresponding author, A.G. All authors have read and agreed to the published version of the manuscript.

Funding: This research received no external funding.

Institutional Review Board Statement: The study was conducted according to the ethics guidelines and approved by the Institutional Review Board (Ethics Committee of the Hebrew University, Jerusalem, Israel; No. 27032018; 2018).

Informed Consent Statement: Informed consent was obtained from all subjects involved in the study.

Data Availability Statement: The dataset generated and analyzed during the current study is available to the first and last authors, but are not publicly available due to ethical guidelines.

Acknowledgments: We are grateful to the parents and children who participated in this study.

Conflicts of Interest: The authors declare no conflict of interest.

References

1. World Health Organization. *International Classification of Functioning, Disability and Health (ICF)*; WHO: Geneva, Switzerland, 2001.
2. Rainey, L.; van Nispen, R.; van der Zee, C.; van Rens, G. Measurement properties of questionnaires assessing participation in children and adolescents with a disability: A systematic review. *Qual. Life Res.* **2014**, *23*, 2793–2808. [CrossRef] [PubMed]
3. American Occupational Therapy Association (AOTA). Occupational therapy practice framework: Domain and process, 4th ed. *Am. J. Occup. Ther.* **2020**, *74*, 7412410010p1–7412410010p87. [CrossRef]
4. Law, M. Participation in the occupations of everyday life. *Am. J. Occup. Ther.* **2002**, *56*, 640–649. [CrossRef] [PubMed]

5. Rodger, S.; Ziviani, J. *Occupational Therapy with Children: Understanding Children's Occupations and Enabling Participation*; Blackwell: Oxford, UK, 2006.
6. Law, M.; Anaby, D.; DeMatteo, C.; Hanna, S. Participation patterns of children with acquired brain injury. *Brain Inj.* **2011**, *25*, 587–595. [CrossRef]
7. Coster, W.; Law, M.; Bedell, G.; Khetani, M.; Cousins, M.; Teplicky, R. Development of the participation and environment measure for children and youth: Conceptual basis. *Disabil. Rehabil.* **2012**, *34*, 238–246. [CrossRef]
8. Coster, W.; Law, M.; Bedell, G.M. *Participation and Environment Measure for Children and Youth (PEM-CY)*; Boston University: Boston, MA, USA, 2010.
9. Granlund, M. Participation–challenges in conceptualization, measurement and intervention. *Child Care Health Dev.* **2013**, *39*, 470–473. [CrossRef]
10. Imms, C.; Adair, B.; Keen, D.; Ullenhag, A.; Rosenbaum, P.; Granlund, M. 'Participation': A systematic review of language, definitions, and constructs used in intervention research with children with disabilities. *Dev. Med. Child Neurol.* **2016**, *58*, 29–38. [CrossRef]
11. Anaby, D.; Law, M.; Coster, W.; Bedell, G.; Khetani, M.; Avery, L.; Teplicky, R. The mediating role of the environment in explaining participation of children and youth with and without disabilities across home, school, and community. *Arch. Phys. Med. Rehabil.* **2014**, *95*, 908–917. [CrossRef]
12. Coster, W.; Bedell, G.; Law, M.; Khetani, M.A.; Teplicky, R.; Liljenquist, K.; Gleason, K.; Kao, Y.C. Psychometric evaluation of the Participation and Environment Measure for Children and Youth. *Dev. Med. Child Neurol.* **2011**, *53*, 1030–1037. [CrossRef]
13. Jeong, Y.; Law, M.; Stratford, P.; DeMatteo, C.; Missiuna, C. Measuring participation of children and environmental factors at home, school, and in community: Construct validation of the Korean PEM-CY. *Phys. Occup. Ther. Pediatr.* **2017**, *37*, 541–554. [CrossRef]
14. Bedell, G.; Coster, W.; Law, M.; Liljenquist, K.; Kao, Y.C.; Teplicky, R.; Anaby, D.; Khetani, M.A. Community participation, supports, and barriers of school-age children with and without disabilities. *Arch. Phys. Med. Rehabil.* **2013**, *94*, 315–323. [CrossRef]
15. Coster, W.; Law, M.; Bedell, G.; Liljenquist, K.; Kao, Y.C.; Khetani, M.; Teplicky, R. School participation, supports and barriers of students with and without disabilities. *Child Care Health Dev.* **2013**, *39*, 535–543. [CrossRef] [PubMed]
16. Law, M.; Anaby, D.; Teplicky, R.; Khetani, M.A.; Coster, W.; Bedell, G. Participation in the home environment among children and youth with and without disabilities. *Br. J. Occup. Ther.* **2013**, *76*, 58–66. [CrossRef]
17. American Psychiatric Association. *Diagnostic and Statistical Manual of Mental Disorders*, 5th ed.; APA: Washington, DC, USA, 2013.
18. Faraone, S.; Asherson, P.; Banaschewski, T.; Biederman, J.; Buitelaar, J.K.; Ramos-Quiroga, J.A.; Rohde, L.A.; Sonuga-Barke, E.J.S.; Tannock, R.; Barbara, F. Attention-deficit/hyperactivity disorder. *Nature Rev. Dis. Prim.* **2015**, *1*, 1–23. [CrossRef] [PubMed]
19. Shimoni, M.A.; Engel-Yeger, B.; Tirosh, E. Participation in leisure activities among boys with attention deficit hyperactivity disorder. *Res. Dev. Disabil.* **2010**, *31*, 1234–1239. [CrossRef] [PubMed]
20. Engel-Yeger, B.; Ziv-On, D. The relationship between sensory processing difficulties and leisure activity preference of children with different types of ADHD. *Res. Dev. Disabil.* **2011**, *32*, 1154–1162. [CrossRef]
21. García-Castellar, R.; Jara-Jiménez, P.; Sánchez-Chiva, D.; Mikami, A.Y. Social skills deficits in a virtual environment among Spanish children with ADHD. *J. Atten. Disor.* **2018**, *22*, 776–786. [CrossRef]
22. Ros, R.; Graziano, P.A. Social functioning in children with or at risk for attention deficit/hyperactivity disorder: A meta-analytic review. *J. Clin. Child Adol. Psych.* **2018**, *47*, 213–235. [CrossRef]
23. Daley, D.; Birchwood, J. ADHD and academic performance: Why does ADHD impact on academic performance and what can be done to support ADHD children in the classroom? *Child Care Health Dev.* **2010**, *36*, 455–464. [CrossRef]
24. Frazier, T.W.; Youngstrom, E.A.; Glutting, J.J.; Watkins, M.W. ADHD and achievement: Meta-analysis of the child, adolescent, and adult literatures and a concomitant study with college students. *J. Learn. Disabil.* **2007**, *40*, 49–65. [CrossRef]
25. Birchwood, J.; Daley, D. Brief report: The impact of attention deficit hyperactivity disorder (ADHD) symptoms on academic performance in an adolescent community sample. *J. Adol.* **2012**, *35*, 225–231. [CrossRef] [PubMed]
26. Kent, K.M.; Pelham, W.E.; Molina, B.S.; Sibley, M.H.; Waschbusch, D.A.; Yu, J.; Gnagy, E.M.; Biswas, A.; Badinski, D.E.; Karch, K.M. The academic experience of male high school students with ADHD. *J. Abnorm. Child Psych.* **2011**, *39*, 451–462. [CrossRef] [PubMed]
27. Harpin, V.A. The effect of ADHD on the life of an individual, their family, and community from preschool to adult life. *Arch. Dis. Child.* **2005**, *90*, i2–i7. [CrossRef] [PubMed]
28. Lavi, G.; Maeir, A.; Traub Bar-Ilan, R.; Levanon-Erez, N. The relationship between executive functions and participation among adolescents with and without attention deficit hyperactivity disorder (ADHD). *Isr. J. Occup. Ther.* **2017**, *26*, H250–H266.
29. Hammel, J.; Magasi, S.; Heinemann, A.; Gray, D.B.; Stark, S.; Kisala, P.; Carlozzi, N.E.; Tulsky, D.; Garcia, S.F.; Hahn, E.A. Environmental barriers and supports to everyday participation: A qualitative insider perspective from people with disabilities. *Arch. Phys. Med. Rehabil.* **2015**, *96*, 578–588. [CrossRef]
30. Rosenberg, L.; Ratzon, N.Z.; Jarus, T.; Bart, O. Perceived environmental restrictions for the participation of children with mild developmental disabilities. *Child Care Health Dev.* **2012**, *38*, 836–843. [CrossRef]
31. Bedell, G.M.; Khetani, M.A.; Cousins, M.A.; Coster, W.J.; Law, M.C. Parent perspectives to inform development of measures of children's participation and environment. *Arch. Phys. Med. Rehabil.* **2011**, *92*, 765–773. [CrossRef]
32. Anaby, D.; Hand, C.; Bradley, L.; DiRezze, B.; Forhan, M.; DiGiacomo, A.; Law, M. The effect of the environment on participation of children and youth with disabilities: A scoping review. *Disabil. Rehabil.* **2013**, *35*, 1589–1598. [CrossRef]

33. Egilson, S.T.; Jakobsdóttir, G.; Ólafsson, K.; Leósdóttir, T. Community participation and environment of children with and without autism spectrum disorder: Parent perspectives. *Scand. J. Occup. Ther.* **2017**, *24*, 187–196. [CrossRef]
34. Izadi-Najafabadi, S.; Ryan, N.; Ghafooripoor, G.; Gill, K.; Zwicker, J.G. Participation of children with developmental coordination disorder. *Res. Dev. Disabil.* **2019**, *84*, 75–84. [CrossRef]
35. De Schipper, E.; Lundequist, A.; Wilteus, A.L.; Coghill, D.; De Vries, P.J.; Granlund, M.; Holtmann, M.; Jonsson, U.; Karande, S.; Levy, F.; et al. Comprehensive scoping review of ability and disability in ADHD using the International Classification of Functioning, Disability and Health-Children and Youth Version (ICF-CY). *Euro. Child Adol. Psych.* **2015**, *24*, 859–872. [CrossRef] [PubMed]
36. Mahdi, S.; Viljoen, M.; Massuti, R.; Selb, M.; Almodayfer, O.; Karande, S.; de Vries, P.J.; Rohde, L.; Bölte, S. An international qualitative study of ability and disability in ADHD using the WHO-ICF framework. *Euro. Child Adol. Psych.* **2017**, *26*, 1219–1231. [CrossRef] [PubMed]
37. Lasky, A.K.; Weisner, T.S.; Jensen, P.S.; Hinshaw, S.P.; Hechtman, L.; Arnold, L.E.; Murray, D.E.; Swanson, J.M. ADHD in context: Young adults' reports of the impact of occupational environment on the manifestation of ADHD. *Soc. Sci. Med.* **2016**, *161*, 160–168. [CrossRef] [PubMed]
38. Dvorsky, M.R.; Langberg, J.M. A review of factors that promote resilience in youth with ADHD and ADHD symptoms. *Clin. Child Fam. Psych. Rev.* **2016**, *19*, 368–391. [CrossRef]
39. IBM. *SPSS Statistics for Macintosh*; Version 25.0; IBM Corp: Armonk, NY, USA, 2016.
40. Stevens, J. *Applied Multivariate Statistics for the Social Sciences*; Lawrence Erlbaum Associates: Mahwah, NJ, USA, 2002.
41. Wehmeier, P.M.; Schacht, A.; Barkley, R.A. Social and emotional impairment in children and adolescents with ADHD and the impact on quality of life. *J. Adol. Health* **2010**, *46*, 209–217. [CrossRef]
42. Guimarães Mendes, C.; Cotta Mancini, M.; Marques Miranda, D. Household task participation of children and adolescents with ADHD: A systematic review. *Brazil. J. Occup. Ther.* **2018**, *26*, 658–667.
43. Dunn, L.; Coster, W.J.; Orsmond, G.I.; Cohn, E.S. Household task participation of children with and without attentional problems. *Phys. Occup. Ther. Pediatr.* **2009**, *29*, 258–273. [CrossRef]
44. Barkley, R.A. Behavioral inhibition, sustained attention, and executive functions: Constructing a unifying theory of ADHD. *Psychol. Bull.* **1997**, *121*, 65. [CrossRef]
45. Brown, T.E. ADD/ADHD and impaired executive function in clinical practice. *Curr. Atten. Disabil. Rep.* **2009**, *1*, 37–41. [CrossRef]
46. Mangeot, S.D.; Miller, L.J.; McIntosh, D.N.; McGrath-Clarke, J.; Simon, J.; Hagerman, R.J.; Goldson, E. Sensory modulation dysfunction in children with attention-deficit-hyperactivity disorder. *Dev. Med. Child Neurol.* **2001**, *43*, 399–406. [CrossRef]
47. Pfeifer, L.I.; Terra, L.N.; dos Santos, J.L.F.; Stagnitti, K.E.; Panúncio-Pinto, M.P. Play preference of children with ADHD and typically developing children in Brazil: A pilot study. *Austr. Occup. Ther. J.* **2001**, *58*, 419–428. [CrossRef] [PubMed]
48. Larson, K.; Russ, S.A.; Kahn, R.S.; Halfon, N. Patterns of comorbidity, functioning, and service use for US children with ADHD, 2007. *Pediatrics* **2011**, *127*, 462–470. [CrossRef] [PubMed]

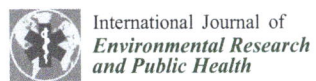

Article

Exploring the Participation Patterns and Impact of Environment in Preschool Children with ASD

Ghaidaa Khalifa [1,*], Peter Rosenbaum [2,3], Kathy Georgiades [4], Eric Duku [4] and Briano Di Rezze [1,3]

1. School of Rehabilitation Science, McMaster University, Hamilton, ON L8S 1C7, Canada; direzzbm@mcmaster.ca
2. Department of Paediatrics, McMaster University, Hamilton, ON L8S 1C7, Canada; rosenbau@mcmaster.ca
3. CanChild Centre for Childhood Disability Research, McMaster University, Hamilton, ON L8S 1C7, Canada
4. Department of Psychiatry and Behavioural Neurosciences, McMaster University, Hamilton, ON L8N 3K7, Canada; georgik@mcmaster.ca (K.G.); duku@mcmaster.ca (E.D.)
* Correspondence: khalifag@mcmaster.ca

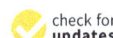

Received: 1 June 2020; Accepted: 3 August 2020; Published: 6 August 2020

Abstract: Participation in everyday activities at home and in the community is essential for children's development and well-being. Limited information exists about participation patterns of preschool children with autism spectrum disorder (ASD). This study examines these participation patterns in both the home and community, and the extent to which environmental factors and social communication abilities are associated with participation. Fifty-four parents of preschool-aged children with ASD completed the Participation and Environment Measure for Young Children and the Autism Classification System of Functioning: Social Communication. The children had a mean age of 48.9 (8.4) months. Patterns of participation were studied using descriptive statistics, radar graphs, and Spearman correlations. Children with ASD participated in a variety of activities at home and in the community, but showed a higher participation frequency at home. Parents identified different barriers (e.g., social demands) and supports (e.g., attitudes) in both settings. There was a moderate positive association between children's social communication abilities and their levels of involvement during participation and the diversity of activities. This study highlights the importance of social communication abilities in the participation of preschool children with ASD, and the need to support parents while they work to improve their child's participation, especially within their communities.

Keywords: autism spectrum disorder; participation; environment; social communication; childhood

1. Introduction

Participation is defined in the WHO's International Classification of Functioning, Disability, and Health (ICF) as "involvement in a life situation" [1]. Since the introduction of the ICF, this definition has evolved and has been given several meanings in the literature [2,3]. Participation has also been described as the intensity of engagement or being involved in a life situation [2], and as the experience of taking part in an everyday activity [4]. Participation has been defined as a multidimensional concept that includes two essential constructs: *Attendance* to an activity, and level of *involvement* [5,6]. Attendance is defined as "being there" and is measured by the frequency and/or diversity of activities in which the person takes part [5]. *Involvement* is defined as "the experience of participation while attending, including elements of motivation, persistence, social connection, and affect" [5]. The definition by Imms and colleagues [5] informed this study, as this multidimensional concept could be applied to any activity or setting, regardless of the ability of the individual [6].

It is believed that participation is a pre-requisite for human development [7] and an indicator of children's health and well-being [8,9]. According to Bandura's social learning theory [10], new skills are acquired by direct experience and engagement with and/or through the observation of others. Therefore, through participation in everyday activities, children develop cognitive, sensory, motor, and social skills [11], form friendships, and develop their sense of self-identity [7]. Overall, participation is associated with positive outcomes for all children, but it could have more significant impact on the development of children with disabilities. Participation has been reported to have an influence on learning, independence, and social inclusion of children with disabilities [9].

Over the last decade, the number of children diagnosed with autism spectrum disorder (ASD) has increased, with 1 in 54 children diagnosed with ASD in the US [12] and 1 in 66 in Canada [13]. Children receive an ASD diagnosis during the preschool years (median age of diagnosis is 4 years) [14]. Parents are usually stressed and overwhelmed following receiving an ASD diagnosis [15] and their children's participation might not be their priority. The preschool years are the period where children first start to learn their roles in a group, gain new skills, and practice these skills in their environments [16]. In addition, participation in the preschool years highly depends on the opportunities offered to children by adults in their everyday environment, typically their parents or caregivers [17,18]. The literature indicates that children with disabilities participate less frequently in domestic, educational, leisure, and social activities when compared to their typically developing peers [11]. Children with ASD are reported to have limited participation, as well as engaging less frequently and in fewer activities when compared to their typically developing peers [19,20]. They participate less frequently in activities of self-care, community mobility, and leisure activities [19]. Families of preschool children with ASD are reported to participate less in special event activities such as family vacations and birthday parties [20]. School-aged children with ASD are also reported to participate less than their typically developed peers in social activities, unstructured activities, and after school activities [21,22].

Many challenges associated with ASD, such as social communication deficits and/or repetitive behaviors, put children with ASD at risk of limited participation. Their social communication difficulties make it a challenge to be involved and engaged with others, which is required for many aspects of participation [19,23]. Furthermore, their restrictive and repetitive behaviors may set them apart from other children and further limit their participation in everyday activities [19]. In addition, parents of children with ASD indicate that their child's participation may also be impacted because parents may avoid participation outside their home due to fears of the negative perceptions of others [24,25].

As indicated above and in the literature, various aspects of the environment-the physical, social, or attitudinal—can have a significant impact on children's participation [1,4,26]. Bronfenbrenner's bioecological systems theory identified the different layers of the environment and their impact on child development [27]. Child development is affected by their interaction with the environment at various levels (directly and indirectly), including their immediate family, community, and society [27]. This emphasizes the need to look at the potential impact of various environments to understand children's development. Parents of children with disabilities consider the environment to be less supportive and believe that their children have more environmental barriers than typically developing children [9,28]. These barriers could relate to the physical, social, or attitudinal aspects of the environment. The environmental features may either support or hinder the participation of children with ASD. Some of these features include sensory issues, such as level of noise and lighting [29]; furthermore, the physical layout of the space, as well as the social and cognitive demands of some activities, may compromise social connections, such as interacting with others [29]. Availability of resources and services may also support participation of children with ASD [29].

Studies of the impact of the environment on participation with various populations of children with disabilities have shown inconsistent findings. In their study of participation of school-aged children with severe physical disabilities, King et al. [30] found that the environment indirectly impacted on participation. For example, unsupportive environments (e.g., inaccessible or less accommodating) were found to be related to a child's reduced functional ability and therefore were associated with limited participation [30]. A study of participation of children with cerebral palsy found that environmental factors failed to predict the child's participation diversity [31]. Moreover, for preschool children with mild developmental disabilities, environmental factors were found to be significant predictors of children's participation [11]. Studies of participation of school-aged children with ASD found the environment to be one of the factors that impacted their participation [26,28]. In their report, Askari and colleagues [26] reviewed the literature on the impact of the different aspect of the environment (i.e., physical, social, and attitudinal) on participation of children with ASD. In this work, social supports from parents, siblings, or friends were highlighted as important for participation, whereas negative attitudes in the community (e.g., church) presented as barriers for participation for children with ASD [26].

Few measures are designed to assess characteristics of the environment that impact participation in different settings. These include the Child and Family Follow-up Survey (CFFS) [32] and the Participation and Environment Measure (PEM) [33]. The CFFS is designed for children 5 years and older with traumatic brain injuries (TBIs) [32]. It has five sections, one of which is the Child and Adolescent Scale of Participation (CASP), to report on the participation of children with TBIs in the home, school, and community [32]. Another scale is the Child and Adolescent Scale of Environment (CASE), which measures the intensity of the physical, social, and attitudinal environment problems experienced by children with TBIs [32]. The PEM has two versions: The Young Children Participation and Environment Measure (YC-PEM) [34] for children aged 0–5 years, and the Participation and Environment Measure for Children and Youth (PEM-CY) for children and youth aged 5–17 years old [33]. They are used to report on participation and the quality of the environment in various activities in three contexts: At home, daycare/school, and community. PEM can be used with children with various disabilities, as well as children without disabilities.

Another factor that affects participation is the child's social functioning [35,36]. Social communication functioning is inconsistently defined in the literature [37]. New perspectives in the field are making the distinction between social deficits, impairment, functioning, and abilities [38]. In an extensive search of the literature, King and colleagues developed a conceptual model of factors affecting participation in recreational and leisure activities for children with disabilities [39]; the child's social functioning was one of the factors identified in this model. Evidence indicated that better-developed social functional ability was associated with better involvement when participating in activities [39]. The Diagnostic and Statistical Manual of Mental Disorders (DSM-5) defines social communication impairment as "deficits in social-emotional reciprocity, non-verbal behavior, and imitative and make-believe play" [40]. Although deficits in social functioning are one of the core symptoms of ASD [39,41], to our knowledge there is a paucity of research on the impact of social functioning on participation for children with ASD.

To date, studies on participation of children with disabilities have focused on school-aged children and adolescents and those with physical disabilities, while there is a lack of research on participation for young children with ASD [24]. A systematic review by Adair et al. [6] found that of the 394 articles on participation that they reviewed, 105 articles focused solely on cerebral palsy, while only 37 articles focused on ASD. Furthermore, these types of studies usually involve comparing a group of children with disabilities to a group of children without disabilities [29,42–45]. There is a need to study, in depth, the patterns of participation and the potential factors associated with participation amongst preschool children with ASD. The aims of this study were to explore the patterns of participation for preschool children with ASD (3–6 years old) and investigate the impact of different environmental and individual factors on their participation.

2. Methods

2.1. Participants and Procedures

This cross-sectional study investigated the patterns of participation in preschool children with ASD and the factors that are associated with them, including the environment and the social communication abilities of the child. The study involved analysis of data relating to a subsample of children who were recruited for a larger project (the Pediatric Autism Research Cohort (PARC) project-pilot phase). The subsample included children who have completed the YC-PEM, and therefore involved children who were 5 years and younger. PARC is a longitudinal inception cohort of children recently diagnosed with ASD from Hamilton, Ontario. The study was approved by the local research ethics board (Hamilton Integrated Research Ethics Board (HiREB)) and all families provided informed consent. The sample included 94 children diagnosed with ASD. The inclusion criteria for participants involved being under age 6 at enrollment and being enrolled in services at the regional autism program.

2.2. Assessment Measures

Sociodemographic questionnaire: This questionnaire was created specifically for the PARC study and included questions about the child, such as their age, sex, and country of birth. It also asked questions concerning the family background, including their educational level and family income.

2.3. Participation and the Environment

Participation and Environment Measure (Young children version—YC-PEM): YC-PEM was developed based on ICF concepts and is a parent- or caregiver-completed questionnaire. The current study explored participation at home and community settings only. Home and community are considered the natural learning environment of daily activities for young children [46]. For each activity, parents reported: (i) Frequency of participation on an 8-point scale from never (0) to daily (7) for 13 age-appropriate activity items at home and 11 items in the community; (ii) level of involvement in specified activities (5-point scale from minimally involved (1) to very involved (5)); and (iii) whether caregiver/parent would like to see changes in their child's participation in this type of activity (yes or no question). For each setting, parents reported on various features of the environment or resources and their impact on their children's participation, such as the sensory qualities of the environment or the cognitive demands of an activity. For each item in the environment, parents chose one of the following: Whether it has no impact, usually helps, sometimes helps, sometimes makes harder, or usually makes harder. Since the study aim was to explore the pattern of participation, questions on caregivers' desire to change participation were not considered.

The YC-PEM has shown sound psychometric properties with children with different disabilities. It has an acceptable internal consistency (>0.70) for three scales: Frequency ($\alpha = 0.72$); Involvement ($\alpha = 0.80$); and Environmental Support ($\alpha = 0.92$) [47]. The test–retest reliability for the frequency scale was fair to good for home (ICC = 0.61–0.63) and community (ICC = 0.55–0.63), and for the level of involvement scale reliability was good to excellent for the home (ICC = 0.79–0.93) and good for the community (ICC = 0.71–0.97). The reliability for the environment scale was good for the home and community (ICC = 0.91–0.94) [47]. PEM-CY/YC-PEM has been used to investigate the pattern of participation for children with ASD in different settings, but mostly for school-aged children [29,42,48].

2.4. Social Communication Functioning

The construct of social communication was explored using the Autism Classification System of Functioning: Social Communication (ACSF:SC) [49]. The ACSF:SC is a strength-based tool that aims to categorize children with ASD who are between 3 to 6 years old into one of five levels of functioning based on their social communication abilities. This descriptive tool was developed by CanChild researchers based on ICF concepts. The social communication abilities range from level V (lowest ability) through level I (highest ability). This classification tool is not meant to replace any diagnostic or assessment tools, but rather provides a simple standardized method to classify the child's social communication abilities in a consistent manner among the health provider teams, teachers, and parents [50]. A rater who is familiar with the child is asked to provide two ratings: The child's capacity level (what the child can do at their best) and the child's typical performance level (what the child can do on a day-to-day basis). The ACSF:SC demonstrates good intra-rater agreement for parents ($k_w = 0.61$–0.69) and good to very good for professionals ($k_w = 0.71$–0.95) [50].

The inter-rater agreement among parents and professionals ranges from fair to moderate agreement (k_w = 0.33–0.53) [50].

2.5. Data Analysis

The data for the current analysis were drawn from the initial time point from the larger PARC study. Data were analyzed using STATA software, version 13 (StataCorp LLC, Texas, TX, USA), and an effect was considered statistically significant at α = 0.05.

Descriptive statistics, including the means, standard deviations, and percentages of child characteristics and their family's sociodemographic information were first calculated for the participants. The distribution of the sample among the five levels of the ACSF:SC was obtained for the best capacity and typical performance scales. To understand the pattern of participation for our sample, the mean and standard deviation were calculated for the frequency and level of involvement scales of the YC-PEM. The percentages of activities in which the children participated were also calculated. Radar graphs were obtained to illustrate the distribution of scores across items. Radar graphs are used to represent the data visually in order to examine patterns of activity and are shaped like histograms. The radar graphs have multiple spokes spreading from the center of the graph, and the longer the spoke, the higher the magnitude of the variable represented by this spoke [51].

To explore the relationships between the ACSF:SC levels and YC-PEM-reported frequency, level of involvement, and the percentage of activity for both settings, scatter plots were created to visualize the data, followed by Spearman's correlation analysis. The same procedure was done to explore the relationships among the ACSF:SC levels and the environmental scales of the YC-PEM, followed by analysis of variance (ANOVA). ANOVA was conducted to explore whether the size of the differences between best capacity and typical performance levels was associated with the presence of environmental supports or barriers.

3. Results

Descriptive statistics: 54 children completed the ACSF:SC and were included in the analysis. Socio-demographic information of the parents, their household, and their child with ASD is summarized in Table 1.

Table 1. Descriptive statistics and sociodemographic features of the sample.

Demographic Variables	(n = 54)
Child Gender	
Boys	45 (83.3%)
Girls	9 (16.7%)
Child Age (in months)	
Mean (SD)	48.9 (8.4)
Language Spoken at Home	
English	53 (98.2%)
Caregiver's Highest Level of Education	
High School	9 (17%)
Secondary education	44 (83%)
Spouse Highest Level of Education	
High School	11 (23.9%)
Secondary education	35 (76.1%)
Family Annual Income	
<$30,000	9 (17.6%)
$30,001–$60,000	14 (27.5%)
$60,001–$80,000	5 (9.8%)
>$80,000	23 (45.1%)

Non-respondent analysis: Six participants did not complete the ACSF:SC and were excluded from the study. There were no significant differences between the respondent and non-respondent children in terms of their age (t (58) = 0.15, p = 0.9), gender (Pearson X^2 (1) = 1.0, p = 0.3), or language spoken at home (Pearson X^2 (1) = 0.36 p = 0.6).

ACSF:SC best capacity and typical performance scores: Parents of 50% of the participants rated their child the same for typical performance and best capacity, and 44.4% of parents judged their children to have lower typical performance abilities than their best capacity ability. Parents of only 5.6% of the participants judged their children to have higher typical performance abilities than their best capacity (Table 2). A total of 46.3% of participants had a ±1-level difference, while only 2% had a 2-level difference.

Table 2. Autism Classification System of Functioning: Social Communication (ACSF:SC) best capacity and typical performance ratings. Agreement between best capacity and typical performance is highlighted.

Best Capacity	Typical Performance					
	I	II	III	IV	V	Total
I	2 3.7%	4 7.4%	0 0.0	0 0.0	0 0.0	6 11.1%
II	1 1.9%	4 7.4%	7 12.9%	0 0.0	0 0.0	12 22.2%
III	0 0.0	0 0.0	10 18.5%	8 14.8%	1 1.9%	19 35.2%
IV	0 0.0	0 0.0	1 1.9%	6 11.1%	4 7.4%	11 20.4%
V	0 0.0	0 0.0	0 0.0	1 1.9%	5 9.3%	6 11.1
Total	3 5.6%	8 14.8%	18 33.3%	15 27.8%	10 18.5%	54 100

YC-PEM

Participation: Overall, parents reported their children as participating in a variety of activities at home and in the community. Frequency and level of involvement are demonstrated in the radar graphs to depict the activities in which children engaged within the home and community settings (Figures 1 and 2).

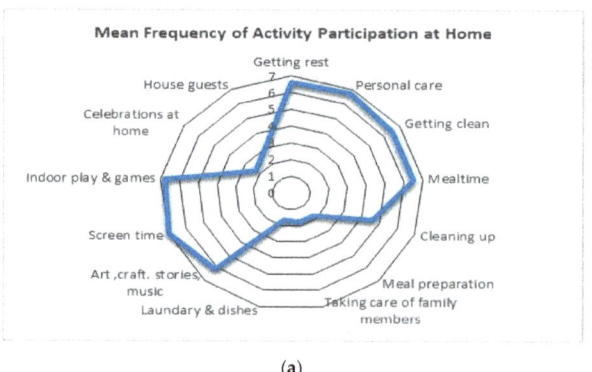

(a)

Figure 1. Cont.

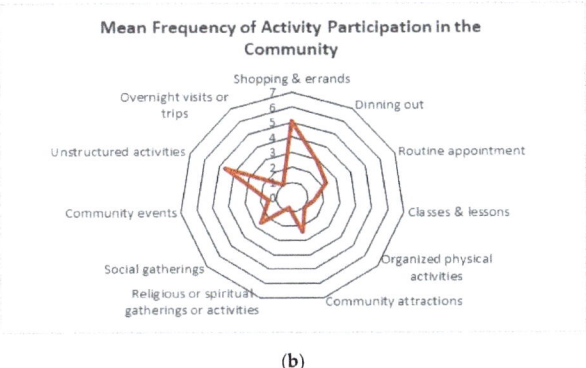

(b)

Figure 1. (a) Mean frequency of activity participation at home, (b) mean frequency of activity participation in the community.

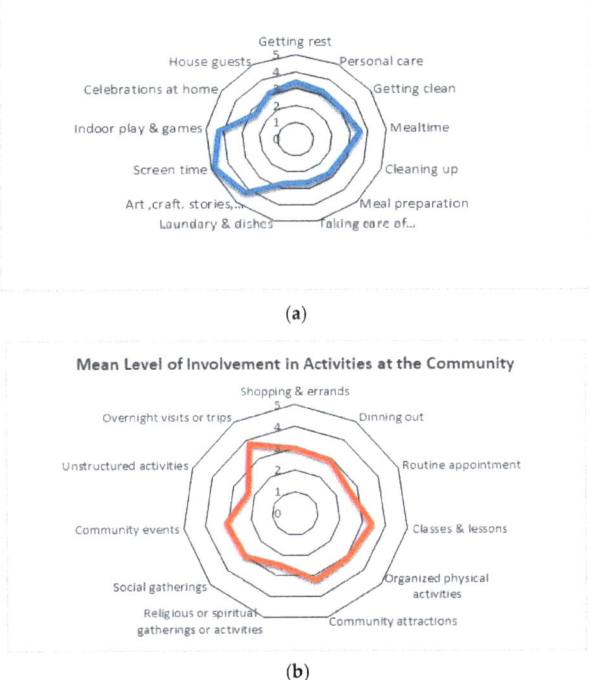

Figure 2. (a) Mean level of involvement in activities at home, (b) mean level of involvement in activities in the Community.

4. Home Setting

Activity frequency and level of involvement: The majority of our sample (>73%) were reported to participate most frequently in basic care routine activities (mean = 6.6) (Figure 1a); 50% were reported to be "somewhat involved" in these activities (Figure 2a). Household chores were reported to have the lowest frequency in the home setting with a mean of 1.8 ("few times in the last four months") in three out of four activities. Participants were reported to have different levels of involvement ranging from "not very involved" to "very involved". Furthermore, up to 65% of the participants were reported to have never participated in these chores. Participants showed high frequency rates in the interactive and organized play with the majority (98%) participating daily in these activities and being very involved. Socializing with friends and family was also reported to have low frequency from "few times in the last four months" (44%) to "a few times a month" (up to 27%). The level of involvement ranged from not very involved to very involved (Supplementary Table S1).

Environmental supports and barriers: Half of the parents reported that the physical layout of their houses supported their children's participation, as shown in Table 3. Sensory qualities were perceived as a support for 37.7% of the parents. Cognitive and social demands were reported to support children's participation for 22.6% and 26.4%, respectively, with a further 24.5% and 30.2% parents considering them as barriers. The attitudes of family were reported as supportive for 34.7% of parents. A total of 46.7% of parents considered money and time to support their children's participation.

Relationship between social communication and participation: Spearman's correlation analyses provided the same correlations for best capacity and typical performance levels and participation. Therefore, we decided to use the typical performance levels as they represent everyday functional performance. There was very low correlation between participation *frequency* and the ACSF:SC (typical performance level) ($r = -0.02$, $p = 0.9$). However, the Spearman's rank correlation showed a low negative correlation between the *level of involvement* and the ACSF:SC ($r = -0.32$, $p < 0.01$), and a moderate negative correlation between the *percentage of activity participation* and the ACSF:SC ($r = -0.42$, $p < 0.01$). Because of the scaling of the ACSF:SC, the correlation was negative, but there was a positive association between the level of involvement, percentage of activity participation, and social communication (i.e., the better the social communication ability on the ACSF:SC, the higher the level of involvement and the wider the variety of activities in which the child participates).

Table 3. Environmental features as perceived by parents at home.

Environmental Features	Home Setting			
	% Supports	% Barriers	% No Impact	% Sometime Helps/Sometime Make Harder
Physical Layout	55.0	0.0	25.0	21.0
Sensory Qualities	37.7	1.8	37.7	22.6
Physical Demands	30.2	9.4	39.6	20.8
Cognitive Demands	22.6	24.5	20.8	32.1
Social Demands	26.4	30.2	20.8	20.8
Relationships with Family Members	51.9	3.8	5.8	38.5
Attitudes	34.7	4.1	26.5	32.7
Policies	25.5	17.6	35.3	21.6
Services	25.5	27.5	13.7	31.4
Supplies	97.7	0.0	0.0	2.2
Information	50.0	2.3	0.0	47.7
Time	46.7	11.1	0.0	42.2
Money	46.7	4.4	0.0	48.9

5. Community Setting

Activity frequency and level of involvement: Overall, the frequency of participation in the community activities was lower than those in the home setting (Figure 1b). Children were reported to participate most frequently in shopping and errands (once a week), followed by unstructured physical activities (a few times a month). The lowest frequency observed was 1 (once in the last four months) for classes and lessons, organized physical activities and overnight trips, vacations and visits. However, even with the low frequency, children were reported as being involved when doing these activities. In all of the activities, there were parents who reported that their children never participated in these activities. For example, 73.4% of parents reported that their children never participated in an organized physical activity.

Environmental supports and barriers: The sensory quality of the environment was reported by parents as a barrier for 23.1% of the participants (Table 4). Cognitive and social demands were reported by parents as supportive for 22% and 11.8% of the participants, respectively, while reported as barriers for 24% and 35.3% of the participants, respectively. Parents reported attitudes and relationships with friends to be supportive for 25% and 24% of the participants, respectively. Personal transportation, equipment, and supplies were reported as supports for more than 60% of participants. Time and money to support their children's participation at the community were also reported by 40% of the parents.

Relationship between social communication level and participation: There was very low correlation between the ACSF:SC (typical performance) level and the participation *frequency* or the percentage of activity participation. There was a moderate negative correlation between the ACSF:SC (typical performance) level and the *level of involvement* ($r = -0.41$, $p = < 0.01$). Once again, although the correlation was negative, there was a positive association between the level of involvement and social communication abilities (i.e., the better the social communication ability on the ACSF:SC, the higher the level of involvement when children participate in activities).

ACSF:SC and the environmental supports and barriers: The Spearman's analysis showed very low correlation ($r \leq 0.03$) between the ACSF:SC levels and the environmental supports or barriers for both the home and community settings.

The sample was then divided into three groups based on the size of differences between the best capacity and typical performance levels of the ACSF:SC. In group 1, differences were ≤ -1, in group 2 there were no differences, and in group 3 the differences were $\geq +1$. The ANOVA showed no difference between the groups in terms of home environmental support ($F (2, 50) = 0.08$, $p = 0.9$). Since the environmental barriers at home, as well as environmental supports and barriers in the community were not normally distributed, the Kruskal–Wallis tank test was conducted but no difference was found between groups ($p > 0.05$).

Table 4. Environmental features as perceived by parents in the community.

Environmental Features	Community Setting			
	% Support	% Barrier	% No Impact	% Sometime Helps/Sometime Make Harder
Physical Layout	30.8	5.8	42.3	21.2
Sensory Qualities	11.5	23.1	19.2	44.2
Physical Demands	19.2	7.8	32.7	38.5
Cognitive Demands	22.0	24.0	16.0	38.0
Social Demands	11.8	35.3	13.7	37.3
Attitudes	25.0	11.5	15.4	48.1
Relationship with Peers	24.0	16.0	18.0	42.0
Weather	7.7	11.5	30.8	50.0
Safety	30.8	9.6	36.5	23.1
Policies	26.0	6.0	34.0	34.0
Personal Transportations	76.5	5.9	11.8	5.9
Public Transportations	21.6	5.9	66.7	5.9
Program & Services	35.3	9.8	5.9	49.0
Equipment or Supplies	86.8	0.0	2.6	10.5
Information	43.6	5.0	0.0	51.3
Time	46.2	7.7	0.0	46.2
Money	43.6	5.0	0.0	51.3

6. Discussion

This descriptive study explored participation patterns of preschool children with ASD and factors associated with participation, including the environment and the social communication abilities of the child.

Participation pattern for preschoolers with ASD in different settings: Overall, preschool children with ASD participated in a variety of activities at home. Organized play activities, such as screen time, indoor play, and games, were reported to have the highest frequency, which was also reported in other studies [19,29,42,52]. In fact, in one study, children with ASD had a higher frequency of participation than their typically developed peers in activities such as watching TV and screen time [29]. These activities usually do not involve socializing or engaging with others. Previous studies found that children with ASD usually participate in activities alone or with few people—usually their families [22,42].

Children in this study were also reported to have the lowest frequency of participation in household chores. For example, the mean frequency of participation in meal preparation was 1.8 (out of 7), for taking care of family members was 1.8, and for laundry and dishes was 1.7. These findings were also evident in the literature with preschool and school-aged children with ASD [19,53]. When asked, parents revealed that they did not consider assigning chores to their children with ASD [19]. Parents reported that offering chores to their children with ASD would require a lot of energy to accommodate their children's behaviors and needs, and therefore they chose not to engage them in these activities [19]. Participating in chores could provide children with ASD with the opportunity to practice their problem-solving skills, increase family socializing, teach them to take responsibilities, and prepare them to take care of themselves and others [54,55].

Our findings also indicated that children with ASD generally have lower rates of participation in community settings (mean = 2.9) when compared to a home setting (mean = 5.9). The same findings were reported for children with various disabilities [56,57]. Parents of children with ASD reported having less control over the environment in the community [11,53]. It is more challenging for parents to manage their children's behavior in the community due to the unpredictability of the situations and sensory stimulation. As such, families reported that their energy is spent trying to think about the environment—what to expect and how their child may react [19]. The whole process is exhausting for them and consequently they avoid participating in activities in the community [53]. When considering participation for children with ASD in the community, this highlights the importance of taking the whole family into consideration as a unit, rather than only focusing on the child and their capabilities. These findings are consistent with Bronfenbrenner's Ecological Theory of Human Development [27], in which the child's developmental outcome is influenced by their interactions with different levels of the environment. At the level of the microsystem, child development is influenced by their immediate environment, which typically includes the family [27]. Parents are responsible for offering opportunities for their children to participate [19,53]. In one study, parents reported avoiding dining out or taking their child to grocery stores because of their risk of a behavioral meltdown [53]. This is supported by our findings that even though these children have generally lower frequency of participation in the community, some were reported to have a high level of involvement of participation in activities in the community. For example, participating in overnight trips and vacations had the lowest frequency (1 out of 7) in the community; however, children who participated had the highest level of involvement (3.8 out of 5) compared to all other community activities. Although there were no control groups in the current study to see how patterns of participation in this cohort compare to those of children without ASD, other studies have reported common findings that children with disabilities have lower participation frequency and involvement than children without disabilities [26,28]. Even when children with and without disabilities participated in the same activities, their levels of involvement are different [26].

Environmental barriers and supports: Parents reported a variety of environmental supports and barriers. However, in some cases what was reported as a support for some parents was considered as a barrier for others. For example, 22% of parents considered the cognitive demands of an activity as a support to their child's participation at home; however, the same percentage of parents considered it as a barrier. The same applies for social demands of the activity and the availability of services, where similar percentages of parents had considered it as either a support or a barrier. This underscores the importance of taking into consideration the individual variations among children with ASD and how the needs of each child vary in different contexts [28]. Furthermore, sensory qualities of the environment were considered mainly as a support at the home, while a higher percentage considered it as a barrier in the community. This lends further support to the fact that parents' lack control over the community environment and its impact on their children's participation. It also supports the findings of another study where atypical sensory processing, such as hyper-responsiveness, was associated with lower frequency of activity participation in the community [58].

Relationship between social communication and participation: Our findings indicated that better social communication abilities were associated with a wider variety of activities in which the child participated at home, and higher levels of involvement when participating in these activities. However, in the community, better social communication abilities were only associated with higher level of involvement, which aligns with the findings that identify the complexity of participation in the community and the different factors that impact it.

Clinical Implications

The study findings provide some insights for clinicians who work with children with ASD and their families. One important implication for service providers is actively to encourage parents of preschoolers to involve their children in as wide a range of daily activities and recreational opportunities as possible from a very young age, so that "participation" becomes part of daily life and is not then seen as a prescribed "add-on". Young children's participation in activities is a reflection of their family choices, available opportunities, as well as their abilities and interest. Whereas typically-developing children often take the initiative to be involved in activities, families of children with ASD need to be supported and encouraged to see opportunities to help improve their children's participation at home and in the community. Considering each child's individual needs, clinicians could provide some strategies to improve their participation. For example, household chores could be modified and broken down into several steps that the child could follow to improve various skills, such as their problem-solving skills. Clinicians could also provide some strategies to manage children's behavior in the community to increase their participation. When recommending interventions, clinicians need to take into consideration the family as a whole and any special situations they might have. Clinicians should also be aware of the community with regard to sensitivities, needs, and vulnerabilities of children with ASD.

7. Limitations and Future Research

Results of this study should be considered in light of possible sampling and data limitations, including the small sample size and the study design. Cross sectional data limits our ability to identify whether social communication ability increases participation or whether the opposite is true. However, the PARC study continues to collect longitudinal data, which will provide the opportunity to further examine this in the future. In addition, only families who are enrolled in ASD services were included, which could be a potential source for sample selection bias (access to service bias). For example, children being seen could have complex issues while children with higher cognitive abilities may not be seen within the clinical setting. Furthermore, this study was based on parents' recall and no direct observation of children's participation was conducted. Future studies could include a qualitative dimension for a deeper understanding of children's participation from parents' perspectives. Other factors that may impact on participation, such as socioeconomic status and maternal education, could also be investigated in future studies. Participation patterns could also be investigated longitudinally in future studies. Simpson and colleagues (2019) studied longitudinally the participation pattern of children with ASD who are transitioning to adolescents (age 9 and 10 years old) [48]. Over three years, they found a trend regarding socializing and participating in physical activities (participation declined as children's ages increased) [48]. Similar studies with different age groups are essential and would highlight the important factors to consider for intervention planning to improve or maintain their participation in various activities.

8. Conclusions

This study adds to the emerging body of literature on participation patterns for preschool-aged children with ASD. In addition, it explores the relationship between social communication and participation, which is a key factor central to ASD. Preschool children with ASD participated in various activities at home and in the community, which are the main environments for participation for this age group. However, parents need support to facilitate and improve their children's participation in both settings. Furthermore, for interventions to be successful, especially those intended to modify the environment, the individuality of children with ASD, with variable abilities, should be acknowledged and considered when planning intervention goals. In addition, interventions should go beyond modifying the environment around the children and consider the environments that support them, including their family.

Supplementary Materials: The following are available online at http://www.mdpi.com/1660-4601/17/16/5677/s1, Table S1: Percentage of children participation frequency and level of involvement.

Author Contributions: G.K. and B.D.R. conceptualized the idea and methodology for this study. Data curation, investigation, and formal analysis of the data were conducted by G.K. and validated by E.D., G.K. was responsible for the original draft preparation. B.D.R., P.R., K.G., and E.D. were responsible for reviewing and editing the manuscript, and B.D.R. supervised the project. All authors have read and agreed to the published version of the manuscript.

Funding: Funding support for this study was provided by the following: The Hamilton Health Science Research Early Career Award (ECA) 2018–2020; the Hamilton Health Sciences New Investigator Fund (NIF) 2019.

Acknowledgments: The authors thank all the children and families who participated in the PARC Project. The authors also acknowledge Stelios Georgiades and Anna Kata from the PARC Project Team for their support, as well as the research staff members and trainees who contributed to this study. This study was supported by the Faculty of Health Sciences and Department of Psychiatry & Behavioural Neurosciences at McMaster University, McMaster Children's Hospital Research Collaborative, Hamilton Health Sciences, and by an award from the Autism Spectrum Disorders Research Project of Grand Master Paul E Todd-2017–19. At the time of writing, G.K. was supported by a scholarship from King Saud University for Health Sciences, Jeddah, Saudi Arabia.

Conflicts of Interest: The authors declare no conflict of interest.

References

1. World Health Organization. *International Classification of Functioning, Disability and Health: ICF*; World Health Organization: Geneva, Switzerland, 2001.
2. Maxwell, G.; Alves, I.; Granlund, M. Participation and environmental aspects in education and the ICF and the ICF-CY: Findings from a systematic literature review. *Dev. Neurorehabilit.* **2012**, *15*, 63–78. [CrossRef] [PubMed]
3. Granlund, M.; Arvidsson, P.; Niia, A.; Björck, E.-A.; Simeonsson, R.; Maxwell, G.; Adolfsson, M.; Eriksson, L.-A.; Pless, M. Differentiating activity and participation of children and youth with disability in Sweden: A third qualifier in the International Classification of Functioning, Disability, and Health for Children and Youth? *Am. J. Phys. Med. Rehabil.* **2012**, *91*, S84–S96. [CrossRef] [PubMed]
4. Coster, W.; Law, M.; Bedell, G.; Khetani, M.; Cousins, M.; Teplicky, R. Development of the participation and environment measure for children and youth: Conceptual basis. *Disabil. Rehabil.* **2012**, *34*, 238–246. [CrossRef]
5. Imms, C.; Adair, B.; Keen, D.; Ullenhag, A.; Rosenbaum, P.; Granlund, M. 'Participation': A systematic review of language, definitions, and constructs used in intervention research with children with disabilities. *Dev. Med. Child Neurol.* **2016**, *58*, 29–38. [CrossRef] [PubMed]
6. Adair, B.; Ullenhag, A.; Rosenbaum, P.; Granlund, M.; Keen, D.; Imms, C. Measures used to quantify participation in childhood disability and their alignment with the family of participation-related constructs: A systematic review. *Dev. Med. Child Neurol.* **2018**, *60*, 1101–1116. [CrossRef] [PubMed]
7. Nina, K.; Sigrid, Ø. A Comparative ICF-CY–Based Analysis and Cultural Piloting of the Assessment of Preschool Children's Participation (APCP). *Phys. Occup. Ther. Pediatr.* **2015**, *35*, 54–72. [CrossRef]
8. Albrecht, E.C.; Khetani, M.A. Environmental impact on young children's participation in home-based activities. *Dev. Med. Child Neurol.* **2017**, *59*, 388–394. [CrossRef]
9. Guichard, S.; Grande, C. The role of environment in explaining frequency of participation of pre-school children in home and community activities. *Int. J. Dev. Disabil.* **2019**, *65*, 108–115. [CrossRef]
10. Bandura, A.; Walters, R.H. *Social Learning Theory*; Prentice-Hall: Englewood Cliffs, NJ, USA, 1977.

11. Rosenberg, L.; Bart, O.; Ratzon, N.Z.; Jarus, T. Personal and environmental factors predict participation of children with and without mild developmental disabilities. *J. Child Fam. Stud.* **2013**, *22*, 658–671. [CrossRef]
12. Data and Statistics on Autism Spectrum Disorder|CDC. Centers for Disease Control and Prevention. 2020. Available online: https://www.cdc.gov/ncbddd/autism/data.html (accessed on 1 July 2020).
13. Public Health Agency of Canada. Autism Spectrum Disorder among Children and Youth with ASD in Canada 2018-Canada.Ca. Canada.ca. 2018. Available online: https://www.canada.ca/en/public-health/services/publications/diseases-conditions/autism-spectrum-disorder-children-youth-canada-2018.html (accessed on 27 March 2020).
14. Shulman, C.; Esler, A.; Morrier, M.J.; Rice, C.E. Diagnosis of Autism Spectrum Disorder across the Lifespan. *Child Adolesc. Psychiatr. Clin.* **2020**, *29*, 253–273. [CrossRef]
15. Meirsschaut, M.; Roeyers, H.; Warreyn, P. Parenting in families with a child with autism spectrum disorder and a typically developing child: Mothers' experiences and cognitions. *Res. Autism Spectr. Disord.* **2010**, *4*, 661–669. [CrossRef]
16. Parten, M.B. Social participation among pre-school children. *J. Abnorm. Soc. Psychol.* **1932**, *27*, 243. [CrossRef]
17. Law, M.; King, G.; Petrenchik, T.; Kertoy, M.; Anaby, D. The assessment of preschool children's participation: Internal consistency and construct validity. *Phys. Occup. Ther. Pediatr.* **2012**, *32*, 272–287. [CrossRef] [PubMed]
18. Kellegrew, D.H. Creating opportunities for occupation: An intervention to promote the self-care independence of young children with special needs. *Am. J. Occup. Ther.* **1998**, *52*, 457–465. [CrossRef]
19. LaVesser, P.; Berg, C. Participation patterns in preschool children with an autism spectrum disorder. *OTJR Occup. Particip. Health* **2011**, *31*, 33–39. [CrossRef]
20. Rodger, S.; Umaibalan, V. The routines and rituals of families of typically developing children compared with families of children with autism spectrum disorder: An exploratory study. *Br. J. Occup. Ther.* **2011**, *74*, 20–26. [CrossRef]
21. Hochhauser, M.; Engel-Yeger, B. Sensory processing abilities and their relation to participation in leisure activities among children with high-functioning autism spectrum disorder (HFASD). *Res. Autism Spectr. Disord.* **2010**, *4*, 746–754. [CrossRef]
22. Reynolds, S.; Bendixen, R.M.; Lawrence, T.; Lane, S.J. A pilot study examining activity participation, sensory responsiveness, and competence in children with high functioning autism spectrum disorder. *J. Autism Dev. Disord.* **2011**, *41*, 1496–1506. [CrossRef]
23. Lawlor, M.C. The significance of being occupied: The social construction of childhood occupations. *Am. J. Occup. Ther.* **2003**, *57*, 424–434. [CrossRef]
24. Coussens, M.; van Driessen, E.; De Baets, S.; van Regenmortel, J.; Desoete, A.; Oostra, A.; Vanderstraeten, G.; Waelvelde, H.V.; van de Velde, D. Parents' perspectives on participation of young children with attention deficit hyperactivity disorder, developmental coordination disorder, and/or autism spectrum disorder: A systematic scoping review. *Child CareHealth Dev.* **2020**, *46*, 232–243. [CrossRef]
25. Thompson, D.; Emira, M. 'They say every child matters, but they don't': An investigation into parental and carer perceptions of access to leisure facilities and respite care for children and young people with Autistic Spectrum Disorder (ASD) or Attention Deficit, Hyperactivity Disorder (ADHD). *Disabil. Soc.* **2011**, *26*, 65–78.
26. Askari, S.; Anaby, D.; Bergthorson, M.; Majnemer, A.; Elsabbagh, M.; Zwaigenbaum, L. Participation of children and youth with autism spectrum disorder: A scoping review. *Rev. J. Autism Dev. Disord.* **2015**, *2*, 103–114. [CrossRef]
27. Bronfenbrenner, U. Toward an experimental ecology of human development. *Am. Psychol.* **1977**, *32*, 513. [CrossRef]
28. Egilson, S.T.; Jakobsdóttir, G.; Ólafsson, K.; Leósdóttir, T. Community participation and environment of children with and without autism spectrum disorder: Parent perspectives. *Scand. J. Occup. Ther.* **2017**, *24*, 187–196. [CrossRef]
29. Egilson, S.T.; Jakobsdóttir, G.; Ólafsdóttir, L.B. Parent perspectives on home participation of high-functioning children with autism spectrum disorder compared with a matched group of children without autism spectrum disorder. *Autism* **2018**, *22*, 560–570. [CrossRef]
30. King, G.; Law, M.; Hanna, S.; King, S.; Hurley, P.; Rosenbaum, P.; Kertoy, M.; Petrenchik, T. Predictors of the leisure and recreation participation of children with physical disabilities: A structural equation modeling analysis. *Child. Health Care* **2006**, *35*, 209–234. [CrossRef]

31. Imms, C.; Reilly, S.; Carlin, J.; Dodd, K.J. Characteristics influencing participation of Australian children with cerebral palsy. *Disabil. Rehabil.* **2009**, *31*, 2204–2215. [CrossRef]
32. Bedell, G.M. Developing a follow-up survey focused on participation of children and youth with acquired brain injuries after discharge from inpatient rehabilitation. *NeuroRehabilitation* **2004**, *19*, 191–205. [CrossRef]
33. Coster, W.; Bedell, G.; Law, M.; Khetani, M.A.; Teplicky, R.; Liljenquist, K.; Gleason, K.; Kao, Y.C. Psychometric evaluation of the Participation and Environment Measure for Children and Youth. *Dev. Med. Child Neurol.* **2011**, *53*, 1030–1037. [CrossRef]
34. Khetani, M.A.; Coster, W.; Law, M.; Bedell, G.M. *Young Children's Participation and Environment Measure (YC-PEM)*; (Copyright to Authors); Colorado State University: Fort Collins, CO, USA, 2013.
35. Law, M. Participation in the occupations of everyday life. *Am. J. Occup. Ther.* **2002**, *56*, 640–649. [CrossRef]
36. Pinquart, M.; Teubert, D. Academic, physical, and social functioning of children and adolescents with chronic physical illness: A meta-analysis. *J. Pediatr. Psychol.* **2012**, *37*, 376–389. [CrossRef] [PubMed]
37. Tajik, D.-P.; Hidecker, M.J.C.; Selvakumaran, S.; Fan, L.; Batth, S.; Fang, H.; Ross, B.; Stone, A.C.; Reed, B.; Kunitz, C.; et al. Operationalizing Social Communication in Autism Research: A Scoping Review over 20 years. *Curr. Dev. Disord. Rep.*. Under review.
38. Bishop, S.; Farmer, C.; Kaat, A.; Georgiades, S.; Kanne, S.; Thurm, A. The need for a developmentally based measure of social-communication skills. *J. Am. Acad. Child Adolesc. Psychiatry* **2019**, *58*, 555. [CrossRef] [PubMed]
39. King, G.; Lawm, M.; King, S.; Rosenbaum, P.; Kertoy, M.K.; Young, N.L. A conceptual model of the factors affecting the recreation and leisure participation of children with disabilities. *Phys. Occup. Ther. Pediatr.* **2003**, *23*, 63–90. [CrossRef]
40. American Psychiatric Association. *Diagnostic and Statistical Manual of Mental Disorders (DSM-5®)*; American Psychiatric Pub: Washington, DC, USA, 2013.
41. Syriopoulou-Delli, C.K.; Agaliotis, I.; Papaefstathiou, E. Social skills characteristics of students with autism spectrum disorder. *Int. J. Dev. Disabil.* **2018**, *64*, 35–44. [CrossRef]
42. Simpson, K.; Keen, D.; Adams, D.; Alston-Knox, C.; Roberts, J. Participation of children on the autism spectrum in home, school, and community. *Child CareHealth Dev.* **2018**, *44*, 99–107. [CrossRef]
43. Khetani, M.; Graham, J.E.; Alvord, C. Community participation patterns among preschool-aged children who have received Part C early intervention services. *Child CareHealth Dev.* **2013**, *39*, 490–499. [CrossRef]
44. Law, M.; Anaby, D.; Teplicky, R.; Khetani, M.A.; Coster, W.; Bedell, G. Participation in the home environment among children and youth with and without disabilities. *Br. J. Occup. Ther.* **2013**, *76*, 58–66. [CrossRef]
45. Ullenhag, A.; Krumlinde-Sundholm, L.; Granlund, M.; Almqvist, L. Differences in patterns of participation in leisure activities in Swedish children with and without disabilities. *Disabil. Rehabil.* **2014**, *36*, 464–471. [CrossRef]
46. Dunst, C.J.; Bruder, M.B.; Trivette, C.M.; Hamby, D.W. Everyday activity settings, natural learning environments, and early intervention practices. *J. Policy Pract. Intellect. Disabil.* **2006**, *3*, 3–10. [CrossRef]
47. Khetani, M.A.; Graham, J.E.; Davies, P.L.; Law, M.C.; Simeonsson, R.J. Psychometric properties of the young children's participation and environment measure. *Arch. Phys. Med. Rehabil.* **2015**, *96*, 307–316. [CrossRef] [PubMed]
48. Simpson, K.; Adams, D.; Bruck, S.; Keen, D. Investigating the participation of children on the autism spectrum across home, school, and community: A longitudinal study. *Child CareHealth Dev.* **2019**, *45*, 681–687. [CrossRef] [PubMed]
49. ACSF: SC Tool_User Guide. Canchild.ca. 2016. Available online: https://canchild.ca/en/resources/254-autism-classification-system-of-functioningsocial-communication-acsf-sc (accessed on 28 February 2020).
50. Di Rezze, B.; Rosenbaum, P.; Zwaigenbaum, L.; Hidecker, M.J.; Stratford, P.; Cousins, M.; Camden, C.; Law, M. Developing a classification system of social communication functioning of preschool children with autism spectrum disorder. *Dev. Med. Child Neurol.* **2016**, *58*, 942–948. [CrossRef] [PubMed]
51. Mallinson, T.; Hammel, J. Measurement of participation: Intersecting person, task, and environment. *Arch. Phys. Med. Rehabil.* **2010**, *91*, S29–S33. [CrossRef]
52. Di Marino, E.; Tremblay, S.; Khetani, M.; Anaby, D. The effect of child, family and environmental factors on the participation of young children with disabilities. *Disabil. Health J.* **2018**, *11*, 36–42. [CrossRef]
53. Larson, E.A. The orchestration of occupation: The dance of mothers. *Am. J. Occup. Ther.* **2000**, *54*, 269–280. [CrossRef]

54. DeGrace, B.W. The everyday occupation of families with children with autism. *Am. J. Occup. Ther.* **2004**, *58*, 543–550. [CrossRef]
55. Dunst, C.J.; Hamby, D.; Trivette, C.M.; Raab, M.; Bruder, M.B. Everyday family and community life and children's naturally occurring learning opportunities. *J. Early Interv.* **2000**, *23*, 151–164. [CrossRef]
56. Lim, C.Y.; Law, M.; Khetani, M.; Pollock, N.; Rosenbaum, P. Participation in out-of-home environments for young children with and without developmental disabilities. *OTJR Occup. Particip. Health* **2016**, *36*, 112–125. [CrossRef]
57. Jeong, Y.; Law, M.; Stratford, P.; DeMatteo, C.; Missiuna, C. Measuring participation of children and environmental factors at home, school, and in community: Construct validation of the Korean PEM-CY. *Phys. Occup. Ther. Pediatr.* **2017**, *37*, 541–554. [CrossRef]
58. Little, L.M.; Ausderau, K.; Sideris, J.; Baranek, G.T. Activity participation and sensory features among children with autism spectrum disorders. *J. Autism Dev. Disord.* **2015**, *45*, 2981–2990. [CrossRef] [PubMed]

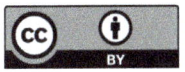

© 2020 by the authors. Licensee MDPI, Basel, Switzerland. This article is an open access article distributed under the terms and conditions of the Creative Commons Attribution (CC BY) license (http://creativecommons.org/licenses/by/4.0/).

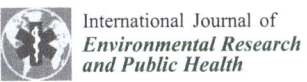

Concept Paper

Definitions and Operationalization of Mental Health Problems, Wellbeing and Participation Constructs in Children with NDD: Distinctions and Clarifications

Mats Granlund [1,2,*], Christine Imms [3], Gillian King [4], Anna Karin Andersson [1,2], Lilly Augustine [2,5], Rob Brooks [6], Henrik Danielsson [2,7], Jennifer Gothilander [8], Magnus Ivarsson [2,7], Lars-Olov Lundqvist [2,9], Frida Lygnegård [1,2] and Lena Almqvist [8]

1. CHILD, School of Health and Welfare, Jönköping University, 55110 Jönköping, Sweden; annakarin.andersson@ju.se (A.K.A.); frida.lygnegard@ju.se (F.L.)
2. The Swedish Institute for Disability Research, 58183 Linköping, Sweden; lilly.augustine@ju.se (L.A.); henrik.danielsson@liu.se (H.D.); magnus.ivarsson@liu.se (M.I.); lars-olov.lundqvist@regionorebrolan.se (L.-O.L.)
3. Department of Paediatrics, The University of Melbourne, Melbourne 3052, Australia; christine.imms@unimelb.edu.au
4. Bloorview Research Institute, Torornto, ON M4G 1R8, Canada; gking27@uwo.ca
5. CHILD, School of Education and Communication, Jönköping University, 55110 Jönköping, Sweden
6. School of Clinical and Applied Sciences, Leeds Beckett University, Leeds LS1 3HE, UK; r.b.brooks@leedsbeckett.ac.uk
7. Department of Behavioural Sciences and Learning, Linköping University, 58183 Linköping, Sweden
8. School of Health, Care and Social Welfare, Mälardalen University, 72123 Vasteras, Sweden; jennifer.gothilander@mdh.se (J.G.); lena.almqvist@ju.se (L.A.)
9. University Health Care Research Center, Faculty of Medicine and Health, Örebro University, 70185 Örebro, Sweden
* Correspondence: mats.granlund@ju.se; Tel.: +46-36-10-12-21

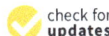

Citation: Granlund, M.; Imms, C.; King, G.; Andersson, A.K.; Augustine, L.; Brooks, R.; Danielsson, H.; Gothilander, J.; Ivarsson, M.; Lundqvist, L.-O.; et al. Definitions and Operationalization of Mental Health Problems, Wellbeing and Participation Constructs in Children with NDD: Distinctions and Clarifications. *Int. J. Environ. Res. Public Health* **2021**, *18*, 1656. https://doi.org/10.3390/ijerph18041656

Academic Editor: Paul B. Tchounwou
Received: 2 December 2020
Accepted: 2 February 2021
Published: 9 February 2021

Publisher's Note: MDPI stays neutral with regard to jurisdictional claims in published maps and institutional affiliations.

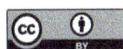

Copyright: © 2021 by the authors. Licensee MDPI, Basel, Switzerland. This article is an open access article distributed under the terms and conditions of the Creative Commons Attribution (CC BY) license (https://creativecommons.org/licenses/by/4.0/).

Abstract: Children with impairments are known to experience more restricted participation than other children. It also appears that low levels of participation are related to a higher prevalence of mental health problems in children with neurodevelopmental disorders (NDD). The purpose of this conceptual paper is to describe and define the constructs mental health problems, mental health, and participation to ensure that future research investigating participation as a means to mental health in children and adolescents with NDD is founded on conceptual clarity. We first discuss the difference between two aspects of *mental health problems*, namely mental disorder and mental illness. This discussion serves to highlight three areas of conceptual difficulty and their consequences for understanding the mental health of children with NDD that we then consider in the article: (1) how to define mental health problems, (2) how to define and assess mental health problems and mental health, i.e., wellbeing as separate constructs, and (3) how to describe the relationship between participation and wellbeing. We then discuss the implications of our propositions for measurement and the use of participation interventions as a means to enhance mental health (defined as wellbeing). Conclusions: Mental disorders include both diagnoses related to impairments in the developmental period, i.e., NDD and diagnoses related to mental illness. These two types of mental disorders must be separated. Children with NDD, just like other people, may exhibit aspects of both *mental health problems* and wellbeing simultaneously. Measures of wellbeing defined as a continuum from flourishing to languishing for children with NDD need to be designed and evaluated. Wellbeing can lead to further participation and act to protect from mental health problems.

Keywords: concept; mental health problems; mental health; wellbeing; participation; concept

1. Introduction

Children with impairments are known to experience more restricted participation than other children [1]. It also appears that low levels of participation are related to a higher prevalence of mental health problems in children with neurodevelopmental disorders (NDD) [2,3]. NDD is a group of early onset conditions associated primarily with the functioning of the neurological system and brain, including diagnoses such as attention-deficit/hyperactivity disorder, autism, and intellectual disability [4]; sometimes, cerebral palsy is also seen as an example of NDD, although it is primarily presented as a motor disorder in DSM-V. NDDs lead to impairments in physical, social, or academic functioning, which affect different aspects of participation.

In the Family of Participation Related Constructs (fPRC) framework, participation is described as consisting of two dimensions: physical or virtual attendance in activities, which is seen as a necessary prerequisite for the second dimension, involvement while attending the activity [5]. The fPRC framework builds on the International Classification of Functioning, Disability, and Health (ICF) definition of participation [6] by specifying two separate dimensions of attendance and involvement. It has been suggested that participation is a determinant of mental health [7]; however there is not currently a deep understanding of the relationships between mental health and participation within NDD.

While a higher prevalence of mental health problems is reported for children with impairments [3,8], especially for children with NDD, the suppositions behind the higher prevalence are implicit rather than explicit. In medical literature, mental health is commonly defined as the absence of mental health problems [9], but without a clear definition of the construct of mental health being provided. Based on Jahoda [10], Westerhof and Keyes [11] suggest that mental health is a positive phenomenon that is more than the absence of mental health problems. They define mental health in terms of hedonistic and eudaimonic wellbeing, which is also the definition we will defend in this article.

Children and adolescents with NDD seldom receive non-pharmacological mental health interventions specifically aimed at reducing mental health problems [12], although studies aimed at increasing subjective wellbeing with the help of mindfulness intervention exist [13]. We suggest that participation interventions—that is, those that aim to improve attendance or involvement in varied life situations—can be implemented to strengthen mental health as well as indirectly prevent or decrease mental health problems in children and adolescents with NDD. Thus, interventions aimed at increasing participation may be a means to increase perceived mental health [14,15]. To test this proposal, the conceptual relations between mental health problems, mental health (defined as wellbeing), and participation need to be clarified. The purpose of this paper is to describe and define these constructs to ensure that future research investigating participation as a means to mental health is founded on conceptual clarity.

To achieve our purpose, we first discuss the difference between two aspects of mental health problems, namely mental disorder and mental illness. This discussion serves to highlight three areas of conceptual difficulty and their consequences for understanding the mental health of children with NDD that we then consider in the remainder of this article: (1) how to define mental health problems (and delimit them from mental disorders and mental illness), (2) how to define and assess mental health problems and mental health (i.e., wellbeing) as separate constructs, and (3) how to describe the relationship between participation and wellbeing. We then discuss the implications of our propositions for measurement and the use of participation interventions as a means to enhance mental health (defined as wellbeing), thus proposing a way forward.

2. Issues of Classification of Mental Disorders and NDD in Diagnostic Manuals

In the ICF, aspects of functioning disability and health are classified as body structure and function, activity, and participation, thereby building on a bio-psycho-social model. The ICF is supposed to be a supplement to the diagnostic manuals used in medicine disorders, the International Classification of Diseases (ICD-11) [4], and mental disorders, the Diagnostic Systems Manual (DSM 5) [16]. These diagnostic systems include NDD, for example, intellectual disability and ADHD, within the classification of types of mental disorder, along with schizophrenia, depression, and disorders due to substance abuse [6]. In the ICD-11, mental disorders are defined and described in chapter 6: Mental, behavioral, or neurodevelopmental disorders. This chapter states:

> *"Mental, behavioral and neurodevelopmental disorders are syndromes characterized by clinically significant disturbance in an individual's cognition, emotional regulation, or behavior that reflects a dysfunction in the psychological, biological, or developmental processes that underlie mental and behavioral functioning. These disturbances are usually associated with distress or impairment in personal, family, social, educational, occupational, or other important areas of functioning."* (Chapter 6, p.1 ICD-11, 2020)

In this description, the relationship between mental disorders and everyday functioning is emphasized. The definition provides core aspects to look for when diagnosing mental disorders (cognitive, emotional, or social abilities and behavior), but it is only in the subclassifications that a distinction is made between NDD and mental illnesses such as depression or general anxiety disorder. In discriminating between different mental disorders, the ICD-11 states that NDD is characterized by symptoms that emerge in the developmental period; however, this characteristic is not unique to NDD, as other mental disorders may also present in the developmental period.

Because classification systems like ICD-11 and DSM-V are designed to define "disease" or "condition", they do not define positive mental health and do not explicitly make a distinction between bio-psycho-social levels. Unless outcomes in terms of mental health are clearly defined, it is difficult to assess mental health other than as the absence of a disease or condition. Unless mental health outcomes are clearly defined, it is difficult to plan interventions aimed at improving mental health for children and adolescents with NDD, because no positive outcome other than lack of mental health problems is described. In Table 1, definitions of the terms used in this paper are presented.

Table 1. Definitions of key terms.

Mental disorder	Mental, behavioral, and neurodevelopmental disorders are syndromes characterized by clinically significant disturbance in an individual's cognition, emotional regulation, or behavior that reflects a dysfunction in the psychological, biological, or developmental processes that underlie mental and behavioral functioning. These disturbances are usually associated with distress or impairment in personal, family, social, educational, occupational, or other important areas of functioning. ICD 11, version 09/2020, chapter 6 (http://id.who.int/icd/entity/334423054) [4]
Neurodevelopmental disorder	Neurodevelopmental disorders are behavioral and cognitive disorders that arise during the developmental period that involve significant difficulties in the acquisition and execution of specific intellectual, motor, language, or social functions. Although behavioral and cognitive deficits are present in many mental and behavioral disorders that can arise during the developmental period (e.g., Schizophrenia, Bipolar disorder), only disorders whose core features are neurodevelopmental are included in this grouping. The presumptive etiology for neurodevelopmental disorders is complex, and in many individual cases is unknown. ICD 11, version 09/2020, chapter 6 (http://id.who.int/icd/entity/1516623224) [4]
Mental illness	Mental illness (mental ill health) includes severe mental health problems and strain, impaired functioning associated with distress, symptoms and diagnosable mental disorders (e.g., schizophrenia, bipolar disorder) (European Commission, 2005) [17]
Mental health problems	A broad concept covering both less serious mental strain and more severe symptoms, fulfilling criteria for a diagnosable mental illness [9]

Table 1. Cont.

Mental health	"is a state of wellbeing in which an individual realizes his or her own abilities, can cope with the normal stresses of life, can work productively and fruitfully, and is able to make a contribution to his or her community" [18] (p. 2). Mental health defined as wellbeing vary over the life course. The description of wellbeing below is here used as an operationalization of mental health.
Wellbeing as mental health	Wellbeing's positive emotional states include the two different ideas of happiness: hedonic (happiness or pleasure), that is living a pleasant life, or eudemonic (striving for, achieving something more—either personal growth or something outside the self), that is, living a goal directed or meaningful life [19,20].
Flourishing	"Adults with complete mental health are flourishing in life with high levels of wellbeing. To be flourishing, then, is to be filled with positive emotion and to be functioning well psychologically and socially." [20]
Languishing	A state of a low level of wellbeing described as unhappiness and experiencing difficulties: "Adults with incomplete mental health are languishing in life with low wellbeing. Thus, languishing may be conceived of as emptiness and stagnation, constituting a life of quiet despair that parallels accounts of individuals who describe themselves and life as "hollow", "empty", "a shell", and "a void" [20]. The definition focuses on low levels of wellbeing rather than expressions of mental health problems.
Participation	Involvement in a life situation comprising of two dimensions: attendance and involvement [5].
Participation as attendance	"Being there", that is being present (physically or virtually) in the life situation [5].
Participation as involvement	The "experience of participation while attending the life situation" [5].

3. Core Difficulties with the Definition and Operationalization of the Constructs Defined for Children with NDD

We identify three core difficulties with definitions and operationalization of these constructs:

Problem 1. How to define mental health problems in children with NDD and delimit them from mental disorders and mental illness.

Problem 2. How to define and assess mental health problems and wellbeing as separate constructs in children with NDD.

Problem 3. How to describe the relationship between participation and wellbeing in children with NDD.

3.1. Problem 1: Distinguishing Mental Health Problems from Mental Illness and Mental Disorders in Children with NDD

We propose that any construct and measure of mental health problems should be equally applicable for children and adolescents, regardless of cognitive and physical impairment, and without defining mental illness as equal to the impairment

The constructs mental disorders, mental illness, and mental health problems all concern problems related to mental function. In this section, we first discuss the relationship between mental disorders and mental illness and thereafter the relationship between mental illness and mental health problems.

3.1.1. Mental Disorders and Mental Illness—The Example of NDD

The World Health Organization [6] provides a general definition of a health condition as: "an umbrella term for disease (acute or chronic), disorder, injury or trauma. A health condition may also include other circumstances such as pregnancy, ageing, stress, congenital anomaly, or genetic predisposition" [6], (p. 228). The definition of a mental disorder seems to build on the general definition of a health condition [4]. Mental illness is not formally defined in the ICD-11 but is, in everyday language, used to describe mental disorders other than NDD, such as mood disorders, anxiety, and fears [9]. In the ICD-11, NDD diagnoses are included as examples of mental disorders. The definition of NDD (see Table 1) stresses that NDD concerns cognitive and behavioral problems that arise during the developmental period. This implies that NDD has qualities distinct from other mental disorders and is, therefore, a sub-category of its own. One could argue, however, that there is a good case for not separating different diagnoses based on whether they indicate cognitive difficulties or not, since, for example, cognitive impairments are also a part of the clinical picture in severe depression (in that case time-limited), schizophrenia (more permanent in nature), and addiction. The fact that NDD primarily concern intellectual, motor, and/or social functions that are more or less permanent, compared to mental health problems, and arise during the developmental period provides an argument for separating NDD from mental disorders that can be described as mental illness.

3.1.2. Mental Illness and Mental Health Problems

In their conceptual analysis of mental health, mental disorders, and mental health problems, Bremberg and Dalman [9] illustrate the overlap between the constructs using a figure. We have adapted their figure by making a distinction between mental disorders and mental illness to illustrate our argument (made above) that NDD does not necessarily involve mental illness (see Figure 1).

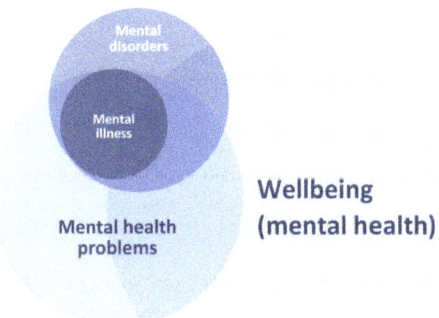

Figure 1. Relations between different concepts used when discussing mental health.

As Figure 1 illustrates, in many cases mental health problems overlap with wellbeing: mental health problems are a normal part of people's lives, but so is wellbeing. However, mental health problems also partly overlap with mental illness: having persistent mental health problems in childhood increases the probability of being diagnosed with a mental illness in adulthood [21]. Figure 1 also shows that mental illness is completely subsumed within mental health problems, but some mental disorders (e.g., NDD) do not automatically overlap with mental illness or mental health problems.

3.1.3. Difficulties in Defining and Operationalizing Mental Health Problems Following from Conceptual Diffuseness

When definitions of constructs or diagnoses, such as mental health and NDD, are restricted to separate and different levels of the bio-psycho-social model, there is no risk for confusion or overlap, e.g., between traumatic brain injury, which is defined primarily on basis of etiology on the biological level, and behavior problems (as measured by CBCL). However, the risk for confusion between symptom-based diagnoses, such as NDDs, and mental health constructs operating at the same level(s) of the model, is more probable.

An example of a very practical consequence of the conceptual overlap between a mental disorder and a mental health problem, which may create conceptual confusion, is how authors define mental health problems when screening children with NDD. A study by Bailey et al. [22] used two indexes of mental health difficulties, as suggested for typical populations [23], namely internalizing (emotional and peer problems) and externalizing (conduct and hyperactivity) mental health difficulties, based on the definition of a mental disorder. The same type of indices is used with other "problem behavior" screening instruments, such as the Child Behavior Checklist (CBCL) [24]. Using this operationalization, children with intellectual disability have significantly more mental health problems than typically functioning children. However, this fusion of what may be factors related to cognitive impairments (i.e., communication/peer problems and hyperactivity) and behavior problems (i.e., emotion and conduct problems) may in fact lead to an overestimation of the prevalence of externalizing and internalizing mental health problems among children and adolescents with diagnoses of NDDs.

Longitudinal studies of behavior problems involving children and adolescents with diagnosed NDD [21] and children with self-reported NDD problems [25] suggest that there is a continuum of chronicity for common mental disorders. These studies suggest that problems not necessarily related to mental illness but to consequences of cognitive impairments (hyperactivity and peer problems) have stronger stability over time than mental disorders that can be described as mental illness (i.e., anxiety and depression).

Mental illness is seen as a severe and intensive type of mental health problem, situated completely within the broader circle of mental health problems (see Figure 1). The point at which mental health problems are severe enough to be diagnosed as a mental illness is debatable and somewhat arbitrary [9]. Most mental health problems have a shorter duration and less severity than a mental illness. Mental illnesses are primarily identified through diagnostic interviews where the person is required to meet certain criteria regarding the severity and persistence of problems to receive a diagnosis.

Longitudinal studies of mental health problems are needed to investigate relationships between mental health problems, such as conduct problems, anxiety, and sadness/depression (mental illness), and NDD, a mental disorder separate from mental illness.

3.1.4. Mental Health Problems and Wellbeing (Mental Health) over the Life Course

Mental health problems vary over the life course with certain periods, such as adolescence, having both biological change and changes in life role expectations that increase the likelihood of mental health problems. Periods of more, or fewer, mental health problems exist in life for all people. We have used Halfon et al.'s [26] illustration, originally intended to describe changes in "health" over the life span, to visualize the life span trajectories of mental health problems and mental health (see Figure 2). Figure 2 illustrates that mental health problems can vary over time on a continuum from no problems to severe mental health problems. It is possible that neither complete wellbeing nor severe mental health problems/mental illness occur frequently. The same figure can be used to illustrate variations over the life span in mental health, defined as a state of wellbeing (see Table 1). When studying the trajectories of mental health problems in children with NDD, we are primarily interested in how mental health problems vary over time. Studying the occurrence of mental health problems may, however, not be enough—wellbeing is also important.

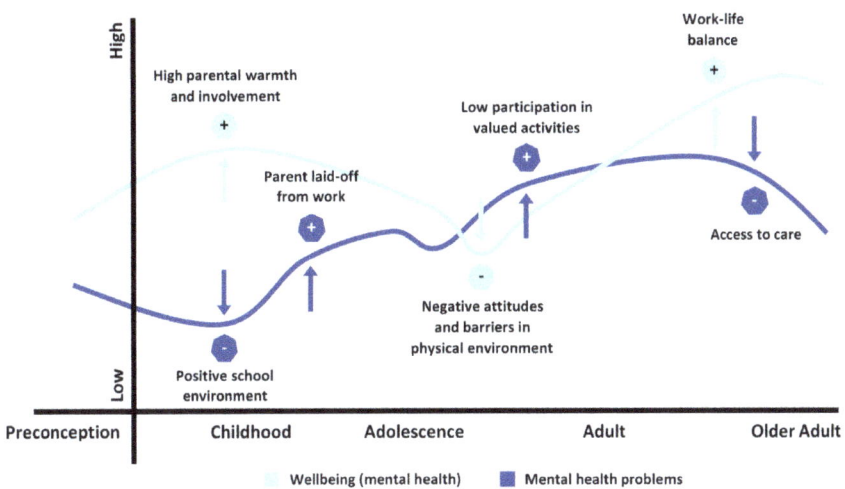

Figure 2. Wellbeing in a life span perspective, adapted from Halfon et al. (2014) [26].

3.2. Problem 2: Distinguishing Mental Health Problems and Wellbeing as Separate Constructs in Children with NDD

We propose that mental health should not be reduced to the absence of mental illness, but should encompass variations in mental health on a continuum from low to high levels of wellbeing.

Research in positive psychology and related fields have employed numerous conceptualizations of positive mental health and wellbeing [27,28]. Each understanding of the concept may present advantages and disadvantages, and arguments for each definition could be based on validity, pragmatic aspects, logic, and so forth. One characteristic of a construct that is sometimes overlooked is whether its definition is equally valid for the full width of human experience and functioning. If the overarching goal in wellbeing research is to describe universal as well as unique aspects of human functioning, then there is relatively little utility for concepts that are only valid for a subgroup of humanity, such as typically developed adults in western countries.

3.2.1. Mental Health—A Multidimensional Wellbeing Concept

The WHO's definition of mental health [18] explicitly equates mental health with wellbeing. The WHO's definition can be used easily when working with adults without severe cognitive impairments. It is not as easy to apply to children and adolescents within the NDD spectrum, because their ability to meet aspects of the definition—"realizing abilities, cope with stress, work productively, and make a contribution to society"—may, by definition, preclude a determination of "wellbeing".

Usually, wellbeing is seen as comprising positive emotional states (feeling good) [29–32] and as having fewer/lower negative emotional states [31,33]. Some authors also describe good functioning as being a part of wellbeing [29,30], including having a command over resources or achieving a balance between resources and challenges [34]. In a study of student perspectives, wellbeing was found to be related to being (e.g., happy, satisfied), having (e.g., rights, relationships, resources, voice), and doing (e.g., looking after self and others, having goals, and making good decisions) [35]. The three dimensions of being, having, and doing can apply to all people, including children with NDD, and can be linked to two dominating, broad perspectives in wellbeing research: hedonia and eudaimonia [36]. Thus, wellbeing's positive emotional states include the two different ideas of happiness: hedonic (happiness or pleasure), that is living a pleasant life, or eudemonic (striving for, achieving something more—either personal growth or something outside the self), that is, living a goal directed or meaningful life [19]. People experience both hedonic and eudemonic happiness but may seek or value one type of wellbeing more than the other. In children and adolescents with significant NDD, the "doing" and edudaimonic elements of wellbeing may have a restricted range of expressions or require substantial support from others; however, they are not by definition excluded from the experience.

It has been suggested that wellbeing may be best understood as a multidimensional phenomenon incorporating both ideas of wellbeing [36]. One attempt at combining hedonic and eudaimonic influences is seen in Keyes et al. [20] work. Keyes argues that mental health consists of three partly overlapping dimensions of wellbeing: emotional wellbeing (entailing positive affect, absence of negative affect, and perceived satisfaction with life), psychological wellbeing (consisting of self-acceptance, positive relations with others, personal growth, purpose in life, environmental mastery, and autonomy), and social wellbeing (social acceptance, social actualization, social contribution, social coherence, and social integration). When testing this suggestion, Keyes et al. [20] found support for a two-factor wellbeing model, corresponding to the two traditions: eudaimonia, comprising psychological and social wellbeing indicators, and hedoninia, comprising subjective (emotional) wellbeing.

3.2.2. A Dual Model of Mental Health and Mental Health Problems

Because the WHO has provided both a definition of mental disorders and a definition of mental health in which mental health is explicitly named as wellbeing, the relationship between wellbeing and mental health problems needs clarifying. Do wellbeing and mental health problems exist on the same continuum? Literature describing wellbeing as the presence of positive feelings towards your own life tends to see wellbeing as a continuum of its own. Keyes [37] considers levels of wellbeing on a scale anchored by languishing (unhappiness and experiencing difficulties) at one end and flourishing (happy and thriving—the most positive state) at the other [37,38]. Several studies provide evidence that mental health problems and wellbeing are two separate but correlated constructs, rather than one (MacArthur Foundation's Midlife in the United States survey) [39]. Studies including children with NDD lend further support to this dual-factor model of mental health [40,41]. The term flourishing is suggested as useful to characterize people with high scores in emotional, psychological, and social wellbeing, whereas languishing can be used to categorize people with low scores on wellbeing. Thus, languishing is seen as indicating a low level of wellbeing that might, or might not, occur in conjunction with mental health problems or illness.

In conclusion, the support for the dual continua model means that we can add another layer to Figure 1. It is theoretically possible for someone to fulfill the criteria for a mental disorder (e.g., autism) and to also experience any level of mental health problems and wellbeing (circles partly overlapping). Mental illness most likely influences a person's wellbeing, but in theory, it is possible to experience aspects of positive mental health such as wellbeing when suffering from a mental health problem. The relationship between mental health problems and the dual continua model is illustrated in Figure 3.

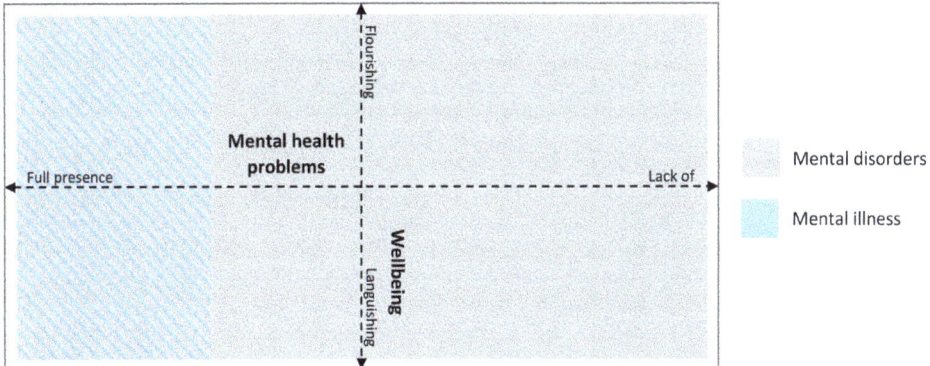

Figure 3. The relation of mental disorders and mental illness to the dual-continua model of wellbeing and mental health problems.

3.3. Problem 3: The Relationship between Participation and Wellbeing in Children with NDD

We propose that participation is a key concept to relate to wellbeing because of its focus on functioning in the context of everyday activities. Participation can be an antecedent of wellbeing as well as a consequence of wellbeing.

In discussing the relationship between wellbeing and participation, we consider the antecedents and consequences of wellbeing and participation as described across diverse literature bases such as children with disabilities, aging populations, and the business literature. Antecedents and consequences provide information about possible causal links between the constructs of wellbeing and participation, although both wellbeing and participation are complexly determined and may have a cascade of effects. First, we provide descriptions of the construct of participation.

3.3.1. How Participation Is Conceptualized in Various Bodies of Literature

Recent research in the child-onset disability field identifies participation as being involvement in a life situation with two dimensions. The first dimension attendance relates to the life situations and the second dimension to the involvement or engagement while being there. The dimensions are situated within the fPRC, which is neutral about the activity or life situation in which participation occurs, that is, participation can be considered in relation to any activity [5] and is pertinent for all people.

Although participation can occur in any life situation, the need to identify the situation in which participation is being studied implies that participation is a contextually based construct. Research about participation can be found in diverse literature, for example, business literature that focuses on participation in work (e.g., [42,43], or youth delinquency research that focuses on participation in crime or the legal system [44]. Some participation research implies that participation requires others to be present—thus effectively limiting the types of life situations in which participation can be said to have occurred. For example, in the aged care/adult disability literature, there has been a focus on participation being relevant in "social", "community", or "complex" activities [45,46]. The fPRC describes participation as being relevant to any life situation, including activities done individually, thus providing important conceptual clarity and applicability to all people.

Across various fields of literature are examples of studies in which the term participation is not defined explicitly: presumably based on the assumption that we all know and agree about what it is. When participation is not defined, what is measured is commonly the "attendance" dimension: that is, how often people attend particular activities, or what proportion of people attend particular situations. The notion of involvement is further explored here, because there is greater variation across literature on how involvement is operationalized compared to attendance.

Research about participation in decision making provides one mechanism for exploring involvement. Decision making is a process—whether done collaboratively or independently—and can be relevant to any life situation. Concerning participation in community development, the implied definition of participation is both attendance (in the decision-making activity) and involvement in dialogue [47]. This perspective is consistent with youth delinquency research studies in which participation in the legal proceedings has been considered in relation to involvement in decision making and problem solving around issues directly affecting the individual [48]. A focus on collaboration in decision making is also apparent in some education literature that describes participation as children being listened to by adults and having their views considered in decision making [49]. Puritz and Majd [50] describe involvement as having a meaningful opportunity to be heard.

Participation defined as "taking part", which might include interacting, doing, helping, or contributing [45], or as engagement in (complex) activities [46], also provides ideas about involvement. Operationalizing these ideas, however, often results in "counting occasions of doing (something)" an idea that is closer to the notion of attending than the experience of involvement. Likewise, in the business and education literature, although the term engagement is used more commonly than participation, the focus is frequently related to "engaged time" [51]—once again a measure of attendance. In contrast, engagement defined by Russell et al. [52] as "energy in action, the connection between person and activity" (p. 1), conveys the essence of the experience of participation, and reinforces the need to consider participation in context.

Bringing the ideas of attendance and involvement together, Bergqvist et al. [53] reported that "when a person chooses to attend an activity, it is possible for the person to be involved and that might lead to participation" (p. 1). In this example, participation is seen as a potential outcome of doing something, which suggests that participation cannot be separated from either doing or belonging. This definition of participation is consistent with the fPRC from the perspective that attendance is seen as a necessary but not sufficient condition for involvement.

Hoogsteen and Woodgate's [54] conceptual analysis of participation through the lens of childhood disability resulted in a definition of participation with four elements: "(i) the child must take part in something or with someone; (ii) the child must feel included or have a sense of inclusion in what they are partaking in; (iii) the child must have a choice or control over what they are taking part in; (iv) the child must work towards obtaining a personal or socially-meaningful goal or enhancing the quality of life" (pp. 329–330). The first two elements are consistent with the ideas of attendance and involvement. The third element is problematic as children often participate in activities or situations that they do not choose or control; however, the problematic nature of this element relates specifically to the attendance aspect of participation, as providing children with choices within an activity setting can help them feel involved or engaged [55,56]. This reflects an empowerment approach to the design of participation opportunities. The fourth element proposed seems closer to definitions of wellbeing than participation, but might point to the notion of future participation being driven by past and current participation—i.e., participation as a means.

3.3.2. Antecedents and Consequences to Wellbeing and Participation

The relationship between participation and wellbeing must be considered as a transactional process over time where participation at one point in time may affect wellbeing at a later point in time, and vice versa. To further consider this relationship within a process framework, two concepts that denote a causal order of events will be used: antecedents and consequences. Antecedents concern events that occur before a specified event and consequences concern events that occur after a specified event.

Antecedents to wellbeing have been described as relating to resources or contextual factors and to personal attributes. For example, having social capital and enough income [57] can support wellbeing. From a personal perspective, altruism or volunteering [32,58] and adapting to your own needs for wellbeing and your life circumstances [29] have all been identified as antecedents to wellbeing. Antecedents to low levels of wellbeing (i.e., languishing) may also be resources and contextual factors—for example, family and work variables and life stressors [32,59], limited resources [32], and lack of social engagement [60,61]. Of the factors identified as antecedents to wellbeing, participation is rarely explicitly described, although can be inferred from the literature describing altruistic behaviors, adaptive behaviors, and social engagement. Powell et al. [35] is one exception: they clearly identified participation as an antecedent contributing to wellbeing.

Consequences of wellbeing include protection against mental health problems [62], future resilience and wellbeing [57,63], connectedness with peers [57], improved work/school productivity, engagement and achievement [59], and a sense of meaning in life [28]. Thus, one consequence of wellbeing appears to be participation; other consequences relate to personal attributes of resilience, coping, and future wellbeing.

Antecedents of participation from across the fields of literature can also be summarized as factors related to the person or the context. Person-related antecedents include interest or willingness to take part [54], and past satisfaction [64], as well as antecedents that prevent participation, such as pain [64], depression, mood disorder [32], fatigue, or physical limitations [65]. Age was proposed to shape participation in that it influences capacity for choice. Contextual antecedents of participation included initiatives that influence the physical, attitudinal, and relational environment [33,42,43]; information provided [66]; and peer modelling, family processes, socioeconomic factors, cultural practices, and governance structures [67,68]. These broad-ranging antecedents provide information about how contexts might be shaped or influenced to support participation.

Consequences of participation as attendance included gaining skills, academic or educational achievement, health, development of self-determination or self-efficacy, overall development, and wellbeing [51,69–72]. The consequences of participation as involvement if seen as collaboration in action and decision making included impacts at the level of both person and context. For example, having agency or power and being able to contribute to choices that impact the future are personal consequences; societal transformation to realize rights and more equitable distribution of resources and benefits are contextual consequences [47,71]. Examples of consequences of participation in harmful activities were reported to include poor mental health, substance abuse, cynicism, and societal disengagement and crime [67,68]—again involving both personal and contextual consequences, strongly supporting the reciprocal nature of participation in context.

Consequences of a lack of participation were reported to include deprivation, social injustice, limited wellbeing, lack of dignity, loss of rights [47,66], and a lack of involvement leading to lack of attendance at work or low productivity [33]. A lack of participation can lead to a lack of contribution to building social capital by particular groups in society. For example, if those with disability are not participating, their potential to shape culture, build tolerance to diversity, benefit from and contribute to common resources, and establish valued norms impacts the nature of community/society for all [73]. Additionally, the consequences of imbalanced participation, i.e., not being able to achieve balance in doing all the activities that "need" to be done and resting, included stress and mental fatigue [53].

3.3.3. Relationships between Participation and Wellbeing

The descriptions of wellbeing are primarily focused on the person's summative perception of their feelings about their life in terms of emotions, psychological functioning, and/or social wellbeing or a specific domain of life (e.g., recreation, work), whether focused on pleasure or striving or a combination. In contrast, descriptions of participation focus on the person taking part in context. In relation to the fPRC, wellbeing might be most closely related to ideas of "sense-of-self", which is described as both antecedent and consequent to participation in the fPRC. The broader literature related to participation also clearly (and commonly) links wellbeing as both an antecedent (when poor [i.e., when people are languishing] it limits/reduces participation) and a consequence of participation. When participation is possible, balanced, and not in harmful activities, wellbeing (flourishing) can be enhanced. If participation is not balanced or is predominantly in harmful/negative activities, wellbeing is seen to reduce. Thus, participation and wellbeing are bi-directional: participation can influence wellbeing, and (positive) wellbeing can increase the possibility of participation [59].

Van Campen and Ledema [74] investigated the relationship between participation and wellbeing specifically, providing evidence about the need to understand both dimensions of participation. They focused on the impact of objective participation (attendance) on subjective wellbeing. They hypothesized a linear relationship between duration of illness leading to severity of impairment leading to objective participation leading to subjective wellbeing. Objective participation was measured as the frequency of hours in paid work, frequency of social contacts, number of holidays, and number of museum visits (thus measures of attendance). Subjective wellbeing was measured as health-related quality of life, using scales capturing mental health problems, and a measure of happiness (wellbeing). They found no empirical support for a direct relationship between objective participation and mental health problems or wellbeing. When models were adjusted to include age and socio-economic factors, a better fit was seen. In the discussion, the authors identified the need to understand subjective participation to understand its impact on wellbeing. They cited Csikszentmihalyi's notion of flow and interpreted this finding as follows: "it is not the fact that someone participates but how they participate that determines subjective wellbeing" (p. 643).

4. Implications for Measurement and Intervention with Children with NDD Following from the Three Propositions

The three problems discussed have implications for how mental health problems, wellbeing, and participation are measured in studies focusing on children with NDD. There are also implications for interventions focusing on decreasing mental health problems or enhancing wellbeing. Measurement and intervention are important topics that require consideration beyond the scope of this paper. In this section, we briefly point to some areas that need further discussion and empirical investigation.

4.1. Implications for Measurement: The Risk of Confusion between NDD-Core Symptoms, Mental Health Problems, and Wellbeing

One essential aspect of any instrument aiming to measure mental health problems or screen for mental illness in children with NDD is that it should not tap into core problems associated with the NDD in question. Looking at two of the most widely used behavior problem screening questionnaires for children and adolescents, the Child Behavior Checklist (CBCL) [24] and the Strengths and Difficulties questionnaire (SDQ) [75], it is apparent that both contain several items that risk doing so (e.g., "avoids looking others in the eye" from the CBCL and "easily distracted, concentration wanders" from the SDQ). This suggests that the problem of confusing NDD symptoms and mental health problems may apply to a substantial proportion of the research on mental health problems undertaken with children with NDDs.

This issue is equally important when measuring wellbeing, since the presence of an NDD does not predispose individuals to either languishing or flourishing. This problem does not primarily lay within the rating scales themselves but in how data are treated. For example, concerning mental health problems, the SDQ [75] is commonly used to screen mental health problems in children with NDD, e.g., Bailey et al. [22]. In the SDQ, there are four "problem scales": (i) hyperactivity (covering problems with both hyperactivity and inattention—the basic symptom criteria for Attention Deficit Hyperactivity Disorder), (ii) conduct problems, (iii) emotional problems (sadness, depression), and (iv) peer problems (problems in relating to peers). The subscales hyperactivity and peer problems should not be defined as mental health problems of an individual. Hyperactivity can exist along with good everyday functioning as operationalized as participation in play activities in preschool [76]. Peer problems are related to how other people react to a child and the child's communication skills; thus, this scale is also a measure of communicative and environmental problems. For this reason, we recommend caution when drawing conclusions based on indexes, such as the internalizing or externalizing indices of the SDQ and CBCL, about mental health problems in children and adolescents with NDD diagnoses.

4.2. Implications for Measurement: The Issue of Inclusiveness

A related and equally important aspect of measurement instruments is the matter of inclusiveness at the conceptual level, that is, items and scales should not preclude any level of wellbeing or mental health problems based on normative assumptions of human functioning (it should be a purely empirical question). For example, if working "productively and fruitfully" is considered by WHO [18] as a central part of wellbeing, then the individuals with the severest disabilities, for whom work in the traditional sense will never be an option, are predestined to lower levels of wellbeing. One way of reducing the risk of building conceptual barriers may be to let respondents assess wellbeing in general with a few items or using a single question. There are of course limitations to such approaches that reduce a complex phenomenon to a few items. We recommend that researchers and clinicians consider the inclusiveness of any scale chosen to measure wellbeing and mental health problems in children with NDD. Given our definition of wellbeing as subjective, we realize this recommendation is difficult to follow in the case of individuals with profound intellectual disabilities. This literature tends to use proxy-completed measures of quality of life (not wellbeing), such as the KidsLife Scale [77], which is based on a series of life domains including self-determination, social inclusion, and interpersonal relationships, in addition to material, physical, and emotional wellbeing.

Even after having considered the risk of confusing mental health problems with core symptoms of NDD and inclusiveness, the questions of inclusive measurement design and procedures remain. Many questionnaires have cognitive barriers that may make them inaccessible for children with NDDs. Instruments suited for assessing mental health problems and wellbeing in children with NDD need to be developed or adapted. In addition, manuals for how to set up structured interviews to support individuals in self-rating wellbeing and mental health problems need to be developed. One example of a questionnaire that tries to deal with these issues constructively is the Wellbeing in Special Education Questionnaire [40]. The instrument has been validated with children with mild to moderate intellectual disability and includes generic questions about wellbeing along with questions about mental health problems that could be argued to be relevant for children regardless of the level of functioning.

Conceptual inclusiveness is also pertinent to measures of participation. Following the publication of the International Classification of Functioning, Disability, and Health [6], in which the concept participation was introduced, multiple participation measures were developed. However, the lack of conceptual clarity within the ICF led to considerable variation in approaches to measurement development [78]. One of the key issues was the conflating of the ideas of independence in performing an activity or task, with involvement in life situations (the ICF definition of participation). The problem with this approach is that children with NDD were, by definition, assessed as having poor or restricted participation simply because they were not independent (e.g., they required supports to participate due to intellectual impairment) or had limitations in their activity skills (e.g., poor manual ability). In terms of measuring participation, the inclusion of an assessment of support or aids required to participate has been critiqued in the literature [79,80]. It is considered important to conceptualize participation intrinsically and separately from other factors or variables [79]. Children with NDD may experience participation restrictions, but this should not be determined based on their skills, or attributes associated with their condition [5]. Participation attendance (being there) and involvement (the experience of participation while attending) in life situations are pertinent to all people at all phases of the life course. Measures of participation should reflect one or both these constructs.

4.3. Interventions Focused on Decreasing Mental Health Problems in Persons with NDD

Interventions that address mental health problems with anxiety and sadness/depression in persons with NDD are limited. Pharmacological interventions for severe mental health problems, such as antidepressant medication, may not be effective [81]. Non-pharmacological interventions have focused on talking therapies. Mindfulness (combining talking with meditation) has been shown to be effective for reducing anxiety in persons with autism [82] and a cognitive–behavioral therapy combination of on-line sessions and face to face meetings has been shown to reduce anxiety in adolescents with intellectual disability [83]. Evidence for the effect of psychotherapy is primarily limited to case-studies [84]. There is emerging evidence that talking therapies need to be modified for young people with NDD [85]. There is a dearth of evidence for talking therapies for persons with NDD who may experience more significant motor and communication difficulties. Few studies focusing on decreasing mental health problems measure wellbeing or participation of children and youth with NDD as secondary outcomes of treatment.

4.4. Participation Interventions as a Means to Enhancing Wellbeing in Children and Adolescents with NDD

The childhood disability literature is just beginning to explore the effects of participation interventions on wellbeing. Studies of various participation interventions, including arts-based, physical activity, life skills, coaching, and resilience-focused interventions, have provided preliminary evidence for effects on wellbeing (e.g., psychosocial well-being, self-determination, self-efficacy). For example, a scoping review of arts-based interventions for children with disabilities, which included performance (e.g., music, dance, theatre) and visual (e.g., drawing, painting, sculpting) arts-based programs, indicated that these interventions show potential to positively impact psychosocial wellbeing (i.e., emotional and social functioning), although further investigation is required with broader populations of children with physical and developmental disabilities [86]. Therapeutic horse riding, an example of a physical activity intervention, has been found to positively influence and expand the self-concepts of children with disabilities [87]. A review of the literature on therapeutic horseback riding indicates some evidence for statistically significant decreases in depression and distress, although this evidence is inconsistent and there are methodological problems in this body of research [88]. Youth with disabilities taking part in a transition-oriented life skills program have been found to have significant pre-post changes in their autonomy (as an aspect of self-determination) and self-efficacy [56]. The growing literature on coaching interventions for children and youth with disabilities focuses on engagement and goal attainment [89,90] and has yet to consider longer-term effects on wellbeing. However, the broader coaching literature indicates that participation in a cognitive–behavioral life coaching program is associated with enhanced wellbeing and quality of life [91]. Resilience-focused interventions are another promising area of intervention. A systematic review of universal resilience-focused interventions targeting child and youth wellbeing in the school setting [92] has indicated effects concerning the reduction of mental health problems.

5. Conclusions

This position paper suggests future directions in the scientific study of wellbeing and mental health problems in children with NDD and describes the implications for participation interventions aimed at sustaining wellbeing in children with disabilities following from the propositions:

(1) Mental disorders include both diagnoses related to impairments in the developmental period, i.e., NDD and diagnoses related to mental illness. These two types of mental disorders must be separated when measuring mental health in children with disabilities. Thus, summary indexes such as externalizing and internalizing problems should be avoided, since more stable characteristics related to impairment are conflated with mental health problem indicators. Measures of mental health problems involving

only mental illness indicators and not NDD impairment-related symptoms need to be developed for children diagnosed within the NDD spectrum.
(2) Mental health problems and wellbeing are two related but different continua where one focuses on mental health problems and illness and the other on different degrees of wellbeing; therefore, they must be measured separately. Children with NDD, just like other people, may exhibit aspects of both mental health problems and wellbeing simultaneously. Measures of wellbeing defined as a continuum from flourishing to languishing for children with NDD need to be designed and evaluated.
(3) Wellbeing and participation are distinct from each other. Wellbeing is situated within the person and can be seen as a generalized measure of a person's mental health within generalized contexts, while participation is always situated within a more specific context or activity. The relationship between the constructs can be seen as a spiral, where participation can be both an antecedent to wellbeing and a consequence of wellbeing. Because participation is contextualized, it can be the focus of direct interventions (targeted at the context or the person) that aim to enhance wellbeing. The relationship between participation and mental health problems is hypothesized to be indirect. By increasing or sustaining participation, wellbeing can be affected. Wellbeing will lead to further participation but also act as protection from mental health problems. The proposal that participation interventions can enhance wellbeing and indirectly lessen mental health problems needs to be tested in intervention research.

Author Contributions: M.G., C.I., G.K., A.K.A., L.A. (Lilly Augustine), R.B., H.D., J.G., M.I., L.-O.L., F.L. and L.A. (Lena Almqvist) contributed to the conceptualization, writing the original draft, and the review and editing of the manuscript. M.G. had a leading role in the conceptualization, funding acquisition, writing the original draft, and the review and editing of the manuscript. C.I., G.K., and L.A. (Lena Almqvist) have also had leading roles in the review and editing of the manuscript. The visualizations were adapted (Figures 1 and 2) and created (Figure 3) by M.I. All authors have read and agreed to the published version of the manuscript.

Funding: This research took place within the research program CHILD-PMH (Child Participation and Mental Health), which was funded by the Swedish Research Council (VR) grant number 2018-05824.

Institutional Review Board Statement: Not applicable.

Informed Consent Statement: Not applicable.

Acknowledgments: This conceptual paper was facilitated by the administrative support of Helena Engkvist and by creative discussions with the rest of the researchers involved in CHILD-PMH.

Conflicts of Interest: The authors declare no conflict of interest.

References

1. King, G.; Law, M.; Hurley, P.; Petrenchik, T.; Schwellnus, H. A Developmental Comparison of the Out-of-school Recreation and Leisure Activity Participation of Boys and Girls With and Without Physical Disabilities. *Int. J. Disabil. Dev. Educ.* **2010**, *57*, 77–107. [CrossRef]
2. Carlberg, L.; Granlund, M. Achievement and participation in schools for young adolescents with self-reported neuropsychiatric disabilities: A cross-sectional study from the southern part of Sweden. *Scand. J. Public Health* **2019**, *47*, 199–206. [CrossRef]
3. Missiuna, C.; Moll, S.E.; King, S.; King, G.; Law, M. A trajectory of troubles: Parents' impressions of the impact of developmental coordination disorder. *Phys. Occup. Ther. Pediatr.* **2007**, *27*, 81–101. [CrossRef]
4. World Health Organization. *ICD 11 Version 09/2020 [Internet]*; World Health Organisation: Geneva, Switzerland, 2020. Available online: https://icd.who.int/en (accessed on 3 February 2021).
5. Imms, C.; Granlund, M.; Wilson, P.H.; Steenbergen, B.; Rosenbaum, P.L.; Gordon, A.M. Participation, both a means and an end: A conceptual analysis of processes and outcomes in childhood disability. *Dev. Med. Child Neurol.* **2017**, *59*, 16–25. [CrossRef] [PubMed]
6. World Health Organization. *ICF: International Classification of Functioning, Disability, and Health*; World Health Organization: Geneva, Switzerland, 2001. Available online: https://www.who.int/standards/classifications/international-classification-of-functioning-disability-and-health (accessed on 3 February 2021).

7. Jewett, R.; Sabiston, C.M.; Brunet, J.; O'Loughlin, E.K.; Scarapicchia, T.; O'Loughlin, J. School sport participation during adolescence and mental health in early adulthood. *J. Adolesc. Health* **2014**, *55*, 640–644. [CrossRef]
8. Augustin, L.; Granlund, M.; Lygnegård, F. Trajectories of participation, mental health and mental health problems in adolescents with self-reported neurodevelopmental disorders. Unpublished work, submitted D&R.
9. Bremberg, S.; Dalman, C. *Begrepp, Mätmetoder Och Förekomst Av Psykisk Hälsa, Psykisk Ohälsa Och Psykiatriska Tillstånd: En Kunskapsöversikt. (Constructs, Assessment Methods and Prevalence, Mental Health, Mental Illness and Mental Health Disorders)*; FORTE: Stockholm, Sweden, 2015. Available online: https://forte.se/publikation/begrepp-matmetoder/ (accessed on 3 February 2021).
10. Jahoda, M. *Joint Commission on Mental Health and Illness Monograph Series: Vol. 1. Current Concepts of Positive Mental Health*; Basic Books: New York, NY, USA, 1958. [CrossRef]
11. Westerhof, G.J.; Keyes, C.L. Mental Illness and Mental Health: The Two Continua Model Across the Lifespan. *J. Adult Dev.* **2009**, *17*, 110–119. [CrossRef]
12. Brooks, R.; Lambert, C.; Coulthard, L.; Pennington, L.; Kolehmainen, N. Social participation to support good mental health in neurodisability. *Child. Care Health and Development.* submitted.
13. Hartley, M.; Dorstyn, D.; Due, C. Mindfulness for Children and Adults with Autism Spectrum Disorder and Their Caregivers: A Meta-analysis. *J. Autism Dev. Disord.* **2019**, *49*, 4306–4319. [CrossRef] [PubMed]
14. Anaby, D.; Avery, L.; Gorter, J.W.; Levin, M.F.; Teplicky, R.; Turner, L.; Cormier, I.; Hanes, J. Improving body functions through participation in community activities among young people with physical disabilities. *Dev. Med. Child Neurol.* **2019**, *62*, 640–646. [CrossRef]
15. Nguyen, M.N.; Watanabe-Galloway, S.; Hill, J.L.; Siahpush, M.; Tibbits, M.K.; Wichman, C. Ecological model of school engagement and attention-deficit/hyperactivity disorder in school-aged children. *Eur. Child Adolesc. Psychiatry* **2018**, *28*, 795–805. [CrossRef]
16. American Psychiatric Association. *Diagnostic and Statistical Manual of Mental Disorders*, 5th ed.; American Psychiatric Association: Washington, DC, USA, 2013; p. 5.
17. Improving the Mental Health of the Population. Towards a Strategy on Mental Health for the European Union. Available online: https://ec.europa.eu/health/ph_determinants/life_style/mental/green_paper/mental_gp_en.pdf (accessed on 14 October 2005).
18. World Health Organization. *Promoting Mental Health: Concepts, Emerging Evidence, Practice [Internet]*; World Health Organization: Geneva, Switzerland, 2005. Available online: https://www.who.int/mental_health/evidence/en/promoting_mhh.pdf (accessed on 3 February 2021).
19. Boniwell, I.; Henry, J. Developing conceptions of well-being: Advancing subjective, hedonic and hedonic theories. *Soc. Psychol. Rev.* **2007**, *9*, 3–18.
20. Keyes, C.L.; Shmotkin, D.; Ryff, C.D. Optimizing well-being: The empirical encounter of two traditions. *J. Personal. Soc. Psychol.* **2002**, *82*, 1007–1022. [CrossRef]
21. Copeland, W.E.; Adair, C.E.; Smetanin, P.; Stiff, D.; Briante, C.; Colman, I.; Fergusson, D.; Horwood, J.; Poulton, R.; Costello, E.J.; et al. Diagnostic transitions from childhood to adolescence to early adulthood. *J. Child Psychol. Psychiatry* **2013**, *54*, 791–799. [CrossRef]
22. Bailey, T.; Totsika, V.; Hastings, R.P.; Hatton, C.; Emerson, E. Developmental trajectories of behaviour problems and prosocial behaviours of children with intellectual disabilities in a population-based cohort. *J. Child Psychol. Psychiatry* **2019**, *60*, 1210–1218. [CrossRef]
23. Goodman, A.; Lamping, D.L.; Ploubidis, G.B. When to use broader internalising and externalising subscales instead of the hypothesised five subscales on the Strengths and Difficulties Questionnaire (SDQ): Data from British Parents, Teachers and Children. *J. Abnorm. Child Psychol.* **2010**, *38*, 1179–1191. [CrossRef]
24. Achenbach, T.M.; Ruffle, T.M. The Child Behavior Checklist and Related Forms for Assessing Behavioral/Emotional Problems and Competencies. *Pediatr. Rev.* **2000**, *21*, 265–271. [CrossRef] [PubMed]
25. Will, M.N.; Wilson, B.J. A longitudinal analysis of parent and teacher ratings of problem behavior in boys with and without developmental delays. *J. Intellect. Disabil.* **2014**, *18*, 176–187. [CrossRef] [PubMed]
26. Halfon, N.; Larson, K.; Lu, M.; Tullis, E.; Russ, S. Lifecourse Health Development: Past, Present and Future. *Matern. Child Health J.* **2014**, *18*, 344–365. [CrossRef] [PubMed]
27. Diener, E.; Suh, E.M.; Lucas, R.E.; Smith, H.L. Subjective well-being: Three decades of progress. *Psychol. Bull.* **1999**, *125*, 276–302. [CrossRef]
28. Manderscheid, R.W.; Ryff, C.D.; Freeman, E.J.; McKnight-Eily, L.R.; Dhingra, S.; Strine, T.W. Evolving Definitions of Mental Illness and Wellness. *Prev. Chronic Dis.* **2009**, *7*, A19.
29. Brown, T.M. "Hitting the Streets": Youth Street Involvement as Adaptive Well-Being. *Harv. Educ. Rev.* **2016**, *86*, 48–71. [CrossRef]
30. Halliday, A.J.; Kern, M.L.; Garrett, D.K.; Turnbull, D.A. The student voice in well-being: A case study of participatory action research in positive education. *Educ. Action Res.* **2019**, *27*, 173–196. [CrossRef]
31. Herke, M.; Rathmann, K.; Richter, M. Trajectories of students' well-being in secondary education in Germany and differences by social background. *Eur. J. Public Health* **2019**, *29*, 960–965. [CrossRef] [PubMed]
32. Kahana, E.; Bhatta, T.; Lovegreen, L.D.; Kahana, B.; Midlarsky, E. Altruism, helping, and volunteering: Pathways to well-being in late life. *J. Aging Health* **2013**, *25*, 159–187. [CrossRef]

33. Goetzel, R.Z.; Ozminkowski, R.J.; Sederer, L.I.; Mark, T.L. The business case for quality mental health services: Why employers should care about the mental health and well-being of their employees. *J. Occup. Environ. Med.* **2002**, *44*, 320–330. [CrossRef]
34. Dodge, R.; Daly, A.P.; Huyton, J.; Sanders, L.D. The challenge of defining wellbeing. *Int. J. Wellbeing* **2012**, *2*, 222–235. [CrossRef]
35. Powell, M.A.; Graham, A.; Fitzgerald, R.; Thomas, N.P.; White, N.E. Wellbeing in schools: What do students tell us? *Aust. Educ. Res.* **2018**, *45*, 515–531. [CrossRef]
36. Ryan, R.M.; Deci, E.L. On Happiness and Human Potentials: A review of research on hedonic and eudaimonic well-being. *Annu. Rev. Psychol.* **2001**, *52*, 141–166. [CrossRef] [PubMed]
37. Keyes, C.L.M. Mental health in adolescence: Is America's youth flourishing? *Am. J. Orthopsychiatry* **2006**, *76*, 395–402. [CrossRef] [PubMed]
38. Skrzypiec, G.; Askell-Williams, H.; Slee, P.; Rudzinski, A. Students with Self-identified Special Educational Needs and Disabilities (si-SEND): Flourishing or Languishing! *Int. J. Disabil. Dev. Educ.* **2015**, *63*, 7–26. [CrossRef]
39. Keyes, C.L.M. Mental Illness and/or mental health? Investigating axioms of the complete state model of health. *J. Consult. Clin. Psychol.* **2005**, *73*, 539–548. [CrossRef] [PubMed]
40. Boström, P.; Johnels, J.Å.; Thorson, M.; Broberg, M. Subjective Mental Health, Peer Relations, Family, and School Environment in Adolescents with Intellectual Developmental Disorder: A First Report of a New Questionnaire Administered on Tablet PCs. *J. Ment. Health Res. Intellect. Disabil.* **2016**, *9*, 207–231. [CrossRef]
41. Franken, K.; Lamers, S.M.; Klooster, P.M.T.; Bohlmeijer, E.T.; Westerhof, G.J. Validation of the Mental Health Continuum-Short Form and the dual continua model of well-being and psychopathology in an adult mental health setting. *J. Clin. Psychol.* **2018**, *74*, 2187–2202. [CrossRef] [PubMed]
42. Arnold, K.A.; Turner, N.; Barling, J.; Kelloway, E.K.; McKee, M.C. Transformational leadership and psychological well-being: The mediating role of meaningful work. *J. Occup. Health Psychol.* **2007**, *12*, 193–203. [CrossRef]
43. Donald, I.; Taylor, P.; Johnson, S.; Cooper, C.; Cartwright, S.; Robertson, S. Work environments, stress, and productivity: An examination using ASSET. *Int. J. Stress Manag.* **2005**, *12*, 409–423. [CrossRef]
44. Nagin, D.S.; Smith, D.A. Participation in and frequency of delinquent behavior: A test for structural differences. *J. Quant. Criminol.* **1990**, *6*, 335–356. [CrossRef]
45. Richard, L.; Gauvin, L.; Kestens, Y.; Shatenstein, B.; Payette, H.; Daniel, M.; Moore, S.; Levasseur, M.; Mercille, G. Neighborhood resources and social participation among older adults: Results from the VoisiNuage Study. *J. Aging Health* **2012**, *25*, 296–318. [CrossRef]
46. Vaughan, M.W.; LaValley, M.P.; AlHeresh, R.; Keysor, J.J. Which features of the environment impact community participation of older adults? *J. Aging Health* **2016**, *28*, 957–978. [CrossRef]
47. McEvoy, R.; Tierney, E.; Macfarlane, A.E. 'Participation is integral': Understanding the levers and barriers to the implementation of community participation in primary healthcare: A qualitative study using normalisation process theory. *BMC Health Serv. Res.* **2019**, *19*, 515. [CrossRef]
48. Kupchik, A.; Catlaw, T.J. Discipline and Participation: The long term effects of suspension and school security on the political and civic engagement of youth. *Youth Soc.* **2012**, *47*, 95–124. [CrossRef]
49. Zorec, M.B. Children's Participation in Slovene Preschools: The Teachers' Viewpoints and Practice. *Eur. Educ.* **2015**, *47*, 154–168. [CrossRef]
50. Puritz, P.; Majd, K. ensuring authentic youth participation in delinquency cases: Creating a paradigm for specialized juvenile defense practice. *Fam. Court. Rev.* **2007**, *45*, 466–484. [CrossRef]
51. Sierens, S.; Van Avermaet, P.; Van Houtte, M.; Agirdag, O. Does pre-schooling contribute to equity in education? Participation in universal pre-school and fourth-grade academic achievement. *Eur. Educ. Res. J.* **2020**, *19*, 564–586. [CrossRef]
52. Frydenberg, E.; Ainley, M.; Russell, V. Schooling Issue Digest: Student Motivation and Engagement. In *Australian Government Department of Education*; Australian Government Department of Education: Canberra, Australia, 2005.
53. Bergqvist, L.; Öhrvall, A.-M.; Himmelmann, K.; Peny-Dahlstrand, M. When I do, I become someone: Experiences of occupational performance in young adults with cerebral palsy. *Disabil. Rehabil.* **2017**, *41*, 341–347. [CrossRef]
54. Hoogsteen, L.; Woodgate, R.L. Can I play? A conceptual analysis of participation in children with disabilities. *Phys. Occup. Ther. Pediatr.* **2010**, *30*, 325–339. [CrossRef]
55. King, G.; Rigby, P.; Batorowicz, B. Conceptualizing participation in context for children and youth with disabilities: An activity setting perspective. *Disabil. Rehabil.* **2013**, *35*, 1578–1585. [CrossRef]
56. King, G.; McPherson, A.C.; Kingsnorth, S.; Gorter, J.W.; Avery, L.; Rudzik, A.; Ontario Independence Program Research (OIPR) Team. Opportunities, experiences, and outcomes of residential immersive life skills programs for youth with disabilities. *Disabil. Rehabil.* **2020**, *2020*, 1–11. [CrossRef]
57. Hayslip, J.B.; Blumenthal, H.; Garner, A. Health and Grandparent–Grandchild Well-Being: One-Year Longitudinal Findings for Custodial Grandfamilies. *J. Aging Health* **2014**, *26*, 559–582. [CrossRef] [PubMed]
58. Hanniball, K.B.; Aknin, L.B.; Douglas, K.S.; Viljoen, J.L. Does helping promote well-being in at-risk youth and ex-offender samples? *J. Exp. Soc. Psychol.* **2019**, *82*, 307–317. [CrossRef]
59. Parasuraman, S.; Purohit, Y.S.; Godshalk, V.M.; Beutell, N.J. work and family variables, entrepreneurial career success, and psychological well-being. *J. Vocat. Behav.* **1996**, *48*, 275–300. [CrossRef]

60. Beresford, B.; Clarke, S. *Improving the Wellbeing of Disabled Children and Young People through Improving Access to Positive and Inclusive Activities*; Centre for Excellence and Outcomes in Children and Young People's Services (C4EO): London, UK, August 2009; p. 89.
61. Thoits, P.A. *Social Support and Psychological Wellbeing: Theoretical possibilities*; Sarason, G., Sarason, B.R., Eds.; Springer Nature Switzerland AG: Cham, Switzerland, 1985; pp. 51–72.
62. Torok, M.; Rasmussen, V.; Wong, Q.; Werner-Seidler, A.; O'Dea, B.; Toumbourou, J.; Calear, A. Examining the impact of the good behaviour game on emotional and behavioural problems in primary school children: A case for integrating well-being strategies into education. *Aust. J. Educ.* **2019**, *63*, 292–306. [CrossRef]
63. Reschly, A.L.; Christenson, S.L. Prediction of Dropout Among Students With Mild Disabilities: A Case for the Inclusion of Student Engagement Variables. *Remedial Spéc. Educ.* **2006**, *27*, 276–292. [CrossRef]
64. Dashner, J.; Tello, S.M.E.; Snyder, M.; Hollingsworth, H.; Keglovits, M.; Campbell, M.L.; Putnam, M.; Stark, S. Examination of Community Participation of Adults With Disabilities: Comparing Age and Disability Onset. *J. Aging Health* **2019**, *31* (Suppl. 10), 169S–194S. [CrossRef] [PubMed]
65. Clarke, P.; Twardzik, E.; Meade, M.A.; Peterson, M.D.; Tate, D. Social participation among adults aging with long-term physical disability: The role of socioenvironmental factors. *J. Aging Health* **2019**, *31*, 145S–168S. [CrossRef] [PubMed]
66. Woestehoff, S.A.; Redlich, A.D.; Cathcart, E.J.; Quas, J.A. Legal professionals' perceptions of juvenile engagement in the plea process. *Transl. Issues Psychol. Sci.* **2019**, *5*, 121–131. [CrossRef]
67. Bjerregaard, B.; Smith, C. Gender differences in gang participation, delinquency, and substance use. *J. Quant. Criminol.* **1993**, *9*, 329–355. [CrossRef]
68. Gordon, R.A.; Rowe, H.L.; Pardini, D.; Loeber, R.; White, H.R.; Farrington, D.P. Serious Delinquency and Gang Participation: Combining and Specializing in Drug Selling, Theft, and Violence. *J. Res. Adolesc.* **2014**, *24*, 235–251. [CrossRef]
69. Moon, N.W.; Todd, R.L.; Gregg, N.; Langston, C.L.; Wolfe, G. *Determining the Efficacy of Communications Technologies and Practices to Broaden Participation in Education: Insights from a Theory of Change*; Springer International Publishing: Cham, Switzerland, 2015; pp. 179–188.
70. Roth, B.B.; Asbjørnsen, A.E.; Manger, T. The Relationship Between Prisoners' Academic Self-efficacy and Participation in Education, Previous Convictions, Sentence Length, and Portion of Sentence Served. *J. Prison. Educ. Reentry* **2017**, *3*, 108–121. [CrossRef]
71. Essuman, A.; Akyeampong, K. Decentralisation policy and practice in Ghana: The promise and reality of community participation in education in rural communities. *J. Educ. Policy* **2011**, *26*, 513–527. [CrossRef]
72. Marston, C.; Hinton, R.; Kean, S.; Baral, S.; Ahuja, A.; Costello, A.; Portela, A. Community participation for transformative action on women's, children's and adolescents' health. *Bull. World Health Organ.* **2016**, *94*, 376–382. [CrossRef] [PubMed]
73. Chenoweth, L.; Stehlik, D. Implications of social capital for the inclusion of people with disabilities and families in community life. *Int. J. Incl. Educ.* **2004**, *8*, 59–72. [CrossRef]
74. Van Campen, C.; Iedema, J. Are persons with physical disabilities who participate in society healthier and happier? Structural equation modelling of objective participation and subjective well-being. *Qual. Life Res.* **2007**, *16*, 635–645. [CrossRef]
75. Goodman, R. The Strengths and Difficulties Questionnaire: A Research Note. *J. Child Psychol. Psychiatry* **1997**, *38*, 581–586. [CrossRef]
76. Sjöman, M.; Granlund, M.; Almqvist, L. Interaction processes as a mediating factor between children's externalized behaviour difficulties and engagement in preschool. *Early Child Dev. Care* **2016**, *186*, 1649–1663. [CrossRef]
77. Gómez, L.E.; Alcedo, M.Á.; Arias, B.; Fontanil, Y.; Arias, V.B.; Monsalve, A.; Verdugo, M. A new scale for the measurement of quality of life in children with intellectual disability. *Res. Dev. Disabil.* **2016**, *54*, 399–410. [CrossRef]
78. Adair, B.; Ullenhag, A.; Rosenbaum, P.L.; Granlund, M.; Keen, D.; Imms, C. A systematic review of measures used to quantify participation in childhood disability and their alignment with the family of participation-related constructs. *Dev. Med. Child Neurol.* **2018**, *60*, 1101–1116. [CrossRef] [PubMed]
79. Forsyth, R.; Jarvis, S. Participation in childhood. *Child Care Health Dev.* **2002**, *28*, 277–279. [CrossRef]
80. King, G.; Law, M.; King, S.; Hurley, P.; Hanna, S.; Kertoy, M.; Rosenbaum, P. Measuring children's participation in recreation and leisure activities: Construct validation of the CAPE and PAC. *Child Care Health Dev.* **2006**, *33*, 28–39. [CrossRef]
81. Williams, K.; Brignell, A.; Randall, M.; Silove, N.; Hazell, P. Selective serotonin reuptake inhibitors (SSRIs) for autism spectrum disorders (ASD). *Cochrane Database Syst. Rev.* **2013**, *20*, CD004677. [CrossRef]
82. Luxford, S.; Hadwin, J.A.; Kovshoff, H. Evaluating the Effectiveness of a School-Based Cognitive Behavioural Therapy Intervention for Anxiety in Adolescents Diagnosed with Autism Spectrum Disorder. *J. Autism Dev. Disord.* **2017**, *47*, 3896–3908. [CrossRef] [PubMed]
83. Hronis, A.; Roberts, R.M.; Roberts, L.; Kneebone, I. Fearless Me! ©: A feasibility case series of cognitive behavioral therapy for adolescents with intellectual disability. *J. Clin. Psychol.* **2019**, *75*, 919–932. [CrossRef] [PubMed]
84. Vecchiato, M.; Sacchi, C.; Simonelli, A.; Purgato, N. Evaluating the efficacy of psychodynamic treatment on a single case of autism. A qualitative research. *Res. Psychother. Psychopathol. Process Outcome* **2016**, *19*, 49–57. [CrossRef]
85. Wood, J.J.; Ehrenreich-May, J.; Alessandri, M.; Fujii, C.; Renno, P.; Laugeson, E.; Piacentini, J.C.; De Nadai, A.S.; Arnold, E.; Lewin, A.B.; et al. Cognitive behavioral therapy for early adolescents with autism spectrum disorders and clinical anxiety: A randomized, controlled trial. *Behav. Ther.* **2015**, *46*, 7–19. [CrossRef] [PubMed]

86. Edwards, B.; Smart, E.; King, G.; Curran, C.; Kingsnorth, S. Performance and visual arts-based programs for children with disabilities: A scoping review focusing on psychosocial outcomes. *Disabil. Rehabil.* **2018**, *42*, 574–585. [CrossRef]
87. Martin, R.A.; Graham, F.P.; Taylor, W.J.; Levack, W. Mechanisms of Change for Children Participating in Therapeutic Horse Riding: A Grounded Theory. *Phys. Occup. Ther. Pediatr.* **2017**, *38*, 510–526. [CrossRef] [PubMed]
88. MacKinnon, J.R.; Noh, S.; Laliberte, D.; Allan, D.E.; Lariviere, J. Therapeutic Horseback Riding: A review of the literature. *Phys. Occup. Ther. Pediatr.* **1995**, *15*, 1–15. [CrossRef]
89. Schwellnus, H.; King, G.; Baldwin, P.; Keenan, S.; Hartman, L.R. A Solution-Focused Coaching Intervention with Children and Youth with Cerebral Palsy to Achieve Participation-Oriented Goals. *Phys. Occup. Ther. Pediatr.* **2020**, *40*, 423–440. [CrossRef]
90. Graham, F.; Rodger, S.; Ziviani, J. Enabling Occupational Performance of Children Through Coaching Parents: Three Case Reports. *Phys. Occup. Ther. Pediatr.* **2010**, *30*, 4–15. [CrossRef]
91. Grant, A.M. The impact of life coaching on goal attainment, metacognition and mental health. *Soc. Behav. Pers. Int. J.* **2003**, *31*, 253–263. [CrossRef]
92. Dray, J.; Bowman, J.; Campbell, E.; Freund, M.; Wolfenden, L.; Hodder, R.K.; McElwaine, K.; Tremain, D.; Bartlem, K.; Bailey, J.; et al. Systematic Review of Universal Resilience-Focused Interventions Targeting Child and Adolescent Mental Health in the School Setting. *J. Am. Acad. Child Adolesc. Psychiatry* **2017**, *56*, 813–824. [CrossRef] [PubMed]

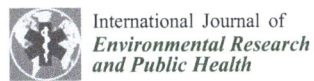

Article

Longitudinal Trends of Participation in Relation to Mental Health in Children with and without Physical Difficulties

Ai-Wen Hwang [1,2], Chia-Hsieh Chang [3], Mats Granlund [4], Christine Imms [5], Chia-Ling Chen [1,2] and Lin-Ju Kang [1,2,*]

1. Graduate Institute of Early Intervention, College of Medicine, Chang Gung University, 259 Wen-Hwa 1st Road, Kwei-Shan, Tao-Yuan City 33302, Taiwan; awhwang@mail.cgu.edu.tw (A.-W.H.); clingchen@gmail.com (C.-L.C.)
2. Department of Physical Medicine and Rehabilitation, Chang Gung Memorial Hospital, Linkou, 5 Fu-Xing St., Kwei-Shan, Tao-Yuan City 33301, Taiwan
3. Department of Pediatric Orthopedics, Chang Gung Memorial Hospital, Linkou, 5 Fu-Xing St., Kwei-Shan, Tao-Yuan City 33301, Taiwan; chiahchang@gmail.com
4. CHILD, Swedish Institute of Disability Research, School of health and welfare, Jönköping University, Gjuterigatan 5, 553 18 Jönköping, Sweden; Mats.Granlund@ju.se
5. Department of Paediatrics, The University of Melbourne, 50 Flemington Road, Parkville, Victoria 3052, Australia; christine.imms@unimelb.edu.au
* Correspondence: linjukang@mail.cgu.edu.tw; Tel.: +886-3-2118800 (ext. 3779); Fax: +886-2-82189072

Received: 5 October 2020; Accepted: 15 November 2020; Published: 18 November 2020

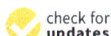

Abstract: Children with physical disabilities (PD) are known to have participation restrictions when in inclusive settings alongside typically developing (TD) children. The restrictions in participation over time may affect their mental health status. This study aimed to investigate the longitudinal relationship between independence in activities (capability) and frequency of attendance in activities, in relation to perceived mental health status in children with and without PD. The participants were a convenience sample of parents of 77 school children with PD and 94 TD children who completed four assessments with a one-year interval between each assessment. Parents of these children were interviewed with the Functioning Scale of the Disability Evaluation System—Child version (FUNDES-Child). Three dimensions of mental health problems—loneliness, acting upset, and acting nervous—were rated by parents with the Child Health Questionnaire (CHQ). Linear trend was tested by repeated-measure ANOVA. The results revealed different longitudinal patterns of independence and frequency of attendance over time for children with PD and TD. Frequency of attending activities may be more important than independence in performing activities for experiencing fewer mental health problems. The findings highlight the need for supporting children's actual attendance in daily activities which may benefit their later mental health.

Keywords: participation; longitudinal study; physical disabilities; inclusion; mental health

1. Introduction

Participation, referring to functioning in everyday life beyond the health condition or disability-related diagnosis, is aligned with inclusive education in the Sustainable Development Goals (SDGs) as part of a United Nations Resolution that are intended to be achieved by 2030. SDGoal 4 states that inclusive and equitable quality education and promotion of lifelong learning opportunities in the home, school, and community "for all" must be ensured. Thus, children with disabilities have the same right to education and learning as other children. This SDG goal supports that all children should be educated within their best-fit environment, providing learning opportunities within participatory learning processes. Therefore, investigating whether the need for positive experiences and learning are met by the unique environmental requirements of children with disabilities will provide critical information for building a society for all.

Physical disability (PD) is one of the categories of disabilities defined in the overall objectives of the United Nations Convention on the Rights of Persons with Disabilities (UNCRPD). Typically, we address the need for safety and equality of school for children with physical difficulty with their peers in an inclusive physical environment [1]. However, the children's mental health, especially in an inclusive setting, is usually not explicitly supported by the surrounding adults and peers. Mental health has been defined as "a state of wellbeing in which every individual realizes his or her own potential, can cope with the normal stresses of life, can work productively and fruitfully and is able to make a contribution to his or her community." [2] School-aged children with physical disabilities [3] and young adults [4] are more likely to develop mental health problems, such as depression and anxiety, than their peers without disabilities.

Research reported increased vulnerability to poor mental health when adolescents make the transition to young adulthood [5]. The mental health of children with a physical disability aged 6–12 years is less well known. In Taiwan, caregivers and professionals focus largely on interventions to improve physical functioning, but mental health is seldom a focus of interest. However, the family costs associated with a mental disorder or mental illness are likely to be higher than those associated with chronic physical disorders [6].

Participation in everyday life activities can be seen as containing two dimensions; physical/virtual attendance and involvement [7]. The life situations in which these dimensions are experienced change over time which influences patterns of attendance and involvement. Long-term outcomes of attendance and involvement may with time affect mental health for children. Mental health may on the other hand affect the probability of adapting to environmental changes following from transition to new life roles. The two dimensions of participation have a bi-directional relation with internal factors within the child as well as external factors in the environment [7]. Internal factors concern activity competence, sense of self, and preferences, while external factors concern physical and social factors in the environment [7]. In earlier research and pediatric rehabilitation intervention, internal factors such as body functions and activity performance have been the focus with the implicit rational that by improving child skills the child will participate more. Thus, activity competence in terms of capability to perform activities in everyday life activities rather than participation in everyday life has been the focus of both assessment and intervention [8–10]. However, the evidence that intervention focusing solely on improving skills leads to enhanced participation is weak [9]. The relationship between activity competence, defined as capability, and the two dimensions of participation needs to be further investigated.

The physical and social activity competence of an individual can be investigated on a continuum from capacity (the ability to perform an activity under ideal circumstances) to capability (the ability to perform an activity in natural environments). In measures of activity competence, e.g., Pediatric Evaluation of Disability Inventory (PEDI) [11] or Child and Adolescent Scale of Participation (CASP) [12], activity competence is operationalized as independence, that is, the level of support needed to perform an activity. The Functioning Scale of the Disability Evaluation System—Child version (FUNDES-Child) [13,14] is a measure containing the further development of CASP to include a measure of frequency of attendance in activities, in addition to the measure of independence in performing an activity (capability). Thus, FUNDES-Child allows us to investigate the relationship between capability and the attendance dimension of participation.

We know that a low frequency of participation in physical activity can lead to a decrease in activity competence defined both as capacity and capability. The International Classification of Functioning, Disability and Health (ICF) framework has been applied in several longitudinal studies that indicate a bi-directional relationship between participation and body function (mental or physical) [15]. For children with severe physical impairments, the longitudinal prediction of participation by body function is stronger than for children with less severe physical impairments [16]. How mental health problems are related to capability as well as participation has been infrequently investigated. A cross-sectional study reported that participation in physical activities can attenuate the odds of depression in children with cerebral palsy (CP) (the Odds Ratio = 1.9; 95%; the Confidence Interval = 0.7–5.3) [3]. Another cross-sectional study reported a bidirectional relationship between mental health problems and participation for children with and without physical disabilities aged 6–14 years [17]. Studies are lacking about how capability and participation can predict or influence later mental health.

It is likely that environmental factors moderate the relationship between capability and participation and mental health, respectively. Barriers in the environment may result in children with disabilities attending activities less frequently than same-aged peers, although they actually have the capability to perform the activity. Kang et al. found that barriers experienced in social support, such as attitudes from family and community, influenced participation more than the physical design of the school for children with physical disabilities [18]. Based on the reported difference between capability and frequency of attending an activity, Hwang et al. proposed that a measure of the gap between independence and frequency of attendance would reflect the closeness of fit between the environment and the person in relation to children with physical impairments [16]. A small gap would indicate a good fit. In Hwang et al.'s study, capability was defined as independence in performing an activity, and frequency of attendance was an operationalization of the attendance dimension of participation [19,20]. Hwang et al. explored the gap between independence and frequency using a nationwide cross-sectional survey with FUNDES-Child [16]. The data showed that the independence–frequency gap of children with cerebral palsy becomes wider with age and that the gap increased more for children with mild compared to severe impairments. The gap may reflect environmental and personal factors that influence individualized service plans or rehabilitation goals aimed at increasing the children's attendance at activities even if they do not have the capability to perform the activities independently.

Studies are needed to reveal the longitudinal influence of participation outcomes and its impacts on other outcomes. Imms and Adair (2016) in a longitudinal study investigated participation in activities outside the school for 93 children with CP for 9 years. Regarding attendance, the diversity of the activities the children attended, as well as the frequency with which the children attended the activities, decreased over time for recreational, active physical, and self-improvement activities; while attendance in social activities increased over time [21]. Anaby et al. (2019), in an intervention study aimed at increasing participation in community activities by adapting the environment, reported that increased self-rated perception of activity performance was related to increased motor capacity (a measure of activity competence) [22].

The purpose of this study was to investigate the longitudinal relationship between independence (capability) and frequency of attendance in relation to perceived mental health status in children with and without physical disabilities. Three specific aims were addressed to reveal the interactions between capability and attendance over time, and how these interactions relate to mental health status. First, the trajectories of independence, frequency of attendance, and the independence–frequency of attendance gap across four years were analyzed for children with and without physical disabilities. Second, the trajectories of independence, frequency of attendance, and the independence–frequency of attendance gap over time were compared in accordance with children's mental health status. Third, the relationships between independence and frequency of attendance across the four years and mental health problems in the last year were examined.

2. Materials and Methods

2.1. Design

A four-year longitudinal descriptive study design was used. We analyzed data from children whose families completed surveys at four time points at one-year intervals. Trained interviewers visited each family to collect data.

2.2. Participants

The proxy–child dyads were recruited from elementary schools in the northern, middle, and southern parts of Taiwan. The inclusion criteria for children with physical disabilities were (1) children from the first to fifth grade; (2) children with the following primary diagnoses or conditions: Amputation, cerebral palsy, cerebral vascular accident/stroke (vascular brain disorders), congenital anomalies, hydrocephalus, juvenile arthritis, nonprogressive muscular disorders, neuropathy, orthopedic conditions (e.g., scoliosis), spinal cord injury, spina bifida, and traumatic brain injury [23], or those who had movement impairments [24] or neuromuscular disabilities [25]; and (3) that parents provided consent. The inclusion criteria for typically developing children were: (1) Children from the first to fifth grade; (2) children without medical diagnosis relating to developmental disabilities; and (3) that parents provided consent. The ethical approval (no. 100-4201A3) was obtained from the Institutional Review Board in the Chang Gung Memorial Hospital in Taiwan. All the participants provided the signed informed consent. The numbers of participants who completed the interviews from the first to the fourth time points were 119, 98, 97, and 94 for TD children, and 93, 78, 78, and 77 for children with PD, respectively (see Table 1 for demographic data). The attrition rates between the first and fourth time points were 21% for TD children and 17% for children with PD.

Table 1. The demographic data for children with typical development (TD) and children with physical disabilities (PD).

	TD (n = 94)				PD (n = 77)			
	Time 1	Time 2	Time 3	Time 4	Time 1	Time 2	Time 3	Time 4
Gestational age (weeks) (SD)	37.5 (2.8)				33.5 (5.4) [a]			
Age (months) (SD)	95.6 (17.7)	109.1 (17.7)	122.9 (18.3)	135.6 (17.9)	92.5 (17.1)	109.2 (19.2)	122.2 (19.7)	134.9 (19.9)
Gender (male) (N, %)	46 (50.5)				53 (68.8) [b]			
Major Diagnosis [c]								
CP					46 (59.7)			
Seizure					16 (20.8)			
Hydrocephalus					3 (3.9)			
Brain hemorrhage					1 (1.3)			
CHD					5 (6.5)			
Down syndrome					1 (1.3)			
Rare disease					1 (2.3)			
GMFCS [d]								
I					7 (15.2)			
II					9 (19.6)			
III					13 (28.2)			
IV					10 (21.7)			
V					7 (15.2)			
MACS [d]								
I					6 (13)			
II					15 (32.6)			
III					8 (17.4)			
IV					13 (28.3)			
V					4 (8.7)			
CFCS [d]								
I					20 (43.5)			
II					8 (17.4)			
III					9 (19.6)			
IV					7 (15.2)			
V					2 (4.3)			
School grade (N, %)								
Kindergarten	14 (15.4)	1 (1.1)	0 (0)	0 (0)	14 (18.2)	1 (1.3)	3 (3.9)	2 (2.6)
First grade	20 (22)	10 (11)	1 (1.1)	0 (0)	23 (29.9)	14 (18.2)	0 (0)	1 (1.3)
Second grade	28 (30.8)	19 (20.9)	9 (9.9)	2 (2.2)	17 (22.1)	17 (22.1)	13 (16.9)	0 (0)
Third grade	19 (20.9)	25 (27.5)	13 (19.8)	8 (8.8)	16 (20.8)	14 (18.2)	15 (19.5)	13 (16.9)

Table 1. Cont.

	TD (n = 94)				PD (n = 77)			
	Time 1	Time 2	Time 3	Time 4	Time 1	Time 2	Time 3	Time 4
Fourth grade	6 (6.6)	17 (18.7)	26 (28.6)	19 (20.9)	6 (7.8)	17 (22.1)	16 (20.8)	15 (19.5)
Fifth grade	2 (2.2)	15 (16.5)	16 (17.6)	25 (27.5)	1 (1.3)	11 (14.3)	17 (22.1)	15 (19.5)
Sixth grade	2 (2.2)	2 (2.2)	17 (18.7)	16 (17.6)	0 (0)	2 (2.6)	10 (13)	18 (23.4)
Seventh grade		2 (2.2)	2 (2.2)	17 (18.7)		1 (1.3)	3 (3.9)	10 (13)
Eighth grade		2 (2.2)	2 (2.2)	2 (2.2)		0 (0)	3 (3.9)	3 (3.9)
Ninth grade				2 (2.2)				0 (0)
School placement (N, %)								
Regular	94 (100)				15 (20.3)	13 (18.1)	17 (22.1)	9 (13.8)
Regular and resource room	0 (0)				20 (27)	23 (31.9)	22 (28.6)	18 (27.7)
Special class in regular school	0 (0)				25 (33.8)	30 (41.7)	30 (39)	26 (40)
Special school	0 (0)				4 (5.4)	4 (5.6)	6 (7.8)	8 (12.3)
Residential school or home	0 (0)				1 (1.4)	1 (1.4)	1 (1.3)	2 (3.0)
Others	0 (0)				9 (12.2)	1 (1.4)	1 (1.3)	2 (3.1)

SD = standard deviation; CP=cerebral palsy; CHD=Congenital Heart Disease. [a] Significant difference between children with TD and PD by independent t-test, alpha set at 0.05; [b] significant difference between children with TD and PD by chi-square, alpha set at 0.05; [c] children's major diagnoses were obtained from physicians; [d] only children with CP were rated by interviewers with the Gross Motor Function Classification System (GMFCS), Manual Ability Classification System (MACS), and the Communication Function Classification System (CFCS) at the first time point test.

2.3. Measure

2.3.1. Functioning Scale of the Disability Evaluation System—Child Version (FUNDES-Child)

The FUNDES-Child utilizes a proxy format in which parents or other caregivers answer questions about their child's activities in the previous 6 months. The FUNDES-Child was translated and modified from the Child and Family Follow-up Survey (CFFS) [12]. The cross-cultural adaption and validation of FUNDES-Child has been reported elsewhere [13,14,18]. The FUNDES-Child contains four parts: Part I: Physical and emotional health (information on health and the way of moving and communication); Part II: Participation (derived from the Child and Adolescent Scale of Participation); Part III: Body function impairment (derived from the Child and Adolescent Factors Inventory); and Part IV: Environmental factors (derived from the Child and Adolescent Scale of Environment). In this study, we only focused on Parts I and II. General mental health status was measured by one question in the FUNDES-Child Part I, which was: "In general, how would you describe your child's emotional health and well-being (i.e., the way he or she feels about himself or herself and his or her life)?" The response was rated as 0 (poor), 1 (fair), 2 (good), 3 (very good), and 4 (excellent).

Participation was assessed using the FUNDES-Child Part II that contains 20 items of children's daily participation in 4 settings: Home, neighborhood/community, school, and home/community living. The scale contains two dimensions: Independence and frequency of attendance [13]. Independence was defined as the child's current level of capability to perform the activity compared to other children of his or her age in the same community. For each item, independence was rated as 0 (independent), 1 (with supervision/mild assistance), 2 (with moderate assistance), 3 (with full assistance). Frequency of attendance was rated with reference to age as 0 (the same or more than expected for age), 1 (somewhat less than expected for age), 2 (much less than expected for age), and 3 (never does). The score was designed to match the coding of the ICF qualifiers, with higher scores indicating more limitations or restrictions in capability and performance. In the FUNDES-Child Part II (participation), therefore, a higher score for independence and frequency of attendance indicates a lower level of independence and a low frequency of attending in the activity. A response of "not applicable" (a child of the same age and in the same community would not be expected to do that activity) was allowed for both dimensions. For example, the item "using transportation to get around in the community" could be rated as not applicable if the child did not need to utilize the transportation system. All items were rated under the condition that children used assistive devices as usual.

As each item in the FUNDES-Child Part II (participation) was on the same ordinal scale with the same anchor points at the extreme end (0–3 points), the two dimensions were comparable based on age-expected independence and frequency of attending. Items rated as "not applicable" were omitted in the scoring [13]. The mean scores for each of the 4 settings of FUNDES-Child Part II (participation) are thus the sum of the scores of all "applicable" items divided by the number of applicable items and then converted to a 0–100 scale for the two dimensions. The trained interviewers could, therefore, interpret the scores within the same directional framework (higher scores represented greater participation restriction and more dependence). A score of 0 on either scale could be interpreted as "doing the same as other children the same age". The reliability of the FUNDES-Child Part II (participation) in children with and without physical disability was examined. Test–retest reliability of 86 parent proxies who were interviewed twice within 2 weeks was established for independence (intraclass correlation coefficient [ICC] = 0.955, $p < 0.001$) and frequency of attendance (ICC = 0.796, $p < 0.001$). Interrater reliability of another 77 parent proxy respondents was established for independence (ICC = 0.994, $p < 0.001$) and frequency of attendance (ICC = 0.860, $p < 0.001$).

2.3.2. Child Health Questionnaire (CHQ)

The CHQ is an internationally recognized general health-related quality of life (HRQOL) instrument that has been rigorously translated into more than 78 languages and standardized for use with children aged 5–18 to assess the child's physical, emotional, and social well-being. There are both parent-reported and child self-completed versions of varying lengths. This study applied the parent-reported 28 (PF28) version at the fourth time point of this study. The CHQ covers three items representing mental health problems: "During the past 4 weeks, how much of the time do you think your child felt lonely?", "During the past 4 weeks, how much of the time do you think your child acted nervous?", "During the past 4 weeks, how much of the time do you think your child acted bothered or upset?" Each item is rated with the Likert scale as 1 (all of the time) to 5 (none of the time); thus, a higher score indicates less frequent mental health problems. The score was then transformed to standardized 0 to 100 scores using the algorithm *(raw score − 1) × 100/4*. The higher standardized score means better mental condition. The whole scale score can be transformed to a Z-score as described in the manual [26].

2.4. Procedure

Study flyers and research invitations were distributed to schools and hospitals. The teachers and clinicians informed the researchers about the families who were interested in this study, and then the research assistants contacted the families. Following signed informed consent from the children's proxies, the trained testers visited families at home or another place convenient to the family, such as schools or hospitals. The trained interviewers conducted structured interviews with the proxies to collect all data. To reduce participant attrition over time, thank you letters and an invitation for the next year were sent to participants' schools and hospitals to be distributed to families every year around the time of Christmas or Chinese New Year.

2.5. Data Analysis

The independence–frequency of attendance gap was analyzed by the score of independence minus the score of frequency of attendance. If the independence–frequency of attendance gap was positive (i.e., independence limitation score > frequency of attendance restriction score, where high scores mean more dependent and restricted), it meant that children attended the activity more frequently than what was expected from their level of independence. If the gap was negative (i.e., independence limitation score < frequency of attendance restriction score), it meant that children attended the activity less frequently than what was expected from their level of independence. The trajectories of independence scores, frequency of attendance scores, and the independence–frequency of attendance gap were graphed to provide a global picture of the changes in patterns across four time points. The mean scores for independence and frequency were plotted on dual Y coordinates (from 0 "as expected for age" to 100 "most dependent" or "most restricted", respectively), illustrating any discrepancy between independence and frequency of attendance scores.

Longitudinal statistical analyses were performed with the Statistical Package for Social Science version 21.0 (SPSS, Inc., Chicago, IL, USA). The changes from the first to the fourth year were examined with a two-way repeated measure ANOVA with a group (PD and TD) by time (the first, second, third, and fourth year) interaction. The trend analysis was performed with repeated measures of ANOVA. The significance of the linear trend was tested by ANOVA for 4 time points, and the between-times sum of squares for the effect of the time point was partitioned into a polynomial trend, namely a linear and higher order trend. The polynomial trend component was tested by an F-ratio (the mean square for linear trend/error term). To deal with the variance inequality, Leven's test for homogeneity was conducted before ANOVA. Welch ANOVA and Games–Howell post hoc analyses were performed if the data failed to meet the equal variance assumption with alpha set at 0.05 (2-tailed). The trajectory of independence score, frequency of attendance score, and the independence–frequency of attendance gap were also graphed.

To address the first and second aims, the above analyses were performed for all children with TD and PD and by the five levels of general mental health status (i.e., excellent, very good, good, fair, and poor) in each group. When analyzing each group based on the level of general mental health status, children with TD who were rated as "very good" and "good" and children with PD who were rated as "very good", "good", and "fair" had adequate sample sizes and thus sufficient statistical power for testing the significance in the trend analysis. For other children, only descriptive statistics were presented. To address the third aim, Pearson or Spearman correlations were used for examining the relationships between independence and frequency of attendance at the first to fourth time points and the mental health problems (i.e., loneliness, upset, and nervous) at the final time point. For exploratory purposes, we focused on correlations that reach a significance level of 0.05.

3. Results

The scores of independence and frequency of attendance measured by the FUNDES-Child Part II (participation) were significantly lower for children with PD than children with TD at each time point ($p < 0.001$). Patterns of change over the four time points showed that the children with PD had increasing scores (i.e., were more dependent and restricted) with age; while children with TD had decreasing scores (i.e., were less dependent and restricted) on the two dimensions (Table 2 and Figure 1). The independence–frequency of attendance gap scores for the TD children were initially negative; they tended to attend activities less frequently although they could perform the activity independently. With time the gap decreased and the change reached significance. For children with PD, the gap was positive, and they tended to be less dependent in the activity, although they attended the activity relatively frequently. With time, the gap increased but did not reach significance (Table 2).

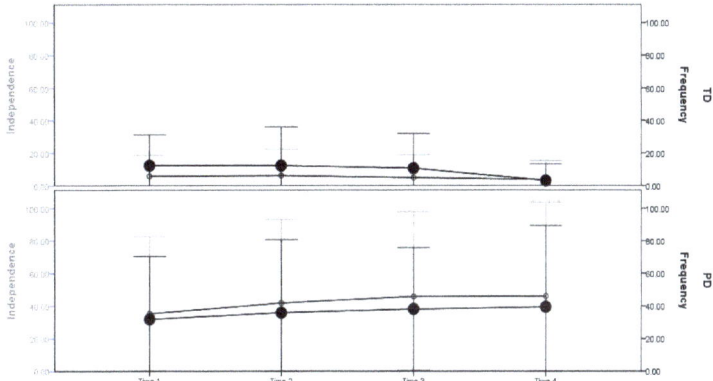

Figure 1. Independence and frequency of attendance gap by groups (TD vs. PD) across the four time points. Note: Dark point (●) and black line with 1 SD error bar illustrate the frequency of attendance scores; open circle point (○) and gray line with 1 SD error bar illustrate the independence scores.

For the change patterns in independence and frequency of attendance across levels of general mental status, the children with PD had increasing scores (more limitations and restrictions) with time, while children with TD had decreasing scores (fewer limitations and restrictions; see Table 2 and Figure 2). The gap scores for the TD children were negative. With time, the gap decreased and the change reached significance for children whose mental health status was "very good" and "good". For children with PD, the gap was positive. With time, the gap increased and the change reached significance only for children whose mental health status was "good" (Table 2). The interaction effects of time and group are available in the Supplementary Materials, Table S1.

Table 2. Results of longitudinal statistical analyses for children with PD and TD children.

	TD					Trend		PD				Trend	
	Mean (SD)							Mean (SD)					
	Time 1	Time 2	Time 3	Time 4	(df = 3)	p		Time 1	Time 2	Time 3	Time 4	F	p
FUNDES-Child total scores for whole participants with typical development (n = 94) and children with disabilities (n = 77).													
Independence	5.74 (6.37)	6.12 (8.14)	4.89 (6.93)	3.65 (5.87)	5.575	0.019		35.28 (23.62)	41.80 (25.68)	45.75 (26.09)	46.01 (28.87)	7.367	0.007
Frequency	12.27 (9.42)	12.25 (11.86)	10.68 (10.57)	3.12 (5.08)	43.193	<0.001		31.85 (19.23)	35.89 (22.37)	38.05 (18.80)	39.39 (25.03)	5.112	0.024
Gap	−6.54 (8.77)	−6.14 (7.97)	−5.79 (7.78)	0.53 (4.00)	40.202	<0.001		3.43 (16.25)	5.92 (15.99)	7.70 (16.66)	6.62 (14.45)	1.978	0.161
Mental health excellent for children with typical development (n = 5) and children with disabilities (n = 5) (NA).													
Mental health very good for children with typical development (n = 69) and children with disabilities (n = 16).													
Independence	5.11 (6.04)	5.41 (7.66)	4.62 (6.51)	2.98 (3.95)	4.648	0.032		27.81 (22.56)	30.31 (23.29)	33.83 (25.53)	34.53 (26.06)	0.753	0.389
Frequency	12.73 (9.71)	11.79 (11.45)	10.40 (10.28)	2.64 (4.28)	39.655	<0.001		26.71 (15.76)	28.09 (19.76)	30.78 (16.83)	23.52 (19.14)	0.117	0.733
Gap	−7.62 (9.55)	−6.39 (8.72)	−5.78 (7.26)	0.34 (3.39)	35.810	<0.001		1.10 (17.57)	−6.39 (8.72)	−5.78 (7.26)	0.34 (3.39)	2.910	0.093
Mental health good for children with typical development (n = 17) and children with disabilities (n = 34).													
Independence	8.34 (7.41)	9.44 (10.32)	7.26 (9.36)	7.04 (10.49)	0.351	0.556		37.06 (24.99)	47.06 (24.81)	49.00 (23.67)	49.79 (28.27)	4.213	0.042
Frequency	12.91 (8.44)	16.60 (14.49)	13.64 (11.36)	4.79 (6.85)	5.559	0.021		32.10 (18.13)	37.25 (22.61)	38.40 (19.16)	42.12 (25.37)	3.577	0.061
Gap	−4.57 (5.37)	−7.16 (5.4)	−6.38 (8.73)	2.25 (4.76)	1.380	0.003		4.96 (18.22)	9.81 (15.02)	10.61 (17.62)	7.67 (14.96)	0.496	0.482
Mental health fair for children with typical development (n = 3) and children with disabilities (n = 18).													
Independence	8.51 (8.67)	5.56 (8.07)	3.51 (0.01)	5.85 (6.16)	NA	NA		35.20 (23.00)	40.24 (27.11)	45.30 (29.06)	44.91 (30.69)	0.138	0.244
Frequency	11.11 (7.41)	8.64 (6.50)	14.65 (16.54)	9.94 (8.65)	NA	NA		31.05 (20.86)	37.81 (22.85)	41.69 (17.09)	46.45 (23.56)	5.008	0.029
Gap	−2.60 (4.33)	−3.09 (5.35)	−11.14 (16.54)	−4.09 (10.72)	NA	NA		4.15 (14.56)	2.44 (13.2)	3.61 (17.23)	−1.55 (15.21)	0.997	0.332

Note: Mental health poor for children with typical development (n = 0) and children with disabilities (n = 4) (NA).

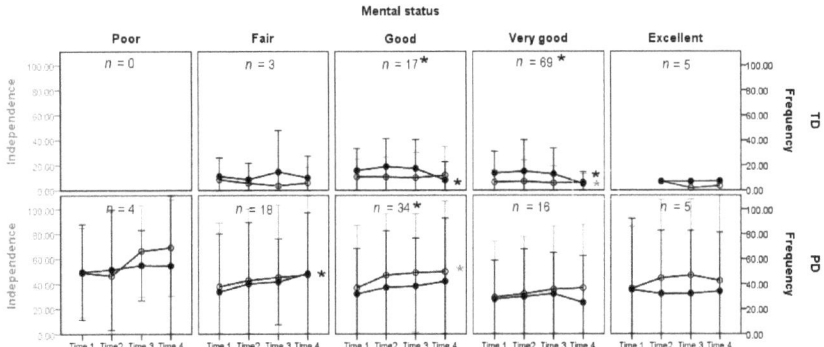

Figure 2. Independence and frequency of attendance gap by groups (TD vs. PD) across four time points by the five mental status of children. Note. TD = typically developing children; PD = physical disability; dark point (•) and black line with 1 SD error bar illustrate the frequency of attendance scores; circle point (○) and gray line with 1 SD error bar illustrate the independence scores; dark star sign (*) beside Time 4 presents a significant trend for frequency of attendance; gray star sign (*) beside Time 4 presents a significant trend for independence. Dark star sign (*) beside the case number presents significant independence–frequency of attendance gap trends in that block.

The correlations between independence scores and frequency of attendance scores across the first to fourth time points and the items of mental health problems at the fourth time point are exhibited in Table 3. Overall, all correlations were in the week-to-moderate range (<±0.4), and all but one was negative. Negative correlation coefficients between the independence and frequency of attendance scores and mental health problems scores indicate that more dependence and higher restrictions in attendance were associated with more mental health problems (i.e., lower scores for loneliness, upset, and nervous). In addition, the correlations between frequency of attendance and mental health problems were in general stronger than those for independence. The independence and frequency of attendance scores were correlated with the score for loneliness only for children with PD, and were also correlated with the score for being nervous only for children with TD. The frequency of attendance, but not independence, was correlated with the score for being upset for both children with TD and PD. When the scores of the three mental health items were aggregated to a Z-score, the frequency of attendance was correlated with the mental health scores at all 4 time points for children with PD, and also at second and third time points for TD children. The correlations between the frequency of attendance and loneliness and being nervous were highlighted by scatter plots of the scores at the fourth time (shown in Figure 3). The plots showed that the TD children who were more restricted in frequency of attendance expressed more feelings of being nervous. The children with PD who were more restricted in frequency of attendance expressed more loneliness.

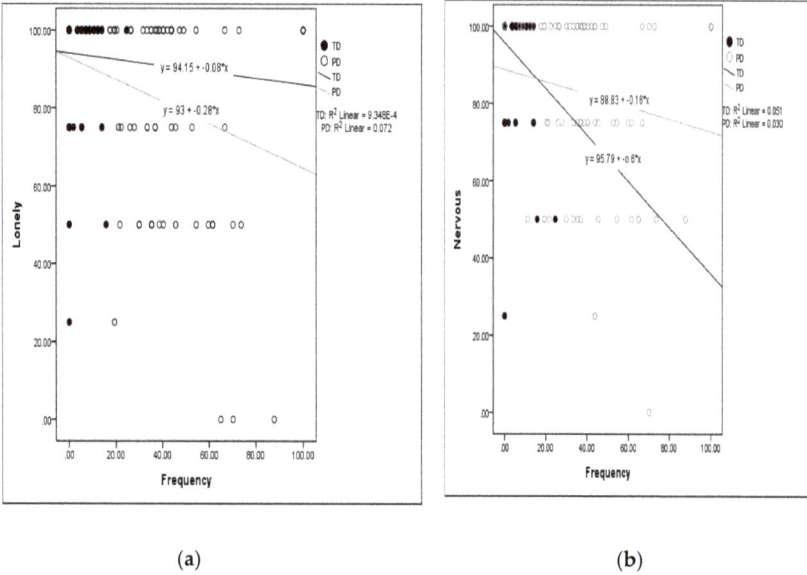

Figure 3. The scatter plots of correlations between (**a**) lonely and frequency; (**b**) nervous and frequency at the fourth time point.

Table 3. Correlation coefficients between mental health problems measured by the Child Health Questionnaire (CHQ) and participation independence and frequency of attendance.

	T4 Lonely		T4 Upset		T4 Nervous		Z-Score	
	TD	PD	TD	PD	TD	PD	TD	PD
T1 Independence	0.025	−0.169	−0.051	−0.142	−0.114	−0.165	−0.050	−0.179
T2 Independence	−0.104	−0.169	−0.172	−0.124	−0.248 *	−0.064	−0.186	−0.137
T3 Independence	−0.072	−0.288 *	−0.139	−0.201	−0.284 **	−0.124	−0.176	−0.235 *
T4 Independence	−0.003	−0.258 *	−0.175	−0.183	−0.301 **	−0.099	−0.170	−0.207
T1 Frequency	−0.029	−0.167	−0.031	−0.231 *	−0.046	−0.204	−0.038	−0.225 *
T2 Frequency	−0.121	−0.332 **	−0.209 *	−0.178	−0.267 **	−0.095	−0.212 *	−0.233 *
T3 Frequency	−0.184	−0.342 **	−0.225 *	−0.281 *	−0.358 **	−0.147	−0.273 **	−0.294 **
T4 Frequency	−0.039	−0.268 *	−0.133	−0.207	−0.232 *	−0.174	−0.144	−0.246 *

* $p < 0.05$; ** $p < 0.01$; T1 to T4 stand for the first to fourth time points.

4. Discussion

This study is unique for using a longitudinal design to investigate long-term changes in two dimensions, capability and frequency of attendance, and the closeness of fit between these two dimensions. This study described participation trajectories for the same group of children, providing strong evidence about their experiences and opportunities over time. The longitudinal investigation on participation for both children with PD and TD added valuable information to what can be deduced from cross-sectional data [16]. In a previous study, cross-sectional data of cohorts of children with PD showed a fluctuating and/or declining trend in participation attendance with age, especially during the transition from elementary school to junior high school [16]. With a longitudinal design, we were able to trace the adaptive process within the same groups of children across different ages.

TD children on average had a decreasing negative gap between independence and frequency of attendance over time. In other words, with age, expected capacity (independence) and performance (participation) were matched. One explanation for this finding is that TD children experienced both increased capability and a stronger self-selection of what activities to attend frequently with age. In contrast, children with PD had decreasing independence over time and relatively stable frequency of attendance, suggesting that, despite a widening gap in age-appropriate independence, participation remained possible. Knowledge about typical and atypical trajectories could inform professionals in how to support children's participation as a means of promoting both physical and mental health.

In terms of children's general mental health status rated by parent proxies, a majority of children with TD were rated as good to very good; while a majority of children with PD were rated as fair to very good. This indicates that parents perceived a relatively good state of mental health status of school-age children in Taiwan. We would expect that when children with and without PD are in an inclusive environment, children with PD may need individualized strategies to enhance learning and socialization to a larger extent than TD children. Caregivers and educators may need supports in providing a learning and socially enhancing environment that helps children maintain an adequate level of mental health. A universal design for learning may be needed to meet the diverse participation needs that occur in inclusive education settings, thus supporting non-discriminatory and inclusive education.

The trajectories identified for independence and frequency of attendance over four years were related to proxy-rated mental health status. Children with TD and PD who were less dependent and less restricted in attendance were also reported to have higher levels of mental health status. In particular, the highest dependence and restrictions in attending the activities were reported for children with PD rated as having poor mental health. However, the positive gap (i.e., attending more than the capability score suggested that a child could do independently) for children with PD remained over time, especially for children with good mental health. The positive gap may indicate the importance of support from the environment to enable frequent participation in the activities. For TD children, a gradual narrowing of the negative gap (due to sustained ability and increased frequency of attending an activity) was related to having good or very good mental health. At the last data collection point, TD children's ability and frequency of attendance were matched. These findings suggest that school-age children with PD may have different lived experiences and adaptive processes from their TD peers as they age. For children with PD, continued environmental supports to enable children to attend more than their capability suggests may be an important support for maintaining good mental health status.

Though the children with disabilities have struggled with physical as well as emotional vulnerability, most children in this study were reported to have less frequent mental health problems, also indicating a relatively good state of mental health status. The relationship between frequency of attendance and later mental health problems was stronger than the relationship between independence and later mental health problems. Our results suggest that in children with PD, attending the activities more frequently was associated with less frequent feelings of loneliness, which is a positive outcome for social well-being. This suggests that it is essential to provide supports for children with PD to keep attending activities over time, regardless of whether they have limited ability to perform the activities independently. In children with TD, attending the activities more frequently was associated with less frequent feelings of nervousness. Experiences and competencies gained through participation may facilitate children's confidence and mastery in performing the activities and is thus associated with positive emotional well-being [27].

Findings of this study have implications for environment-based interventions to achieve a match or even a positive gap between independence and frequency of attendance in activities for a child. Environment-based interventions focus on finding solutions built on the child's strengths and capability that help to remove physical, social, and institutional or activity demands barriers to participation [15]. The active facilitation of participation for children with PD by adapting the environment may further facilitate the maintenance of children's mental health. In particular, building a social-friendly environment relies on responsive relationships with care providers and teachers. For rights-based inclusion, the educator has a role to support the child to develop stable friendships by taking advantage of the positive characteristics of each child [28]. This would make inclusive education offer learning opportunities that engage every child, so they learn together and cope with each other.

This study highlighted the importance of exploring longitudinal patterns of capability and participation frequency in relation to general mental health status. There are, however, some limitations pertaining to the measures used in this study. In terms of mental health measures, only one item of general mental health status and three questions about mental health problems were used. Further research may explore a broader set of mental health issues that reflect emotional, psychological, and social well-being. In terms of the measures of participation, children's involvement in the activities was not investigated. It is likely that personal feelings and experiences when actually engaging in the activities are affecting children's mental health and well-being. The relationship between involvement and mental health warrants further investigation.

5. Conclusions

Children with physical disabilities can, presumably with appropriate supports, sustain a high frequency of attending activities despite difficulties with performing the activities independently. Enriched participation experiences may lead to better mental status of children regardless of disability or not. However, the relationships between frequency of attending, independence, and mental health differed between children with and without PD. Children with TD exhibited fewer mental health problems as rated by proxies, and their negative frequency of attending–independence gap narrowed over time. Children with PD still had a wide positive gap after four years of life experiences. Loneliness was related to less frequent attendance for children with PD, while acting nervously was related to less frequent attendance for children with TD. Interventions for promoting mental health status may be designed based on universal strategies that support participation as well as the characteristics of the individual child.

Supplementary Materials: The following are available online at http://www.mdpi.com/1660-4601/17/22/8551/s1, Table S1: Main and interaction effects of longitudinal statistical analyses for children with PD and TD children.

Author Contributions: Conceptualization, A.-W.H., M.G. and C.I.; data curation, A.-W.H.; formal analysis, A.-W.H., M.G., C.I. and L.-J.K.; funding acquisition, A.-W.H., C.-L.C. and L.-J.K.; investigation, A.-W.H. and L.-J.K.; methodology, A.-W.H., M.G., C.I. and L.-J.K.; resources, C.-H.C., C.I., and C.-L.C.; writing—original draft, A.-W.H.; writing—review and editing, C.-H.C., M.G., C.I., C.-L.C. and L.-J.K. All authors have read and agreed to the published version of the manuscript.

Funding: This research was funded by the Ministry of Science and Technology in Taiwan (MOST 101-2314-B-182-088-, NSC 102-2628-B-182-001-MY3) and Chung Gung Memorial Hospital Medical Research (CMRPD1J0071). The APC was funded by Chung Gung Memorial Hospital (BMRPE09).

Acknowledgments: The researchers thank all the families for their time participating in the interviews, and all the research assistants.

Conflicts of Interest: The authors declare no conflict of interest.

Abbreviations

TD	Typical development
CP	Cerebral palsy
CHD	Congenital heart disease
GMFCS	Gross Motor Function Classification System
MACS	Manual Ability Classification System
CFCS	Communication Function Classification System

References

1. Maxwell, G.; Koutsogeorgou, E. Using social capital to construct a conceptual International Classification of Functioning, Disability, and Health Children and Youth version-based framework for stronger inclusive education policies in Europe. *Am. J. Phys. Med. Rehabil.* **2012**, *91*, S118–S123. [CrossRef] [PubMed]
2. World Health Organization. Promoting Mental Health: Concepts, Emerging Evidence, Practice. Summary Report. 2004. Available online: https://www.who.int/mental_health/evidence/en/promoting_mhh.pdf (accessed on 20 March 2020).

3. Whitney, D.G.; Warschausky, S.A.; Peterson, M.D. Mental health disorders and physical risk factors in children with cerebral palsy: A cross-sectional study. *Dev. Med. Child Neurol.* **2019**, *61*, 579–585. [CrossRef] [PubMed]
4. Hanes, J.E.; Hlyva, O.; Rosenbaum, P.; Freeman, M.; Nguyen, T.; Palisano, R.J.; Gorter, J.W. Beyond stereotypes of cerebral palsy: Exploring the lived experiences of young Canadians. *Child Care Health Dev.* **2019**, *45*, 613–622. [CrossRef] [PubMed]
5. Goodman, R. The longitudinal stability of psychiatric problems in children with hemiplegia. *J. Child Psychol. Psychiatry* **1998**, *39*, 347–354. [CrossRef]
6. Solmi, F.; Melnychuk, M.; Morris, S. The cost of mental and physical health disability in childhood and adolescence to families in the UK: Findings from a repeated cross-sectional survey using propensity score matching. *BMJ Open* **2018**, *8*, e018729. [CrossRef]
7. Imms, C.; Granlund, M.; Wilson, P.H.; Steenbergen, B.; Rosenbaum, P.L.; Gordon, A.M. Participation, both a means and an end: A conceptual analysis of processes and outcomes in childhood disability. *Dev. Med. Child Neurol.* **2017**, *59*, 16–25. [CrossRef]
8. Adair, B.; Ullenhag, A.; Rosenbaum, P.; Granlund, M.; Keen, D.; Imms, C. Measures used to quantify participation in childhood disability and their alignment with the family of participation-related constructs: A systematic review. *Dev. Med. Child Neurol.* **2018**, *60*, 1101–1116. [CrossRef]
9. Adair, B.; Ullenhag, A.; Keen, D.; Granlund, M.; Imms, C. The effect of interventions aimed at improving participation outcomes for children with disabilities: A systematic review. *Dev. Med. Child Neurol.* **2015**, *57*, 1093–1104. [CrossRef]
10. Adair, B.; Shields, N.; Froude, E.; Kerr, C.; Imms, C. Patterns of participation in activities outside school in Australian children: A normative study. *Physiotherapy* **2015**, *101*, e741–e742. [CrossRef]
11. Haley, S.M.; Coster, W.J.; Ludlow, L.H.; Haltiwanger, J.T.; Andrellos, P.J. *Pediatric Evaluation of Disability Inventory (PEDI)*; Trustees of Boston University: Boston, MA, USA, 1992.
12. Bedell, G. Developing a follow-up survey focused on participation of children and youth with acquired brain injuries after discharge from inpatient rehabilitation. *NeuroRehabilitation* **2004**, *19*, 191–205. [CrossRef]
13. Hwang, A.W.; Liou, T.H.; Bedell, G.M.; Kang, L.J.; Chen, W.C.; Yen, C.F.; Chang, K.H.; Liao, H.F. Psychometric properties of the Child and Adolescent Scale of Participation-Traditional Chinese Version. *Int. J. Rehabil. Res.* **2013**, *36*, 211–220. [CrossRef] [PubMed]
14. Hwang, A.W.; Yen, C.F.; Liou, T.H.; Bedell, G.; Granlund, M.; Teng, S.W.; Chang, K.H.; Chi, W.C.; Liao, H.F. Development and validation of the ICF-CY based Functioning Scale of the Disability Evaluation System-Child version (FUNDES-Child) in Taiwan. *FJMA* **2015**, *114*, 1170–1180.
15. Anaby, D.R.; Law, M.C.; Majnemer, A.; Feldman, D. Opening doors to participation of youth with physical disabilities: An intervention study. *Can. J. Occup. Ther.* **2016**, *83*, 83–90. [CrossRef] [PubMed]
16. Hwang, A.W.; Yen, C.F.; Liou, T.H.; Simeonsson, R.J.; Chi, W.C.; Lollar, D.J.; Liao, H.F.; Kang, L.J.; Wu, T.F.; Teng, S.W.; et al. Participation of children with disabilities in Taiwan: The gap between independence and frequency. *PLoS ONE* **2015**, *10*, e0126693. [CrossRef]
17. King, G.; Law, M.; Petrenchik, T.; Hurley, P. Psychosocial Determinants of Out of School Activity Participation for Children with and without Physical Disabilities. *Phys. Occup. Ther. Pediatr.* **2013**, *33*, 384–404. [CrossRef]
18. Kang, L.J.; Yen, C.F.; Bedell, G.; Simeonsson, R.J.; Liou, T.H.; Chi, W.C.; Liu, S.W.; Liao, H.F.; Hwang, A.W. The Chinese version of the Child and Adolescent Scale of Environment (CASE-C): Validity and Reliability for Children with Disabilities in Taiwan. *Res. Dev. Disabil.* **2015**, *38*, 64–74. [CrossRef]
19. Morris, C. Measuring participation in childhood disability: How does the capability approach improve our understanding? *Dev. Med. Child Neurol.* **2009**, *51*, 92–94. [CrossRef]
20. Imms, C. Review of the Children's Assessment of Participation and Enjoyment and the Preferences for Activity of Children. *Phys. Occup. Ther. Pediatr.* **2008**, *28*, 389–404. [CrossRef]
21. Imms, C.; Adair, B.; Keen, D.; Ullenhag, A.; Rosenbaum, P.; Granlund, M. 'Participation': A systematic review of language, definitions, and constructs used in intervention research with children with disabilities. *Dev. Med. Child Neurol.* **2016**, *58*, 29–38. [CrossRef]
22. Anaby, D.; Avery, L.; Gorter, J.W.; Levin, M.F.; Teplicky, R.; Turner, L.; Cormier, I.; Hanes, J. Improving body functions through participation in community activities among young people with physical disabilities. *Dev. Med. Child Neurol.* **2019**, *62*, 640–646. [CrossRef]

23. King, G.; Law, M.; Hanna, S.; King, S.; Hurley, P.; Rosenbaum, P. Predictors of the leisure and recreation participation of children with physical disabilities: A structural equation modeling analysis. *Child Health Care* **2006**, *35*, 209–234. [CrossRef]
24. Egilson, S.T.; Traustadottir, R. Participation of students with physical disabilities in the school environment. *Am. J. Occup. Ther.* **2009**, *63*, 264–272. [CrossRef] [PubMed]
25. Simeonsson, R.J.; Carlson, D.; Huntington, G.S.; McMillen, J.S.; Brent, J.L. Students with disabilities: A national survey of participation in school activities. *Disabil. Rehabil.* **2001**, *23*, 49–63. [PubMed]
26. HealthActCHQ. *The CHQ Scoring and Interpretation Manual*; HealthActCHQ: Boston, MA, USA, 2013.
27. Eime, R.M.; Young, J.A.; Harvey, J.T.; Charity, M.J.; Rayne, W.R. A systematic review of the psychological and social benefits of participation in sport for children and adolescents: Informing development of a conceptual model of health through sport. *Int. J. Behav. Nutr. Phys. Act.* **2013**, *10*, 98. [CrossRef]
28. Paulus, F.W. A bio-psycho-social view of cerebral palsy: Friendships reduce mental health disorders. *Dev. Med. Child Neurol.* **2019**, *61*, 862. [CrossRef]

Publisher's Note: MDPI stays neutral with regard to jurisdictional claims in published maps and institutional affiliations.

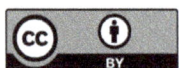

© 2020 by the authors. Licensee MDPI, Basel, Switzerland. This article is an open access article distributed under the terms and conditions of the Creative Commons Attribution (CC BY) license (http://creativecommons.org/licenses/by/4.0/).

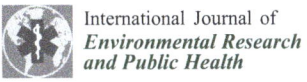

International Journal of *Environmental Research and Public Health*

Article

Exploring the Impacts of Environmental Factors on Adolescents' Daily Participation: A Structural Equation Modelling Approach

Yael Fogel [1,*], Naomi Josman [2] and Sara Rosenblum [2]

1 Department of Occupational Therapy, School of Health Sciences, University of Ariel, 40700 Ariel, Israel
2 The Laboratory of Complex Human Activity and Participation (CHAP), Department of Occupational Therapy, Faculty of Welfare and Health Sciences, University of Haifa, 3498838 Mount Carmel, Israel; naomij@research.haifa.ac.il (N.J.); rosens@research.haifa.ac.il (S.R.)
* Correspondence: yfogel@gmail.com

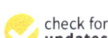

Citation: Fogel, Y.; Josman, N.; Rosenblum, S. Exploring the Impacts of Environmental Factors on Adolescents' Daily Participation: A Structural Equation Modelling Approach. *Int. J. Environ. Res. Public Health* **2021**, *18*, 142. https://dx.doi.org/10.3390/ijerph18010142

Received: 5 November 2020
Accepted: 23 December 2020
Published: 28 December 2020

Publisher's Note: MDPI stays neutral with regard to jurisdictional claims in published maps and institutional affiliations.

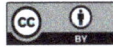

Copyright: © 2020 by the authors. Licensee MDPI, Basel, Switzerland. This article is an open access article distributed under the terms and conditions of the Creative Commons Attribution (CC BY) license (https://creativecommons.org/licenses/by/4.0/).

Abstract: Adolescents with neurodevelopmental difficulties struggle to perform daily activities, reflecting the significant impact of executive functions on their participation. This research examines an integrated conceptual model wherein supportive environmental factors in the community, school and home settings explain the children's participation (involvement and frequency) with their daily activities performance as a mediator. Parents of 81 10- to 14-year-old adolescents with and without executive function deficit profiles completed the Participation and Environment Measure for Children and Youth and the Child Evaluation Checklist. A secondary analysis was conducted to examine the structural equation model using AMOS software. The results demonstrated support for the hypothesised model. Supportive environmental demands in school predicted 32% of home participation, and the adolescents' daily performance reflected that executive functions mediated the relationship between them. Together, these findings highlight the school environment as the primary contributor that affects the children's functioning according to their parents' reports and as a predictor of high participation at home in terms of frequency and involvement. This study has implications for multidisciplinary practitioners working with adolescents in general, and in the school setting specifically, to understand meaningful effects of executive functions on adolescents' daily functioning and to provide accurate assistance and intervention.

Keywords: daily activities performance; executive function deficit (EFD); home; school; community; supportive factor; structural equation modelling

1. Introduction

Participation in daily activities naturally occurs when individuals involve themselves in occupations (daily life activities) that have significance and purpose [1]. Within contemporary theory, participation results from the dynamic transactions between an individual and their environment [2]. The World Health Organization's [3] International Classification of Functioning, Disability and Health: Child and Youth (ICF-CY) version also demonstrated that personal and environmental factors affect interactions among body structure and function, performing daily activities and participating in the community. Adolescents who participate in daily activities form strong bonds with their communities and develop their roles in society, which then helps them prepare for adulthood [4].

Since the ICF-CY was developed, there has been a continued effort to refine the understanding of participation and environmental factors that support or inhibit children both with and without disabilities over time [5]. Maciver et al. [6] reviewed the association among environmental and psychosocial factors with participation in school of children aged 4 to 12 years. Their findings supported the hypothesis that participation outcomes are influenced by known contexts and mechanisms. Specifically, Maciver et al. showed that school routines and structures, objects and spaces and peers and adults are representations of the environment (context). Concerning identified mechanisms, Fogel et al. [7] showed that children with executive function deficits (EFD) faced more barrier factors in the environment than did their peers and found the activities' social and cognitive demands to be the most challenging.

Executive functions (EFs) are a neuropsychological concept referring to a skillset that composes the cognitive process. This skillset allows people to forsake immediate demands to instead achieve long-term goals and thus to organise their behaviour over time [8]. These EFs influence participation and performance in daily life [9], and the performance of most daily activities requires using different EF components. The literature indicated that EFs might serve as an underlying mechanism in neurodevelopmental disorders such as attention deficit hyperactive disorder (ADHD), specific learning disorder and developmental coordination disorder. The contribution of EFs to adolescents' participation [7], scholastic achievements [10] and daily functioning has been reported [11]. The transition from childhood into adolescence often brings a new set of responsibilities and self-regulatory requirements (e.g., in school and social environments) [12] that necessitate adolescents to rely more on this emerging cognitive control.

Recently, Fogel et al. [13] described adolescents with EFD profiles. These adolescents are characterised as impaired when performing complex daily living activities. They often struggle to achieve everyday life goals as efficiently as their peers without EFD. That is, they require considerably more help from adults, need substantially more time to complete tasks and exhibit behaviours that are far more dangerous [13]. Since adolescents with EFD profiles tend to focus on immediate timeframes, they find planning to be a challenge. They also struggle to shift between activities, prioritise essential tasks, manage their time and meet deadlines [14]. These difficulties hinder their effective participation and performance in everyday life, creating a functioning gap between them and adolescents without EFD [11,13,15].

In the existing literature, discussion of the relationships among performance of daily activities, environmental factors and participation is scarce, and the overall picture—including clinical implications—is still unclear. Noreau and Boschen [16] dealt with the complex environment of participation interaction. Their results indicated that despite the environment's obvious theoretical impact on participation, its contribution to restricting or facilitating participation has yet to be demonstrated scientifically. King et al. [17] reported the environment's indirect impact on participation by referring to its direct effects. Specifically, their results showed the adolescent's activity preferences and functional abilities, as well as the family's orientations, to be the most important predictors of participation. Moreover, they indicated the need for a more in-depth look at indirect effects to broaden viewpoints and to consider the roles that other environmental and family factors play in what had been presumed to be causal, developmental sequences.

In contrast, Anaby et al. [18] found that the environment played a mediating role. Their findings explained the participation of young children with or without disabilities across community, school and home settings. Anaby et al. proposed and tested one model for each setting using structural equation modelling (SEM). These models explained 50% to 64% of the variance in both involvement and frequency of participation. According to these results, supports and barriers in the environment significantly mediate between the adolescent's personal factors (e.g., health and functional issues or income) and participation outcomes.

Likewise, most other studies on participation showed that children and adolescents with disabilities participate less in daily activities in terms of level of involvement and frequency in all three settings [19–21] and face more inhibiting environmental factors [7,18]. However, questions about the impact of the child's everyday expression of daily activities performance, and how it relates to participation, are still unanswered and need additional research.

This lack of a documented, compelling association between participation and environmental factors denotes how difficult it is to operationalise these constructs [16]. Therefore, this study examines the extent to which factors that support adolescents' environment also influence their participation. It assumes the mediating factor is adolescents' daily activities performance. To that end, this research uses the Participation and Environment Measure for Children and Youth (PEM-CY) [20,22], which is a reliable, valid and well-documented tool for assessing both participation and environmental factors. Additionally, the study uses the Child Evaluation Checklist (CHECK) questionnaire, which was also found to be valid and reliable, to examine the daily activities performance that reflects EF in young children [23,24] and adolescents [25]. Combining these two questionnaires (completed by the adolescents' parents) connects the current concept presented by the ICF-CY [3], which views children's and adolescents' functioning holistically. It also reflects previous studies' recommendations to examine the complexity of the relationship between participation and environmental requirements and abilities.

This study assumes that support factors in all three environments (community, school and home) may improve adolescents' daily activities performance and thus affect their participation (involvement and frequency) in the various environments. Figure 1 depicts the proposed theoretical model underlying the direct and indirect factors impacting participation. This conceptual model assumes that if the environment is supportive, then the adolescent's daily activities performance will be better and thus will affect their participation.

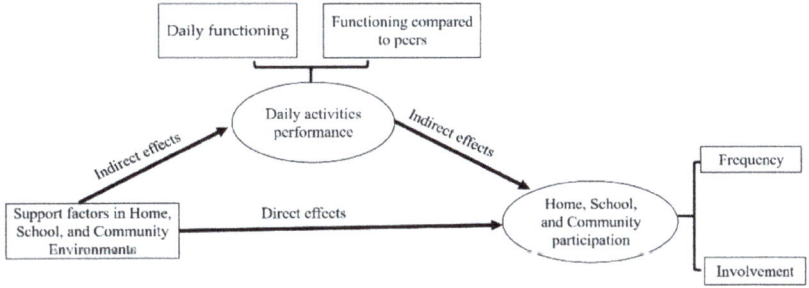

Figure 1. Conceptual model.

2. Materials and Methods

2.1. Participants

This study refers to a secondary analysis using data from a previously published study, which detailed the participant inclusion and exclusion criteria [7,13]. In the current study, the data refer to all participants as one group with no separation between adolescents with and without EFD profiles. Specifically, the participants were 81 early adolescents, 10 to 14 years old ($M = 12.07$ years, $SD = 1.17$). Of them, 57 (70.4%) were boys and 24 (29.6%) were girls. In the original study, 41 participants presented with EFD profiles and 40 with typical development (i.e., without EFD profiles). The EFD profiles were defined using the Behavior Rating Inventory of Executive Function (BRIEF) parent [26] and self-reports [27] and WebNeuro assessments [28]. The parents of all 81 adolescent respondents were invited to participate in the study.

2.2. Procedure

The University of Haifa Ethics Committee approved this study. Both the parents and the participating adolescents signed informed consent forms. Once accepted into the study, the parents completed a demographic questionnaire. The CHECK provided data regarding the daily activities performance reflecting EF and the PEM-CY as the outcome measure.

We tested two proposed theoretical models. Only one SEM fit the data well and successfully tested both the direct and mediated effects of environmental support factors as an observed (measurable) variable in the community, school and home on the theoretical latent variable, participation. It identified the level of involvement and frequency (10 indicators/items for community, 5 for school, 10 for home) as observed variables, as well as the theoretical latent variable, daily activities performance (consisting of daily functioning and functioning compared to peers).

2.3. Measurement Instruments

2.3.1. Demographic Questionnaire

Parents completed the demographic questionnaire, providing data on their education and socioeconomics and on the adolescents' age and gender.

2.3.2. Child Evaluation Checklist

A brief screening instrument used to identify children at risk for under-recognised, invisible neurodevelopmental conditions, the Child Evaluation Checklist (CHECK) [24], emphasises small nuances in the performance features of children's daily activities as related to the children's EFs. The CHECK tool includes two parts. The CHECK-A addresses the current level of daily activities performance, especially frequency. Respondents rate agreement with 30 statements on a Likert scale that ranges from 1 (never) to 4 (always). For example, the statements address whether the adolescents properly estimate the task difficulty and whether they complete tasks they take upon themselves. After exploratory factor analysis, four factors were obtained: organisation (body, essentials and social), self-regulation, performance/expression management and activities of daily living. Cumulatively, these four factors produced a 54.05 variance percentage and $\alpha = 94$ internal consistency.

The CHECK-B compares the adolescents' general daily function to peers. Using ranks from 1 (low) to 5 (high), parents respond to statements that contain phrases such as, "Compared to other children, my child … " or "In work habits, my child's overall functioning is … ".

We calculated an average score for each part and determined internal consistency (CHECK-A, $\alpha = 0.96$; CHECK-B, $\alpha = 0.94$). Construct validity was established and documented in [11].

2.3.3. Participation and Environment Measure for Children and Youth

Although parents completed the primary outcome measure, the Participation and Environment Measure for Children and Youth (PEM-CY) [20,22], herein we present the results in terms of the adolescents as the "participants". Part A of the PEM-CY includes 25 items focusing on participation in a diverse range of activities in community (10 items), school (five items) and home (10 items) settings. For each item, parents report the child's participation through three dimensions: (a) level of involvement on a 5-point scale from 1 (minimally involved) to 5 (very involved); (b) participation frequency on an 8-point scale from 0 (never) to 7 (daily); and (c) parents' desire for a change (e.g., in either involvement or frequency) of their child's participation (yes or no). If parents respond yes to a desire for change, they then select whether they want that change in the child's level of involvement or frequency or a wider variety of activities. However, this study did not include the parents' desire for change.

In this study, participation level of involvement and frequency were calculated as the average of all ratings, except those (either involvement or frequency) for which the parent answered never. The PEM-CY's summary score internal consistency for both participation involvement ($\alpha = 0.72$–0.83) and frequency ($\alpha = 0.59$–0.70) was moderate to good. Test–retest reliability for all participation and environment summary scores (interclass correlation (ICC) from 0.58 to 0.95) and across items within the instrument's community, school and home sections (ICC = 0.68–0.96) was also reported as moderate to good [29].

The PEM-CY's Part B asked parents if specific environmental features aided or hindered their children's participation in activities in each (community, school or home) setting. When parents reported a feature as an aid, we coded that item as a support factor. If parents reported the feature made things harder (sometimes or usually), then we coded the item as a barrier factor. The PEM-CY's summary scores internal consistency for both participation involvement (α = 0.72–0.83) and frequency (α = 0.59–0.70) was moderate to good. Test–retest reliability was reported for all participation and environment summary scores (ICC α = 0.58–0.95) and across items within the instrument's community, school and home sections (α = 0.68–0.96) as moderate to good [22].

2.4. Data Analysis

Using the bootstrapping method, SEM was conducted to examine the mediation model. The bootstrapping procedure's value lies in its ability to process repeated simulations of subsamples from an original database. With this, we could assess the parameter estimate stability and report their values with increased accuracy. Bootstrapping estimates each resampled dataset's indirect effects and determines a confidence interval for these specific indirect effects [30,31]. We analysed the data using SPSS (version 25) and AMOS software. Indices to evaluate the model included chi-square (acceptable when the value is not significant); comparative fit (CFI); non-normed fit (NNFI; adequate values > 0.90 and excellent fit > 0.95); root-mean-square error of approximation (RMSEA; adequate values < 0.08 and excellent fit < 0.06); and standardised root-mean-square residual (SRMR; <0.08) [32]. Level of significance (p value) was 5%.

3. Results

Table 1 presents descriptive statistics and Pearson correlations among the study variables. Results show that significant correlations were found between the participation variables (involvement and frequency) as measured by the PEM-CY and daily activities performance reflecting EF as measured by the CHECK (r = 0.22–0.88; $p < 0.050$ to $p < 0.001$).

The SEM provided excellent goodness of fit indices ($\chi^2(21)$ = 32.08; $p > 0.05$; NFI = 0.95; CFI = 0.98; RMSEA = 0.08; SRMR = 0.08). As depicted in Figure 2, results of this model showed that higher support of environmental demands at school leads to higher daily activities performance (β = 0.61, $p < 0.001$) and relates positively with home participation (β = 0.53, $p < 0.05$). The indirect effect found between support from the school environment and home participation (β = 0.32, $p < 0.01$) means that the daily activities performance is a mediator between environmental demands at school and home participation. The model explained 58% of home participation.

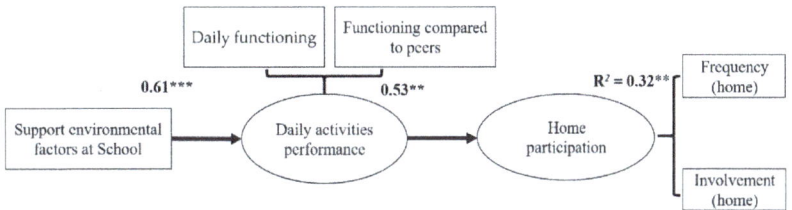

Figure 2. Analysis results of conceptual model mediation. Coefficients in bold are significant at $p < 0.05$. ** $p < 0.01$, *** $p < 0.001$.

Table 2 supports Figure 2. It represents the regression coefficients among all model components to describe the size and direction of the relationship between a predictor and the response variable.

Table 1. Means, standard deviations and correlations among study variables.

Variable	M	SD	1	2	3	4	5	6	7	8	9	10
1. Frequency (home)	5.91	0.57										
2. Involvement (home)	3.79	1.04	0.45 ***									
3. Frequency (school)	4.52	1.33	0.29 **	0.11								
4. Involvement (school)	3.47	1.34	0.34 **	0.54 ***	0.67 ***							
5. Frequency (community)	3.92	1.11	0.15	0.35 **	0.30 **	0.36 **						
6. Involvement (community)	3.52	1.16	0.26 *	0.69 ***	0.09	0.42 ***	0.74 ***					
7. Support (Home)	9.31	2.50	0.38 ***	0.37 **	0.25 *	0.38 **	0.23 *	0.28 *				
8. Support (School)	13.16	3.25	0.40 ***	0.36 **	0.38 ***	0.40 ***	0.10	0.17	0.68 ***			
9. Support (Community)	12.85	2.96	0.27 *	0.39 ***	0.17	0.36 **	0.18	0.28 *	0.58 ***	0.65 ***		
10. Daily functioning	3.40	0.51	0.40 **	0.46 **	0.22 *	0.43 **	0.27 *	0.34 **	0.55 ***	0.72 ***	0.59 ***	
11. Functioning compared to peers	3.60	1.02	0.44 **	0.39 **	0.39 **	0.48 **	0.28 *	0.30 **	0.55 ***	0.72 ***	0.53 ***	0.88 ***

Note. * $p < 0.05$, ** $p < 0.01$, *** $p < 0.001$.

Table 2. Model coefficients.

Latent and Observed Variable			β	p
Daily activities performance	<---	Support (school)	0.609	***
Daily activities performance	<---	Support (home)	0.064	0.547
Daily activities performance	<---	Support (community)	0.151	0.156
Home	<---	Daily activities performance	0.531	0.016
School	<---	Daily activities performance	0.061	0.398
Community	<---	Daily activities performance	0.262	0.061
School	<---	Support (school)	−0.978	·0.879
Home	<---	Support (home)	0.292	0.099
School	<---	Support (community)	0.040	0.803
Home	<---	Support (school)	−0.063	0.778
Community	<---	Support (school)	−0.126	0.702
School	<---	Support (home)	0.424	0.878
Community	<---	Support (home)	0.144	0.395
Home	<---	Support (community)	0.113	0.512
School	<---	Support (community)	0.395	0.897
Frequency (home)	<---	Home	0.594	
Involvement (home)	<---	Home	0.644	***
Frequency (school)	<---	School	1.664	
Involvement (school)	<---	School	7.697	0.331
Frequency (community)	<---	Community	0.625	
Involvement (community)	<---	Community	1.190	***
Daily functioning	<---	Daily activities performance	0.945	
Functioning compared to peers	<---	Daily activities performance	0.935	***

Note. *** $p < 0.001$.

4. Discussion

This study examined the effects of supportive environment factors upon participation among adolescents with and without EFD through an SEM approach. Applying SEM allowed us to isolate both the direct and indirect paths by which the environmental (community, school and home) settings affect the adolescents' participation across the three settings. Specifically, our results show that supportive environmental factors in school have indirect effects on home participation, while the adolescents' daily activities performance serves as a mediator of this relationship. That is, no *direct* connection was found between environment and participation; rather, they are connected through the adolescents' daily activities performance. These results may indicate that as long as there is no improvement in the adolescents' daily activities performance following the supports they receive at school, we cannot expect a change in the home environment—not in leisure activities, household chores, school preparation or homework.

4.1. Supportive School Environment Demands

Role performance in the complex high school environment is critical for academic success; poor role performance in academic and social participation creates high risk for student dropout [33]. The school environment can also often create one of the greatest perceived barriers [34,35]. Unlike several prior studies that described participation barriers without considering the environment's facilitating aspects [16], this study focused on supportive factors. According to the current findings, a supportive school setting can encourage students with and without EFD to more effectively express their daily activities performance and increase participation in the home environment. For instance, Wehlage [36] gathered information from 14 secondary schools that were selected based on their successful dropout prevention programmes. His key findings were relevant to the current study's findings. The results suggested that successful schools create a supportive environment that helps students overcome impediments to membership and engagement. Successful programmes matched students' needs and problems and took advantage of students' interests and strengths. Recently, Mann and Snover [15] argued that to maximise role performance, environmental influence should be viewed as a means to scaffold and develop EF skills. They mentioned the school environments of interest, including administrative and classroom policies, especially regarding their effects on the interplay between person and role performance (both for students and teachers).

Students and teachers' social interactions, as influenced by educational and social values, create the school climate [37]. Increasingly, research has documented the association of prosocial and academic motivation, conflict resolution, altruistic behaviours and self-esteem with positive school climates. As do teacher–student interactions, the social and educational values that influence children's psychological, social and cognitive development also affect the school climate [38]. Such values include the physical environment [39] and safety [40].

In a previous study, Fogel and colleagues [7] highlighted the environmental factors that, according to parents' reports, best predicted adolescents with EFD. For the school environment, these factors include the activity's cognitive and social demands and staff and teachers' attitudes. Fogel et al. found these factors to substantially aid classification of the study population characteristics (i.e., with or without EFD) and prediction of participants' daily functioning. Since adolescents spend a significant amount of time in school, school activities constitute a significant part of their daily routine both academically and socially.

According to the U.S. Department of Education's [41] Safe and Supportive Schools model, the school climate includes three interrelated domains: (a) the school environment (disciplinary, wellness, physical and academic), (b) student engagement (school participation, respect for diversity and relationships) and (c) safety (substance use/abuse, physical and social-emotional). Bradshaw et al. [37] explored this model. Their findings added to the growing research regarding associations between student outcomes and school climates, indicating that the school climate can significantly predict student achievement.

In 1935, Lewin [42] studied environmental influences on people's (especially children's) behaviour. He suggested that all elements of a child's behaviour, such as the environment where the child lives or how the child plays, influence the child's voluntary behaviour and emotions. Lewin expressed that relationships influence which behaviours a child exhibits, and that those behaviours equate to the child's function and environment.

4.2. Daily Activities Performance Reflecting EF

Executive dysfunction may be one among many contributors to difficulties adolescents experience [43]. Impaired EFs can lead to compromised self-regulation and decision making, as well as difficulty performing complex or novel tasks. This, in turn, can negatively affect academic performance across the adolescents' life span, leading them to become frustrated when their efforts prove ineffectual and unsuccessful and the outcomes are unsatisfactory (e.g., [44,45]). For example, Mann and Snover [15] measured academic performance to examine how EFs can affect students' role performance and found a significant correlation between poor executive functioning and low academic performance, regardless of setting.

Due to the complexity of recognising such difficulties, children with EFD are most often perceived as having behavioural problems, lazy, lacking motivation, manipulating, "doing it on purpose" and other misleading negative descriptors [9]. Unlike cases of cerebral palsy or intellectual disabilities, for example, the condition of adolescents with EFD is not as clear cut—it may seem invisible. There is a discrepancy between what others can see and what is really happening to these individuals. There are no physical signs, and the adolescents have average or above average intelligence. Nevertheless, the children and their families sense "something different than other children" but do not know what it is or why it is occurring [11]. Unrecognised EFD can compound these effects on daily occupational performance, which then can create secondary issues [46]. Thus, adolescents with EFD must be viewed through the expression of their daily activities performance—seen past their externalising behaviours to understand their daily functioning and recognise

4.3. Home Participation

Adolescence is marked by increased autonomy and access to adult activities and decreased dependence on primary individuals (e.g., parents) and organisational supports [47]. Despite the natural processes occurring in adolescence, this study's results show that the model explained 58% of specific at-home setting participation. Previous studies have identified the environment where the child lives and develops [48] as a critical context in which EFs develop [49], suggesting that individual differences in EFs are also associated with the home environment. Typically, this home environment is measured by the nature, frequency and amount of activities parents create for their children to learn [50]. However, few studies have dealt with the relationship between participation in the home setting and EFs among young children. Korucu et al. [51] investigated potential associations among general parenting practices, EF-related activities in the home and children's EFs beyond the home environment. They discussed the potential importance for pre-schoolers to be exposed in the home environment to EF-specific activities. In 2020, Korucu et al. [52] demonstrated a positive association between more enriching home literacy environments with pre-schoolers' EFs, which then relate to mathematic skills and readiness for general academics.

According to the PEM-CY, this home participation includes leisure and play activities, such as video or computer games, indoor games and play, arts and crafts and other hobbies, listening to music or watching TV, and activities that require social interaction, including getting together with others. Activities such as school preparation (e.g., gathering and packing materials, school bags and lunches or reviewing schedules) and doing homework (e.g., assignments, readings and projects) are also included. This is illustrated through a homework example. The process to finish homework assignments is multifaceted. To successfully complete an assignment, the student must initially record it accurately, bring home the materials needed (e.g., textbooks, handouts), allot after-school time to work on (and ultimately complete) the project, possess the skills needed to finish the work and then bring the finished assignment back to school and turn it in. For assignments that require long-term planning (e.g., long-term projects or preparing for exams), that process becomes even more complex [53]. Such typical assignments can overload the weakened EFs of children with disabilities. To finish a homework assignment, students must (a) keep their attention on the task at hand, (b) ignore distractions, (c) make a plan and set objectives, (d) decide on milestones, such as "where to start" and when to complete, (e) consider details as well as the big picture and (f) organise the relevant materials [54]. Children and adolescents with EFD profiles struggle with those kinds of daily activities, similar to previous findings among students with learning disabilities [55]. For instance, Langberg et al.'s [53] findings suggested that the latter task—organising materials—is critical for students with ADHD in their process to complete homework and thus should be prioritised in interventions.

4.4. Limitations and Future Studies

Despite its important results, this study has limitations. It included only a small sample in a narrow age range. Larger samples with broader age ranges among adolescents with different disabilities might have expanded the information about the relationship between participation and environment factors across settings. Further, this research did not address parental attitudes towards their children's daily functioning, all factors that may affect functioning perspectives or perspectives other than the parents'. Future studies might incorporate the adolescents' perspectives about their daily activities performance, participation and environmental factors. Future research should analyse the school environment factors for efficient assessment and evaluation processes.

5. Conclusions

The negative, widespread effects of EFD on occupational performance interfere with adolescents' independence in occupations from self-care routines and social interactions to finishing homework and extend into the classroom. Consistently, adolescents with EF issues have been considered as struggling to start a task, understand what the task requires of them, realise they need, and then ask for, help and recognise when they do not have all the necessary information [9].

This study's findings add to the theoretical and practical evidence of components that can assist and improve participation for adolescents both with and without EFD in general and at home specifically. From the users' viewpoint, supportive school environments may include, for example, physically organising the classroom, providing quiet work areas for children who are distracted by various environmental stimuli, establishing small work groups and dividing tasks into stages with increasing levels of difficulty (to give the children a sense of success and motivation for tasks at higher challenge levels). The emphasis should be on allowing the children to acquire self-management skills in academic and day-to-day tasks (work on problem-solving, planning and, especially, control abilities) and adapting the children's abilities (i.e., allowing the children to recognise their strengths and abilities and understand their difficulties). School procedures can be modified to provide relevant adjustments for each child, to be in constant contact with the children's parents and to envision the children and their needs beyond the school framework.

Improved daily activities performance by adolescents with or without EFD can be possible through involvement in a supportive school environment. Assessing the adolescents' daily activities performance can help determine their level of independence in performing everyday activities. It can educate the entire interdisciplinary team, caregivers and families for optimal intervention, discharge coordination and long-term planning.

Author Contributions: Conceptualisation, Y.F., S.R. and N.J.; methods, software and formal analysis, Y.F.; preparing original draft, Y.F.; reviewing and editing, N.J. and S.R.; supervision, N.J. and S.R. All authors have read and agree to the published version of the manuscript.

Funding: This research received no external funding.

Institutional Review Board Statement: The study was approved by the Faculty of Social Welfare and Health Sciences, University of Haifa ethics committee (approval numbers 253/13).

Informed Consent Statement: Informed consent was obtained from all subjects involved in the study.

Data Availability Statement: The data presented in this study are available on request from the corresponding author. The data are not publicly available due to ethical restrictions.

Acknowledgments: We thank Reanna Hirsh for her help with data collection and Liron Lamash for her useful advice.

Conflicts of Interest: The authors declare no conflict of interest.

References

1. American Occupational Therapy Association. Occupational therapy practice framework: Domain and process 3rd ed. *Am. J. Occup. Ther.* **2014**, *68*, S1–S48. [CrossRef]
2. Bartko, W.T.; Eccles, J.S. Adolescent participation in structured and unstructured activities: A person-oriented analysis. *J. Youth Adolesc.* **2003**, *32*, 233–241. [CrossRef]
3. World Health Organization. *International Classification of Functioning, Disability and Health: Child and Youth Version*; World Health Organization: Geneva, Switzerland, 2007.
4. Gorter, J.W.; Stewart, D.; Woodbury-Smith, M. Youth in transition: Care, health and development. *Child Care Health Dev.* **2011**, *37*, 757–763. [CrossRef] [PubMed]
5. Coster, W.; Khetani, M.A. Measuring participation of children with disabilities: Issues and challenges. *Disabil. Rehabil.* **2008**, *30*, 639–648. [CrossRef] [PubMed]
6. Maciver, D.; Rutherford, M.; Arakelyan, S.; Kramer, J.M.; Richmond, J.; Todorova, L.; Romero-Ayuso, D.; Nakamura-Thomas, H.; Velden, M.T.; Finlayson, I.; et al. Participation of children with disabilities in school: A realist systematic review of psychosocial and environmental factors. *PLoS ONE* **2019**, *14*, e0210511. [CrossRef] [PubMed]

7. Fogel, Y.; Rosenblum, S.; Josman, N. Environmental factors and daily functioning levels among adolescents with executive function deficits. *Br. J. Occup. Ther.* **2020**, *83*, 88–97. [CrossRef]
8. Dawson, P.; Guare, R. *Executive Skills in Children and Adolescents: A Practical Guide to Assessment and Intervention*; Guilford Press: New York, NY, USA, 2010.
9. Cramm, H.; Krupa, T.; Missiuna, C.; Lysaght, R.M.; Parker, K.C.H. Broadening the occupational therapy toolkit: An executive functioning lens for occupational therapy with children and youth. *Am. J. Occup. Ther.* **2013**, *67*, e139–e147. [CrossRef]
10. Jacob, R.; Parkinson, J. The potential for school-based interventions that target executive function to improve academic achievement: A review. *Rev. Educ. Res.* **2015**, *85*, 512–552. [CrossRef]
11. Josman, N.; Rosenblum, S. A metacognitive model for children with neurodevelopmental disorders. In *Cognition, Occupation, and Participation across the Life Span: Neuroscience, Neurorehabilitation and Models for Intervention in Occupational Therapy*; Katz, N., Toglia, J., Eds.; AOTA Press: Bethesda, MD, USA, 2018; pp. 273–294.
12. Burnett, A.C.; Scratch, S.E.; Anderson, P.J. Executive function outcome in preterm adolescents. *Early Hum. Dev.* **2013**, *89*, 215–220. [CrossRef]
13. Fogel, Y.; Rosenblum, S.; Hirsh, R.; Chevignard, M.; Josman, N. Daily performance of adolescents with executive function deficits: An empirical study using a complex-cooking task. *Occup. Ther. Int.* **2020**. [CrossRef]
14. Otero, T.M.; Barker, L.A.; Naglieri, J.A. Executive function treatment and intervention in schools. *Appl. Neuropsychol. Child* **2014**, *3*, 205–214. [CrossRef] [PubMed]
15. Mann, D.P.; Snover, R. Executive functioning: Relationship with high school student role performance. *Open J. Occup. Ther.* **2015**, *3*, 1–7. [CrossRef]
16. Noreau, L.; Boschen, K. Intersection of participation and environmental factors: A complex interactive process. *Arch. Phys. Med. Rehabil.* **2010**, *91*, S44–S53. [CrossRef] [PubMed]
17. King, G.; Law, M.; Hanna, S.; King, S.; Hurley, P.; Rosenbaum, P.; Kertoy, M.; Petrenchik, T. Predictors of the leisure and recreation participation of children with physical disabilities: A structural equation modeling analysis. *Child. Health Care* **2006**, *35*, 209–234. [CrossRef]
18. Anaby, D.R.; Law, M.; Coster, W.J.; Bedell, G.; Khetani, M.; Avery, L.; Teplicky, R. The mediating role of the environment in explaining participation of children and youth with and without disabilities across home, school, and community. *Arch. Phys. Med. Rehabil.* **2014**, *95*, 908–917. [CrossRef] [PubMed]
19. Bedell, G.M.; Coster, W.J.; Law, M.; Liljenquist, K.; Kao, Y.-C.; Teplicky, R.; Anaby, D.; Khetani, M.A. Community participation, supports, and barriers of school-age children with and without disabilities. *Arch. Phys. Med. Rehabil.* **2013**, *94*, 315–323. [CrossRef]
20. Coster, W.J.; Law, M.; Bedell, G.; Khetani, M.; Cousins, M.; Teplicky, R. Development of the participation and environment measure for children and youth: Conceptual basis. *Disabil. Rehabil.* **2012**, *34*, 238–246. [CrossRef]
21. Law, M.; Anaby, D.; Teplicky, R.; Khetani, M.A.; Coster, W.J.; Bedell, G. Participation in the home environment among children and youth with and without disabilities. *Br. J. Occup. Ther.* **2013**, *76*, 58–66. [CrossRef]
22. Coster, W.J.; Bedell, G.; Law, M.; Khetani, M.A.; Teplicky, R.; Liljenquist, K.; Gleason, K.; Kao, Y.-C. Psychometric evaluation of the Participation and Environment Measure for Children and Youth. *Dev. Med. Child Neurol.* **2011**, *53*, 1030–1037. [CrossRef]
23. Ogundele, M. Profile of neurodevelopmental and behavioural problems and associated psychosocial factors among a cohort of newly looked after children in an English local authority. *Adopt. Fostering* **2020**, *44*, 255–271. [CrossRef]
24. Rosenblum, S.; Zandani, I.E.; Deutsch-Castel, T.; Meyer, S. The Child Evaluation Checklist (CHECK): A screening questionnaire for detecting daily functional "red flags" of underrecognized neurodevelopmental disorders among preschool children. *Occup. Ther. Int.* **2019**. [CrossRef] [PubMed]
25. Fogel, Y.; Josman, N.; Rosenblum, S. Functional abilities as reflected through temporal handwriting measures among adolescents with neuro-developmental disabilities. *Pattern Recognit. Lett.* **2018**, *121*, 13–18. [CrossRef]
26. Gioia, G.; Isquith, P.; Guy, S.; Kenworthy, L. *Brief Rating Inventory of Executive Function: Professional Manual*; Psychological Assessment Resources: Lutz, FL, USA, 2020.
27. Guy, S.C.; Isquith, P.K.; Gioia, G.A. *Behavior Rating Inventory of Executive Function: Self-Report Version Professional Manual*; Psychological Assessment Resources: Lutz, FL, USA, 2004.
28. Silverstein, S.M.; Berten, S.; Olson, P.; Paul, R.; Williams, L.M.; Cooper, N.; Gordon, E. Development and validation of a world-wide-web-based neurocognitive assessment battery: WebNeuro. *Behav. Res. Methods* **2007**, *39*, 940–949. [CrossRef] [PubMed]
29. Khetani, M.; Marley, J.; Baker, M.; Albrecht, E.; Bedell, G.; Coster, W.J.; Anaby, D.; Law, M. Validity of the Participation and Environment Measure for Children and Youth (PEM-CY) for Health Impact Assessment (HIA) in sustainable development projects. *Disabil. Health J.* **2014**, *7*, 226–235. [CrossRef]
30. Byrne, B.M. *Structural Equation Modeling with EQS: Basic Concepts, Applications and Programming*, 2nd ed.; Routledge: Mahwah, NJ, USA, 2013.
31. Preacher, K.J.; Hayes, A.F. Asymptotic and resampling strategies for assessing and comparing indirect effects in multiple mediator models. *Behav. Res. Methods* **2008**, *40*, 879–891. [CrossRef]
32. Arbuckle, J.L. *Amos 22 User's Guide*; SPSS: Chicago, IL, USA, 2013.
33. Hammond, C.; Linton, D.; Smink, J.; Drew, S. *Dropout Risk Factors and Exemplary Programs: A Technical Report*; National Dropout Prevention Center/Network: Anderson, SC, USA, 2007.

34. Coster, W.J.; Law, M.; Bedell, G.; Liljenquist, K.; Kao, Y.-C.; Khetani, M.; Teplicky, R. School participation, supports and barriers of students with and without disabilities. *Child Care Health Dev.* **2013**, *39*, 535–543. [CrossRef]
35. Law, M.; Petrenchik, T.; King, G.; Hurley, P. Perceived environmental barriers to recreational, community, and school participation for children and youth with physical disabilities. *Arch. Phys. Med. Rehabil.* **2007**, *88*, 1636–1642. [CrossRef]
36. Wehlage, G.G. *Reducing the Risk: Schools as Communities of Support*; Falmer Press: Philadelphia, PA, USA, 1989.
37. Bradshaw, C.P.; Waasdorp, T.E.; Debnam, K.J.; Johnson, S.L. Measuring school climate in high schools: A focus on safety, engagement, and the environment. *J. Sch. Health* **2014**, *84*, 593–604. [CrossRef]
38. Haynes, N.M.; Emmons, C.L.; Ben-Avie, M. School climate as a factor in student adjustment and achievement. *J. Educ. Psychol. Consult.* **1997**, *8*, 321–329. [CrossRef]
39. Wilson, D. The interface of school climate and school connectedness and relationships with aggression and victimization. *J. Sch. Health* **2004**, *74*, 293–299. [CrossRef]
40. Cohen, J.; McCabe, L.; Michelli, N.M.; Pickeral, T. School climate: Research, policy, practice, and teacher education. *Teach Coll. Rec.* **2009**, *111*, 180–213.
41. U.S. Department of Education. Safe and Supportive Schools Model. 2009. Available online: http://safesupportiveschools.ed.gov/index.php?id=33 (accessed on 11 March 2013).
42. Lewin, K. *Environmental Forces in Child Behavior and Development: A Dynamic Theory of Personality*; McGraw-Hill: New York, NY, USA, 1935.
43. Dirette, D.; Kolak, L. Occupational performance needs of adolescents in alternative education programs. *Am. J. Occup. Ther.* **2004**, *58*, 337–341. [CrossRef] [PubMed]
44. Connor, L.T.; Maeir, A. Putting executive performance in a theoretical context. *OTJR* **2011**, *31*, S3–S7. [CrossRef] [PubMed]
45. Ziviani, J.; Copley, J.; Ownsworth, T.; Campbell, N.E.; Cummins, K.L. Visual perception abilities and executive functions in children with school-related occupational performance difficulties. *J. Occup. Ther. Sch. Early Interv.* **2008**, *1*, 246–262. [CrossRef]
46. Wolf, T. Participation in work: The necessity of addressing executive function deficits. *Work* **2010**, *36*, 459–463. [CrossRef] [PubMed]
47. Arnett, J.J. *Emerging Adulthood: The Winding Road from the Late Teens through the Twenties*; Oxford University Press: Oxford, UK, 2014.
48. Zelazo, P.D.; Blair, C.B.; Willoughby, M.T. *Executive Function: Implications for Education: NCER 2017–2000*; National Center for Education Research: Washington, DC, USA, 2016.
49. Bradley, R.H.; Corwyn, R.F. Socioeconomic status and child development. *Annu. Rev. Psychol.* **2002**, *53*, 371–399. [CrossRef] [PubMed]
50. Son, S.H.; Morrison, F.J. The nature and impact of changes in home learning environment on development of language and academic skills in preschool children. *Dev. Psychol.* **2010**, *46*, 1103–1118. [CrossRef]
51. Korucu, I.; Rolan, E.; Napoli, A.R.; Purpura, D.J.; Schmitt, S.A. Development of the Home Executive Function Environment (HEFE) scale: Assessing its relation to preschoolers' executive function. *Early Child Res. Q.* **2019**, *47*, 9–19. [CrossRef]
52. Korucu, I.; Litkowski, E.C.; Purpura, D.J.; Schmitt, S.A. Parental executive function as a predictor of parenting practices and children's executive function. *Infant Child Dev.* **2020**, *29*, e2152. [CrossRef]
53. Langberg, J.M.; Epstein, J.N.; Girio-Herrera, E.; Becker, S.P.; Vaughn, A.J.; Altaye, M. Materials organization, planning, and homework completion in middle-school students with ADHD: Impact on academic performance. *Sch. Ment. Health* **2011**, *3*, 93–101. [CrossRef]
54. Stockall, N. Designing homework to mediate executive functioning deficits in students with disabilities. *Interv. Sch. Clin.* **2017**, *53*, 3–11. [CrossRef]
55. Watson, S.M.; Gable, R.A.; Morin, L.L. The role of executive functions in classroom instruction of students with learning disabilities. *Int. J. Sch. Cogn. Psychol.* **2016**, *3*. [CrossRef]

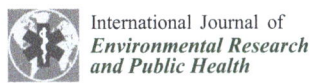

Article

Structural Validity of an ICF-Based Measure of Activity and Participation for Children in Taiwan's Disability Eligibility Determination System

Ai-Wen Hwang [1,2], Chia-Feng Yen [3,*], Hua-Fang Liao [4,*], Wen-Chou Chi [5], Tsan-Hon Liou [6,7], Ben-Sheng Chang [8], Ting-Fang Wu [9], Lin-Ju Kang [1,2], Shu-Jen Lu [10], Rune J. Simeonsson [11], Tze-Hsuan Wang [12] and Gary Bedell [13]

1. Graduate Institute of Early Intervention, College of Medicine, Chang Gung University, Taoyuan 33302, Taiwan; d93428001@ntu.edu.tw (A.-W.H.); lydiakang1003@gmail.com (L.-J.K.)
2. Department of Physical Medicine and Rehabilitation, Chang Gung Memorial Hospital, Linkou 33305, Taiwan
3. Department of Public Health, Tzu Chi University, Hualien 97004, Taiwan
4. School and Graduate Institute of Physical Therapy, National Taiwan University, Taipei 10055, Taiwan
5. Department of Occupational Therapy, College of Medicine, Chung Shan Medical University, Taichung 40201, Taiwan; y6312002@gmail.com
6. Department of Physical Medicine and Rehabilitation, Shuang Ho Hospital, Taipei Medical University, Taipei 11031, Taiwan; peter_liou@shh.org.tw
7. Graduate Institute of Injury Prevention and Control, Taipei Medical University, Taipei 11031, Taiwan
8. Department of Psychology, Soochow University, Taipei 11102, Taiwan; ben306@scu.edu.tw
9. Graduate Institute of Rehabilitation Counseling, National Taiwan Normal University, Taipei 10610, Taiwan; tfwu@ntnu.edu.tw
10. College of Medicine, School of Occupational Therapy, National Taiwan University, Taipei 10055, Taiwan; sjl470924@yahoo.com.tw
11. School Psychology and Early Childhood Education, University of North Carolina at Chapel Hill, Chapel Hill, NC 27599-3500, USA; rjsimeon@email.unc.edu
12. Graduate Institute of Physical Education, National Taiwan Sport University, Taoyuan 33301, Taiwan; wanda@thrct.org
13. Department of Occupational Therapy, Tufts University, Medford, MA 02155-5539, USA; gary.bedell@tufts.edu
* Correspondence: mapleyeng@gmail.com (C.-F.Y.); hfliao@ntu.edu.tw (H.-F.L.)

Received: 7 July 2020; Accepted: 13 August 2020; Published: 24 August 2020

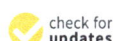

Abstract: To assess activity and participation for children in Taiwan's Disability Eligibility Determination System (DEDS), we developed a questionnaire, the Functioning Disability Evaluation Scale (FUNDES-Child), based on the Child and Adolescent Scale of Participation (CASP). The study follows a methodology research design to investigate the construct validity of the frequency and independence dimensions of FUNDES-Child 7.0. Two samples were randomly stratified from the databank of 13,835 children and youth with disabilities aged 6.0–17.9 years to examine structural validity by exploratory factor analysis (EFA, n = 4111, mean age of 11.3 ± 3.5) and confirmatory factor analysis (CFA, n = 4823, mean age of 11.4 ± 3.5)). EFA indicated a 4-factor structure for the frequency dimension (51.3% variance explained) and a 2-factor structure for the independence dimension (53.6% variance explained). The CFA indicated that the second-order factor structures of both dimensions were more parsimonious with adequate fit indices (Goodness fit Index, GFI; Normed Fit Index, NFI; Comparative Fit Index, CFI; and Tucker-Lewis Index, TLI ≥ 0.95, Root Mean Square Error of Approximation, RMSEA < 0.06). Results provide evidence that the participation part of FUNDES-Child 7.0 has acceptable structural validity for use in Taiwan's DEDS. Utility of FUNDES-Child 7.0 in rehabilitation, welfare, and educational services needs further study.

Keywords: participation; disability; measurement; children; adolescence

1. Introduction

According to Taiwan's People with Disabilities Rights Protection Act (promulgated in 2007), the local government in Taiwan was charged with developing a system to identify and classify disability and determine eligibility for provision of welfare services based on the framework of the International Classification of Functioning, Disability, and Health (ICF) and its child and youth version (ICF-CY) [1,2]. After five years of preparation, including the development and psychometric examination of measures for the eligibility determination and training of testers, the ICF-based Disability Eligibility Determination System (DEDS) was launched nationwide in July 2012. The disability identification is issued based on the results of the ICF-based disability evaluation by a medical team from authorized hospitals and needs assessment from the local social welfare department. The content of the disability evaluation includes physical examinations and assessments related to body function and structure (b/s) codes as well as activity and participation (A & P) components of the ICF and the ICF-CY. To assess the status of activity and participation in the ICF-based DEDS, Taiwan's ICF taskforce group started to develop the Functioning Disability Evaluation Scale (FUNDES) from 2007 until it was formally implemented in July 2012 [3–6]. There is an adult version (FUNDES-Adult) and a child version (FUNDES-Child). To develop a reliable A & P measures in a timely manner, the FUNDES-Adult was developed and modified from the 36-item version of the WHO Disability Assessment Schedule 2.0 (WHODAS 2.0) [7] and the FUNDES-Child from the Child and Family Follow-up Survey (CFFS) [8–10].

The Functioning Scale of the Disability Evaluation System-Child version (FUNDES-Child) has been developed since 2007 as the tool for assessment of functioning (body function, activity and participation) and environmental factors in the DEDS for children aged 6–18 years. Details of the development and initial validation of FUNDES-Child have been described elsewhere [4,11–13]. In brief, the FUNDES-Child is an adapted version of the Child and Family Follow-up Survey (CFFS) [10] translated into traditional Chinese and back translated into English with approval and collaboration from the original author (Dr. Gary Bedell). The FUNDES-Child utilizes a proxy format in which parents or caregivers answer questions about their child's activities in the previous 6 months. In keeping with the format used in the FUNDES-Adult version interview [3,5,6], flash cards with scoring options were used to assist parents in answering questions.

The participation part of FUNDES-Child has two dimensions, "independence" and "frequency". "Independence" or "capability" describes the children's ability to participate in age-expected life situations or to execute age-expected tasks or activities in daily settings as rated. "Frequency" refers to how often children engage in specific tasks or activities. Both dimensions are rated by children's caregivers, who are familiar with the children as compared to same-age peers [14]. The items and response scale of the independence dimension of the participation section of FUNDES-Child was translated and modified from the Child and Adolescent Scale of Participation (CASP) [8,15], which was one part of the Child and Family Follow-up Survey (CFFS). The frequency dimension was designed by the Taiwan ICF team and added to each item of the participation section of FUNDES-Child [3,13] because the original CASP seemed to focus on the concept of ability (independence or capability of FUNDES-Child) and execute activities. The factor structure has been investigated for the independence dimension, but has not been examined for the frequency dimension [8,11]. The development of the FUNDES adult and child versions were completed in 2012, the formal implementation year of the current DEDS. Therefore, we used the data of the FUNDES-Child 7th version (FUNDES-Child 7.0) of the Taiwan Databank of People with Disabilities, which begins in 2013 and is relatively stable and mature, compared to the previous version, to examine the factor structures of both the independence and frequency dimensions in this study. Understanding the internal factor structure helps to manage datasets with large numbers of observed variables that are thought to reflect a smaller number of underlying/latent variables.

Psychometric properties have been examined in previous FUNDES-Child versions [12,13,16–18]. Internal consistency of the independence and frequency dimensions were adequate to excellent for the total score of the participation section of FUNDES-Child (Cronbach's alpha = 0.81–0.96) [13]. Test-retest and inter-rater reliabilities were also found to be adequate to excellent (ICC = 0.85–0.99) [11,13]. Independence and frequency scores based on parent/caregiver reports about the child's school participation were not significantly different from scores based on teacher reports [13]. Known-groups validity evidence was found for the participation independence dimension of FUNDES-Child based on significantly different scores between children with less severe and more severe intellectual disabilities [12]. In addition, prior confirmatory factor analysis yielded a two-factor structure contributing to 64.1% of explained variance for the independence dimension based on a sample of about 200 children with disabilities (ages 6–18) in Taiwan. The two factors were named as the "daily living" and "social/leisure/communication" [11].

Due to the need for cultural adaptation and the practical demands of nationwide application, revisions to FUNDES-Child have been ongoing and are based on feedback from field testers and experts as well as results from data analyses conducted nearly every year. Several versions of the FUNDES have been developed. The cultural adaptations included that the 19th item is about "using transportation to get around in the community (e.g., to and from school, work, social or leisure activities) (driving vehicle or using public transportation), we used bicycle to replace vehicle due to the act regulation for an age limit to drive a vehicle is different from that of other countries) and the item 20th is about "work activities and responsibilities (e.g., completion of work tasks, punctuality, attendance and getting along with supervisors and co-workers). We treat the objects in vocational schools who were working because of the internship and teaching cooperation classes as students in the Taiwan education system. The other reason is about the format of FUNDES-Child, which should be consistent with FUNDES-Adult [3,5]. The construct validity of the two-factor structure of the independence dimension of the participation part of FUNDES-Child has been examined and supported by exploratory factor analysis. The structure factor of the frequency dimension has not yet been examined. The construct validity of a measure, especially the structural validity, is important [19]. The purpose of this study was to examine the structural validity of participation part (both the independence and frequency dimensions) of FUNDES-Child. All processes of FUNDES-Child development are listed in Table 1.

Table 1. The process of the Functioning Scale of the Disability Evaluation System-Child version (FUNDES-Child) tools development.

FUNDES-Child Versions	The Date of Design Completion and Start Training Program	Subscales and Dimensions or Illustrates
Has been developing	2010–2011 • Concept formation and design • The tool was being developing	• CASP has been bi-directionally translated. • Four subscales: (1) home participation, (2) community participation, (3) school participation, and (4) home and community living activities. • One independence (capability) dimension.
FUNDES-Child 5.0 *	2011/09	• Four subscales: (1) home participation, (2) community participation, (3) school participation, and (4) home and community living activities. • Two dimensions of participation: "independence" and "frequency". • The format of FUNDES-Child should be consistent with FUNDES-Adult. • Add flash cards. • To develop the scoring based on ICF.

Table 1. Cont.

FUNDES-Child Versions	The Date of Design Completion and Start Training Program	Subscales and Dimensions or Illustrates
FUNDES-Child 6.0	2012/07-12	Developing the manuals. The adult and children's training programs and versions are combined in the same manual.
FUNDES-Child 7.0	2014/06-12-2017	To separate adult and children's manual and add evidence of the reliability and validity of FUNDES 7.0 (adult and child versions) into the manual. Due to the need for cultural adaptation and the practical demands of nationwide application, revisions to FUNDES-Child have been ongoing based on feedback from field testers and experts as well as results after 2017.

* To match the naming of the FUNDES-Adult version.

2. Materials and Methods

2.1. Design

This cross-sectional study was part of a larger national survey conducted in Taiwan by the Taiwan ICF team [6]. The present study was approved by the Research Ethics Committee of the Hualien Tzu Chi Hospital, Buddhist Tzu Chi Medical Foundation (IRB104-04-A;IRB107-46-B) and Joint Institutional Review Board Taipei Medical University (TMU- Joint Institutional Review Board), Taiwan. The deidentified data were retrieved from the Taiwan Databank of People with Disabilities, which included 14,835 children and youth (aged 6.0–17.9 years) who received the DEDS assessment in 201 authorized hospitals from November 2013 to January 2015 [3,12,16,17,20]. All children and youth were assigned a diagnosis with specific codes of the International Classification of Disease, 9th Revision, Clinical Modification (ICD-9-CM) (http://www.cdc.gov/nchs/icd/icd9cm.htm) to be eligible for the DEDS.

2.2. Participants

Deidentification of information of the seventh version of the FUNDES in the Taiwan Databank of People with Disabilities was used in this study [20]. The FUNDES 7th version was used to collect information related to "activity and participation" of people with disabilities from July 2013 to January 2015 when the current ICF-based disability evaluation system was launched. There is one item pertaining to work in FUNDES-Child participation part. Therefore, if the student was not working, this item would be not applicable, and parents/caregivers would only complete 19 of the 20 items in this section. Given that the majority of individuals in the databank were not working, this study only examined 19 items. Therefore, individuals who were employed were excluded from the total sample ($n = 14,835$), resulting in data on 13,835 children and youth aged 6.0–17.9 years left for factor analyses.

The 13,835 children and youth from the larger sample were then randomly allocated into 3 smaller samples of roughly the same size: sample 1 ($n = 4111$), sample 2 ($n = 4824$), and sample 3 ($n = 4900$). Sample 1 was used for exploratory factor analyses (EFA), and sample 2 and 3 were to be used for the confirmatory factor analyses (CFA) and potential modifications needed for model fit. Because the CFA results of sample 2 showed good model fit, it was unnecessary to conduct CFA in sample 3.

2.3. Procedures

Individuals with information in the Taiwan Databank of People with Disabilities were evaluated via face-to-face interview by physicians and a qualified physical therapist, occupational therapist, social worker, clinical psychologist, or nurse practitioner in the authorized hospitals. The databank included a record of demographic characteristics (including personal factors), assessments of the individual's body function and body structures, activity and participation functioning, and some environmental conditions.

The severity level of a person's impairment was determined in the medical examination stage of the DEDS. Relevant ICF body function/structure categories for specific diagnoses were coded by physicians trained in using a 0- to 4-point qualifier scale (no problem = 0, mild = 1, moderate = 2, severe = 3, and profound = 4). A final summative severity level was determined based on decision rules for combining levels of severity among the individual body function/structure codes [21]. There were 8 types of impairment in the DEDS based on the 8 Body Functions Chapters of the ICF.

2.4. Measures

FUNDES-Child has 79 items, including 4 parts: physical and emotional health (5 items), participation (40 items), the child and adolescent factors inventory (15 items), and the child and adolescent scale of environment (19 items). The participation part was the focus of this study, which includes 20 items in each of the following dimensions: independence and frequency [4,16]. The participation part measures children's extent of participation frequency and independence in home, school, and community life situations and related activities in the previous 6 months compared to same-age peers. The 20 items are divided into 4 domains: home participation, school participation, community participation, and home and community living activities. Domain 1, home participation, has 6 items (item 1–6) to assess participation in the home setting and includes social, play, or leisure activities; chores; self-care activities; communication; and moving around at home. Domain 2, neighborhood and community participation, has 4 items (item 7–10) to assess activities including social, play, or leisure activities; structured events; moving around; and communicating with others in community; Domain 3, school participation, has 5 items (item 11–15) to assess activities including educational (academic) activities; social, play, or leisure activities; moving around; and using educational material in schools. Domain 4, home and community living activities (HCLA), has 5 items (item 16–20) to assess activities including household tasks, shopping and managing money, managing schedule, using transportation to get around, and work activities and responsibility in home and in the transition to community [15].

The items are rated on a four-point scale for two dimensions, independence (independent (0), supervision or mild assistance (1), moderate assistance (2), and full assistance (3)) and frequency (age-expected frequency (0), somewhat less frequent than expected for age (1), much less frequent than expected for age (2), and did not participate (3)) [4]. A "not applicable" response is allowed when the proxy perceives that the child's peers in the community would not be expected to participate on specific items. All items were rated under the assumption that children used assistive devices as usual. For example, an item would be rated as 0 (independent) if the child could participate in an activity with his/her existing devices and without others' assistance. Higher scores indicate greater restriction in participation, reflecting more difficulty, less independence, and lower frequency of participation. The differences between two dimensions of the "activities and participation" components, frequency and independence of FUNDES-Child, could be used to understand the possible impacts of environmental factors [14]. The purpose of this study was, thus, to examine the factor structures of the independence and frequency dimensions of FUNDES-Child 7.0.

2.5. Data Reduction and Statistical Method

About 30% of the data from all 13,835 children were randomly selected as sample 1 ($n = 4111$) for EFA. About a half of the remaining dataset was selected as sample 2 ($n = 4824$) for CFA. Statistical analyses and EFA were performed using SPSS 20.0 (IBM SPSS Statistics, Chicago, IL, USA, 2016). Since most observed item distributions violated normality assumptions and were inter-correlated, we used the iterative principal axis factoring followed by oblique promax rotation [22]. Factorability of items was examined by the Bartlett test (α was set at 0.05) and the Kaiser–Meyer–Olkin (KMO) measure of sampling adequacy. A value of KMO greater than 0.6 is tolerable for EFA [23]. The number of factors was decided by multiple methods including eigenvalues > 1 and scree tests. Factor loadings ≥ 0.3 were considered salient loadings [22]. The extracted latent factors were then named based on conceptual interpretation of the items. For each factor, the average score, standard deviation, range, and internal consistency were reported. The internal consistency was assessed by Cronbach's alpha coefficient. Values between 0.70 and 0.95 are considered adequate [24].

Based on the results of EFA, the first-order model solutions of the frequency and independence dimensions were examined by maximum-likelihood CFA using sample 2 with AMOS 20.0 (IBM, Inc., Armonk, NY, USA, 2012). Considering the presence of multivariate non-normal data, the Bollen–Stine bootstrap methods were applied [25]. The second-order models for both dimensions were also examined by CFA. The second-order model could be a more parsimonious model with all first-order latent factors loaded onto one second-order factor. To assess model fit, fit indices with their cutoff criteria (goodness-of-fit index (GFI) ≥ 0.95, normed fit index (NFI) ≥ 0.95, comparative fit index (CFI) ≥ 0.95, Tucker–Lewis index (TLI) ≥ 0.95, root mean square error of approximation (RMSEA) < 0.06) were used [24,26].

The Chi-square difference test was used for comparing first-order and second-order models. The target coefficient (T), which is the ratio of the Chi-square of the first-order model to the Chi-square of the higher-order (more restrictive) model, was used to evaluate whether the first- or second-order model is preferable for the data [27]. A value of T close to 1 suggests that a second-order model is preferable.

3. Results

3.1. Characteristics of the Samples

Demographic data and health characteristics of the sample are presented in Table 1. Among the 13,835 children, 66% were male and had a mean age of 11.4 (SD = 3.5) years. The majority of children (91%) were classified as having a single type of impairment, with Chapter 1 (mental functions/structures of the nervous system) being the most common type (88%), followed by Chapter 7 (5%, neuromusculoskeletal and movement-related functions/structures) of the ICF coding system. Children with multiple disabilities comprised less than 9% of the sample. The severity level of disability of 60% of the sample was classified as mild and with children able to live independently in their communities. Similar characteristics were found among the EFA and CFA subsamples and the larger sample (Table 2).

Table 2. Characteristics of the study sample.

Characteristics	All Participants n (%)	Sample 1 for EFA [2]	Sample 2 for CFA [2]
	$n = 13{,}835$	$n = 4111$	$n = 4823$
Gender			
Male	9101 (65.8)	2705 (65.8)	3184 (66.0)
Female	4734 (34.2)	1406 (34.2)	1639 (34.0)
Age (years)			
6–9	4733 (34.2)	1444 (35.1)	1644 (34.1)
10–13	4636 (33.5)	1357 (33.0)	1604 (33.3)
14–17	4466 (32.3)	1310 (31.9)	1575 (32.6)
Mean age	11.4 ± 3.5	11.3 ± 3.5	11.4 ± 3.5
Number of impairments identified [1]			
Single type of disability	12,644 (91.4)	3751 (91.2)	4411 (91.4)
Types of disability based on b/s Chapter			
Chapter 1	11,083 (87.7)	3288 (87.7)	3848 (87.2)
Chapter 2	438 (3.5)	136 (3.6)	169 (3.8)
Chapter 3	107 (0.8)	32 (0.9)	36 (0.8)
Chapter 4	210 (1.7)	64 (1.7)	70 (1.6)

Table 2. Cont.

Characteristics	All Participants n (%)	Sample 1 for EFA [2]	Sample 2 for CFA [2]
Chapter 5	14 (0.1)	7 (0.2)	3 (0.1)
Chapter 6	30 (0.2)	11 (0.3)	12 (0.3)
Chapter 7	584 (4.6)	161 (4.3)	206 (4.7)
Chapter 8	13 (0.1)	3 (0.1)	7 (0.2)
Others (chromosome or gene et al.)	165 (1.3)	49 (1.3)	60 (1.3)
Two types of disabilities	1033 (7.5)	311 (7.6)	360 (7.5)
More than three types of disabilities	158 (1.1)	49 (1.2)	52 (1.1)
Disability severity level			
Mild	8241 (59.6)	2464 (59.9)	2889 (60.0)
Moderate	3949 (28.5)	1171 (28.5)	1367 (28.3)
Severe	1104 (8.0)	325 (7.9)	393 (8.1)
Profound	541 (3.9)	153 (3.7)	174 (3.6)
Living situation			
Independent living in community	8042 (58.1)	2455 (59.8)	2743 (56.9)
Assisted living in community	5616 (40.6)	1609 (39.1)	2016 (41.8)
Not living in community	177 (1.3)	47 (1.1)	64 (1.3)

[1] Type of disability was classified using the International Classification of Functioning, Disability, and Health (ICF) Body Functions and Structures (b/s) Chapter. Chapter 1: mental functions/structures of the nervous system; Chapter 2: sensory functions (b2)/the eye, ear, and related structures (s2); Chapter 3: voice and speech functions/structures; Chapter 4: functions/structures of the cardiovascular, hematological, immunological, and respiratory systems; Chapter 5: functions/structures of the digestive, metabolic, and endocrine systems; Chapter 6: genitourinary and reproductive functions/structures; Chapter 7: neuromusculoskeletal and movement-related functions/structures; Chapter 8: functions/structures of the skin and related structures. Each child might have more than one type of disability. [2] Abbreviations: EFA, exploratory factor analysis; CFA, confirmatory factor analysis.

3.2. Exploratory Factor Analyses and Internal Consistency

For the 19 items of the frequency dimension, the KMO measure of sampling adequacy was 0.912, and the Bartlett test of sphericity was statistically significant ($p < 0.001$). Thus, the data were suitable for EFA. The initial EFA extracted five factors with eigenvalues above 1.0 and explained 54.9% of the variance. However, the eigenvalue of the fifth factor was 1.01, with only two items (items 1 and 6) loading on it. Therefore, the 4-factor model was retained with 51.3% variance explained (Table 3). The factors were named as "daily living participation frequency" (4 items), "mobility participation frequency" (5 items), "learning participation frequency" (6 items), and "community participation frequency" (4 items). The factors correlation matrix in Table 2 showed moderate correlations across all factors ($r = 0.45$–0.59).

For the 19 items of the independence dimension, the KMO measure was 0.951 and the Bartlett test was significant ($p < 0.001$). The initial EFA extracted three factors (eigenvalues = 9.71, 1.37, and 1.01) and explained 57.3% of the variance. However, the Scree plot indicated a two factor solution. Therefore, the 2-factor model was retained with 53.6% variance explained (Table 4). The factors were named as 'daily living independence' (10 items) and 'social participation independence' (9 items). The correlation coefficient between the 2 factors was 0.75.

Table 3. Factor loadings of the frequency dimension of FUNDES-Child by exploratory factor analysis ($n = 4111$).

Item No. and Name	Factor [1,2]			
	1	2	3	4
3. Home: Family chores, responsibilities, and decisions	**0.821**	−0.077	0.012	0.047
16. HCLA: Household activities	**0.810**	−0.005	−0.070	0.061
18. HCLA: Managing daily schedule	**0.403**	**0.322**	0.105	−0.092
17. HCLA: Shopping and managing money	**0.356**	0.279	−0.071	0.127
13. School: Moving around	−0.180	**0.639**	0.278	0.022
9. Community: Moving around	−0.104	**0.617**	−0.207	**0.462**
5. Home: Moving around	0.030	**0.552**	0.138	−0.041
19. HCLA: Using transportation to get around	0.181	**0.480**	−0.063	0.025
4. Home: meals with family	**0.370**	**0.447**	0.116	−0.169
15. School: Communicating with other children and adults	−0.057	−0.018	**0.715**	0.201
11. School: Educational activities with classmates	−0.048	0.115	**0.701**	−0.095
12. School: Social, play, and recreational activities with classmates	−0.063	0.047	**0.633**	0.143
14. School: Using educational materials and equipment	−0.007	**0.367**	**0.479**	−0.136
6. Home: Communicating with other children and adults	0.176	−0.009	**0.470**	0.173
1. Home: Social, play, or leisure activities with family members	0.182	−0.039	**0.431**	0.136
7. Community: Social, play, or leisure activities with friends	−0.024	−0.028	0.028	**0.874**
10. Community: Communicating with other children and adults	0.013	0.063	0.096	**0.696**
8. Community: Structured events and activities	0.111	0.156	−0.069	**0.579**
2. Home: Social, play, or leisure activities with friends	0.064	−0.162	0.265	**0.533**
Variance explained (total = 51.3%)	11.9%	12.8%	14.2%	12.4%
Factors inter-correlation coefficients Factor 1		0.55	0.54	0.46
Factor 2			0.59	0.45
Factor 3				0.56

[1] Salient factor loadings (>0.3) are shown in bold. [2] Factor 1 = daily living participation frequency; Factor 2 = mobility participation frequency; Factor 3 = learning participation frequency; Factor 4 = community participation frequency; FUNDES-Child = Functioning Disability Evaluation Scale-Child version; HCLA = home and community living activities.

The summary scores of the four frequency factors and two independence factors of the FUNDES-Child participation part were the sum of actual ratings for items within a given factor divided by the maximum total ratings for items within that factor, and converted to a 0–100 scale. As an example, a summary score for the 4-item factor of daily living participation frequency might be ratings of 3, 3, 2, 1 = 9 divided by four maximum ratings of 3 = 12 for a score of 9/12 converted to 75 on a 0–100 scale. The range of all factor summary scores was all from 0 to 100. The higher score means higher restriction and lower frequencies. The average summary scores and standard deviations of the four frequency factors were 50.2 ± 24.0 (daily living participation frequency), 29.2 ± 21.7 (mobility participation frequency), 37.4 ± 22.1 (learning participation frequency), 56.6 ± 25.3 (community participation frequency), with Cronbach's α of 0.776, 0.774, 0.835, and 0.833, respectively. For the two independence factors, the mean scores were 36.3 ± 22.3 (daily living independence) and 40.6 ± 24.6 (social participation independence), with Cronbach's α of 0.909 and 0.924, respectively.

Table 4. Factor loadings of the independence dimension of FUNDES-Child by exploratory factor analysis (*n* = 4111).

Item No. and Name	Factor [1,2]	
	1	2
16. HCLA: Household activities	**0.821**	−0.027
4. Home: Self-care activities	**0.812**	−0.048
3. Home: Family chores, responsibilities, and decisions	**0.704**	0.074
5. Home: Moving around	**0.670**	−0.035
18. HCLA: Managing daily schedule	**0.647**	0.064
13. School: Moving around	**0.625**	0.105
19. HCLA: Using transportation to get around	**0.610**	0.018
17. HCLA: Shopping and managing money	**0.602**	0.118
9. Community: Moving around	**0.471**	0.243
14. School: Using educational materials and equipment	**0.425**	**0.300**
7. Community: Social, play, or leisure activities with friends	−0.125	**0.911**
10. Community: Communicating with other children and adults	−0.004	**0.821**
2. Home: Social, play, or leisure activities with friends	−0.078	**0.791**
15. School: Communicating with other children and adults	0.054	**0.759**
12. School: Social, play, and recreational activities with classmates	0.140	**0.648**
6. Home: Communicating with other children and adults	0.124	**0.648**
8. Community: Structured events and activities	0.154	**0.611**
11. School: Educational activities with classmates	0.186	**0.539**
1. Home: Social, play, or leisure activities with family members	0.230	**0.517**
Variance explained (total = 53.6%)	26.6%	27.0%
Factors inter-correlation coefficients	Factor 1	0.75

[1] The salient loadings were usually recognized when they are beyond 0.3, which are shown in bold. [2] Factor 1 = daily living independence; Factor 2 = social participation independence; FUNDES-Child = Functioning Disability Evaluation Scale-Child version; HCLA = home and community living activities.

3.3. Confirmatory Factor Analyses

As the EFA suggested a four-factor solution for the frequency dimension, a CFA using sample 2 was conducted with a first-order 4-factor model allowing the four latent factors to correlate freely (model F-1). All standardized factor loadings were greater than 0.51, and the fit indices indicated a good fit (Table 4). The second CFA using a more parsimonious second-order 4-factor model (model F-2) was performed. All fit indices showed a good fit. Comparing the first-order model with the second-order model using the likelihood ratio test resulted in a non-significant Chi-square test ($\chi^2(9) = 8.4$, $p = 0.49$). In addition, the target coefficient (T) of 0.95 supported the second-order construct. Therefore, the more parsimonious second-order 4-factor model was preferred (Figure 1). All 19 items have factor loadings greater than 0.61 on their corresponding factors, supporting the construct validity of the frequency dimension (Figure 1).

For the independence dimension, a CFA using sample 2 with 2 factors emerging from the EFA was conducted. The two latent factors were allowed to correlate freely (model I-1). All standardized factor loadings were greater than 0.61, and the fit indices indicated a good fit (Table 5). For the second-order model (model I-2), all fit indices showed a good fit and the likelihood ratio test yielded a non-significant Chi-square test ($\chi^2(1) = 0.4$, $p = 0.53$). The target coefficient (T) of 0.998 also supported the second-order construct. As shown in Figure 2, all items have factor loadings greater than 0.66.

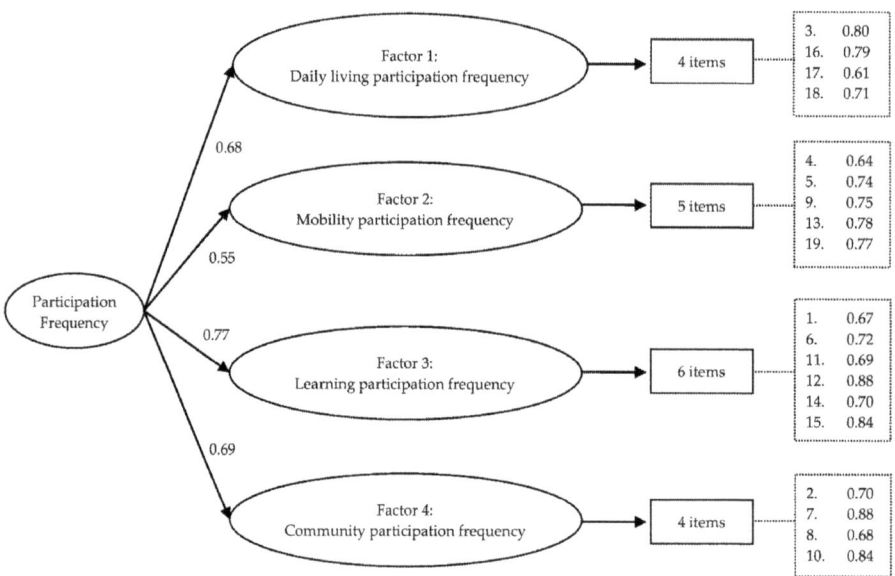

Figure 1. Second-order confirmatory factor analysis model of the frequency dimension of the participation part of the Functioning Disability Evaluation Scale-Child version ($n = 4823$).

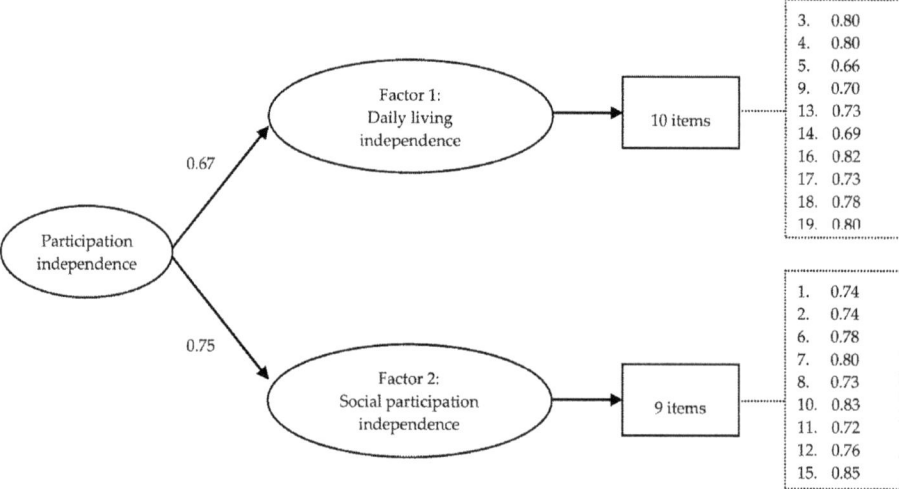

Figure 2. Second-order confirmatory factor analysis model of the independence dimension of the participation part of the Functioning Disability Evaluation Scale-Child version ($n = 4823$).

Table 5. Model fit indices for the frequency and independence dimensions of FUNDES-Child [1] by confirmatory factor analyses ($n = 4823$).

CFA Model	BSχ^2	df	GFI	NFI	CFI	TLI	RMSEA
Frequency dimension							
F-1. First-order 4-factor model	175.2	149	0.996	0.996	0.999	0.996	0.006
F-2. Second-order 4-factor model	183.6	158	0.996	0.996	0.999	0.997	0.006
Independence dimension							
I-1. First-order 2-factor model	190.6	151	0.997	0.997	0.999	0.994	0.007
I-2. Second-order 2-factor model	191.0	152	0.997	0.997	0.999	0.994	0.007

[1] FUNDES-Child = Functioning Disability Evaluation Scale-Child version; BSχ2 = Bollen–Stine Chi-square; GFI = goodness-of-fit index; NFI = normalized fit index; CFI = comparative fit index; TLI = Tucker–Lewis index; RMSEA = root mean square error of approximation.

4. Discussion

Participation is one of the most significant outcomes of rehabilitation, social, and educational interventions [28]. Using a large nationwide Disability Eligibility Determination System (DEDS) sample, the results of this study provided evidence of construct (structural) validity and internal consistency of the participation part of FUNDES-Child for children and youth aged 6 to 18 years old. The results of this study confirmed that the 19 items of the independence dimension of the participation part of FUNDES-Child had distinct factor loadings on the two derived factors (daily living independence and social participation independence) with one higher-order construct of participation independence. These two derived factors are the same as those found in a previous Taiwan study based on a sample of 200 children with various disabilities ages 6–18 years [11]. A new finding from this study suggested a four-factor solution for the frequency dimension along with one higher-order construct of participation frequency. The items loading on each of the four factors reflected the following domains: daily living participation frequency, mobility participation frequency, learning participation frequency, and community participation frequency. The factor summary scores calculated on the basis of the factor structure are important for disability practices, research, and policies.

There were 6 items loaded in the learning participation frequency factor of FUNDES-Child. Four items are activities related to communication, social, leisure, and education in school settings, two items are activities related to communication, social, and leisure in home settings. It is possible that the factors that influence interaction frequency with other persons is similar for children with disabilities, regardless of whether they happen at home or at school. One of our previous studies demonstrated that Taiwan's school and home settings provided relatively sufficient support for children with disabilities to participate [14].

There are some similarities in the findings on the independence dimension in this study and earlier research. The factor structure of the initial (English language) version of the CASP that was the forerunner of FUNDES-Child has been studied using different samples. As mentioned, the initial CASP has the same items and as is likely assessing components of the independence dimension of FUNDES-Child, has been explored by using EFA in one sample of 60 children with acquired brain injury (ABI) aged 3–27 years [9], in 313 children with varied diagnoses (56% children with ABI) aged 3–27 years [8], in 409 youth with varied diagnoses and aged 11–18 years [29], and in 926 children with traumatic brain injury and isolated arm injury aged 0–18 years [30]. The results of the US samples indicated a two-factor solution [9], three-factor solution [8,29] or four-factor solution [30]. Except for one subsample of Golos and Bedell's study (2016), many items had cross loading on two or three factors in U.S. samples. Recently, a one-factor structure of the German version of the CASP was reported [31]. Therefore, the two-factor structure of the CASP in two Chinese samples as well as the independence dimension of FUNDES-Child in the study of Hwang et al. and this study are stable with more distinct factor loadings [11].

The possible reasons for somewhat different factor structures among the studies include differences in samples, influence of cultural and language differences, and testing procedures between the initial

US CASP and Chinese FUNDES-Child. In addition, the more stable and distinctive factor structure found in two Chinese samples might be due to the standardized interview procedure used in collecting participation data. As mentioned before, the FUNDES-Child and FUNDES-Adult questionnaires were developed for the purposes of the ICF-based Disability Eligibility Determination System (DEDS) to respond to the regulation mandated by the People with Disabilities Rights Protection Act. To increase the utility of the questionnaires in the DEDS and fit Taiwan's culture and to ensure confidence of applicants and the government officials, the FUNDES team gradually examined their reliability and validities during implementation, and modified the FUNDES-Child and FUNDES-Adult to have a similar format and fit Taiwan's culture [3,5,6]. For example, flash cards with scoring options were used to assist parents in answering questions in FUNDES-Child.

The distinct factor loading on two derived factors of the independence dimension allows for the calculation of two factor summary scores: daily living independence score and social participation independence score. Most items of daily living independence domain come from the home setting and home and community living activities, and are related to mobility and daily care tasks, while items of social participation independence domain are from community and school setting, and are related to communication and social tasks. Similarly, the participation dimension yields four factor summary scores: daily living participation frequency score, mobility participation frequency score, learning participation frequency score, and community participation frequency score. The items of learning participation frequency and community participation frequency are the same as daily living independence. The items of daily living participation frequency and mobility participation frequency are almost the same as social participation independence except item 4 (home meals with family). For the frequency dimension, item 4 cross-loaded on Factor 2 (mobility participation frequency) and on Factor 1 (Daily living participation frequency), with factor loading of 0.447 and 0.370, respectively. As mentioned before, each frequency item was modified from the independence item of the CASP. Item 4 of the CASP is "self-care activities (e.g., eating, dressing, bathing, combing or brushing hair, using the toilet)". Such self-care activities are basic needs for every child with disabilities and they are involved in those activities almost every day at home in Taiwan. However, for children with disabilities, parents tend to feed them before family meals. We thought that children's experiences of attending family mealtime and interacting with family members are important home participation activities. Therefore, we designed the frequency dimension of item 4 as "how frequently the child has meals with family". Thus, children with greater mobility restriction participation may participate in family meals less frequently.

The results of this study also provide internal consistency evidence related to the FUNDES-Child participation part. The strong internal consistency evidence found for the two subscales in the independence dimension is similar to what has been found in prior studies [8,11,29,30,32]. Overall, these results suggest that the items were inter-related and related to the factor and the whole scale. The other important benefits of our findings of the factor summary scores for disability practices, research, and policies are (1) to allow exploration of which aspects of the gaps of "independence" and "frequency" may be due to environmental factors, which can help us to address the environmental issues to affect child's development; (2) our new factor summary scores in Factor 1 "daily living independence" and Factor 2 "social participation independence" can help policymakers to allocate social welfare resources. Family support and resources should be inducted more for subjects who get higher summary scores in daily living or to figure out the barriers of social participation in the subgroups with higher scores in the Social participation domain.

As mentioned before, in Taiwan's DEDS system, the proxy report of FUNDES-Child has been used. However, the scores between the parent/caregiver report version and youth self-report version of the CASP or of FUNDES-Child are significantly different [8,13,29,33,34]. Children and parents do not only show differences in the perception of participation, they also identify different priorities for participation goals in the individualized educational plan [13,35]. Therefore, stakeholders need to consider their specific research or practice purposes in determining whether to use one or both versions.

Taiwan has used an ICF-based measure of activity and participation successfully in the DEDS. The first stage of needs assessment in Taiwan's DEDS applies the scores for FUNDES to determine the social welfare supports related to mobility restriction, the necessity of accompaniment (that means there is one attendant that can accompany the person with a disability with free tickets to participate in social activities if the activities are paid), and RehabBus. The application of FUNDES by clinicians or social welfare service providers in order to understand what are the restrictions and to enhance the social participation for people with disabilities has also been proposed [4,5,13,34]. In Taiwan, the ICF framework has been applied in early intervention and special education services [34–37]. However, FUNDES-Child requires additional testing and validation. We hope the main theme of ICF—enhancing the full participation of people with disabilities in society—could be reached through the application of FUNDES-Child.

There are a few limitations of this study that must be noted. First, although the large sample size of this study provided sufficient statistical power, the majority of children in the sample had intellectual disabilities. Thus, further study would be needed for children who were less represented in the sample.

Second, this study did not use a theoretical construct of participation for children with disabilities. In ICF, the definition of participation is "involvement in a life situation" [1]. However, there is no clear international consensus on the participation construct in pediatric settings. Imms et al. (2017) have proposed a family of participation-related constructs (fPRC), indicating that participation has two essential components: attendance, defined as "being there" and measured as frequency of attending and/or the range or diversity of activities; and involvement, the experience of participation [38]. The two dimensions of the participation part of FUNDES-Child, independence and frequency, belong to different components of the fPRC. The frequency dimension belongs the attendance component and the independence dimension may be seen as belonging to performance competence component of the fPRC. Further studies are needed to examine the utility of the summary factor scores of these two dimensions in disability determination systems as well as rehabilitation and special education services.

5. Conclusions

The FUNDES-Child participation part was adapted to Taiwanese culture and includes an independence and frequency dimension across the home, preschool, school, and community settings for children and youth. The results from the exploratory and confirmatory factor analyses provide evidence for the structural validity of FUNDES-Child based on samples drawn from the larger Taiwan population of children ages 6.0–17.9 years with disabilities. The evidence was strong for the independence 2-factor solution with strong internal consistency of the two domains, showing promise for use as subscales, since the findings provide preliminary psychometric evidence to inform the application of FUNDES-Child to assess children's "activity and participation" independence or capabilities and frequencies of attendance and, also, to inform how scores can be used for different purposes in Taiwan.

Author Contributions: Each author has participated in the concept and design; analysis and interpretation of data; drafting or revising of the manuscript and that each author has approved the manuscript as submitted. H.-F.L., A.-W.H. and C.-F.Y. were mainly responsible for the conception and design of the article, interpretation of data, drafting the article and final approval of the version to be published. W.-C.C., B.-S.C., T.-F.W., L.-J.K. and S.-J.L. were responsible for acquisition of data mainly. T.-H.L., R.J.S. and G.B. were responsible for the conceptualization and design and scaling of the items used in FUNDES-Child. A.-W.H., T.-H.W. and C.-F.Y. were mainly responsible for data analysis and drafting the method section of the article. H.-F.L., A.-W.H., and C.-F.Y. were mainly responsible for drafting the article and final approval of the version to be published. All authors have read and agreed to the published version of the manuscript. All individuals listed as authors meet the appropriate authorship criteria. We also declare that we have no financial interests related to the material in the manuscript.

Funding: This research was funded by the Ministry of Health and Welfare, Executive Yuan, Taiwan, grant number 98M8178, 99M4080, 99M4073, 100M4145, 101M4100, 102M4022, M03F2194, and M04F5018 and the Ministry of Science and Technology, grant number NSC 102-2628-B-182-001-MY3 and NSC 101-2314-B-182-088.

Acknowledgments: We would like to thank the Taiwanese ICF team members and all the data collectors of each hospital, particularly the following people: Yen-Nan Chiu, Tien-Chen Liu, Lu Lu, Shyh-Dye Lee, Fu-Sung Lo, Tai-Lung Cha, Ti-Li Kao, and Kuo-Lung Lee. International experts Christine Imms and Granlund Mats are also acknowledged for their contribution to the development of FUNDES-Child.

Conflicts of Interest: The authors declare no conflict of interest.

Abbreviations

DEDS	Disability Eligibility Determination System
FUNDES	Functioning Disability Evaluation Scale
CASP	Child and Adolescent Scale of Participation
HCLA	home and community living activities

References

1. World Health Organization. *International Classification of Functioning, Disability, and Health (ICF)*; World Health Organization: Geneva, Switzerland, 2001.
2. World Health Organization. *International Classification of Functioning, Disability and Health: Children & Youth Version (ICF-CY)*; World Health Organization: Geneva, Switzerland, 2007.
3. Chiu, W.T.; Yen, C.F.; Teng, S.W.; Liao, H.F.; Chang, K.H.; Chi, W.C.; Wang, Y.H.; Liou, T.H. Implementing disability evaluation and welfare services based on the framework of the International Classification of Functioning, Disability and Health: Experiences in Taiwan. *BMC Health Serv. Res.* **2013**, *13*, 416. [CrossRef] [PubMed]
4. Liao, H.F.; Yen, C.F.; Hwang, A.W.; Liou, T.H.; Chang, B.S.; Wu, T.F.; Lu, S.J.; Chi, W.C.; Chang, K.H. Introduction to the application of the Functioning Scale of the Disability Evaluation System. *Formos. J. Med.* **2013**, *17*, 317–331. [CrossRef]
5. Liao, H.F.; Yen, C.F.; Liou, T.H.; Chi, W.C. The development and application of the Functioning Disability Evaluation Scale. In *Community Development Quarterly*; Social and Family Affairs Administration, Ministry of Health and Welfare: Taipei, Taiwan, 2015; Volume 105, pp. 77–98.
6. Teng, S.W.; Yen, C.F.; Liao, H.F.; Chang, K.H.; Chi, W.C.; Wang, Y.H.; Liou, T.H. Evolution of system for disability assessment based on the International Classification of Functioning, Disability, and Health: A Taiwanese study. *J. Formos. Med. Assoc.* **2013**, *112*, 691–698. [CrossRef] [PubMed]
7. Üstün, T.B.; Chatterji, S.; Kostanjsek, N.; Rehm, J.; Kennedy, C.; Epping-Jordan, J.; Saxena, S.; von Korff, M.; Pull, C. Developing the World Health Organization Disability Assessment Schedule 2.0. *Bull. World Health Organ.* **2010**, *88*, 815–823. [CrossRef]
8. Bedell, G. Further validation of the Child and Adolescent Scale of Participation (CASP). *Dev. Neurorehabil.* **2009**, *12*, 342–351. [CrossRef]
9. Bedell, G.M. Developing a follow-up survey focused on participation of children and youth with acquired brain injuries after discharge from inpatient rehabilitation. *NeuroRehabilitation* **2004**, *19*, 191–205. [CrossRef]
10. Bedell, G.M.; Dumas, H.M. Social participation of children and youth with acquired brain injuries discharged from inpatient rehabilitation: A follow-up study. *Brain Inj.* **2004**, *18*, 65–82. [CrossRef]
11. Hwang, A.W.; Liou, T.H.; Bedell, G.M.; Kang, L.J.; Chen, W.C.; Yen, C.F.; Chang, K.H.; Liao, H.F. Psychometric properties of the child and adolescent scale of participation—Traditional Chinese version. *Int. J. Rehabil. Res.* **2013**, *36*, 211–220. [CrossRef]
12. Hwang, A.W.; Yen, C.F.; Liou, T.H.; Bedell, G.; Granlund, M.; Teng, S.W.; Chang, K.H.; Chi, W.C.; Liao, H.F. Development and validation of the ICF-CY-Based Functioning Scale of the Disability Evaluation System—Child Version in Taiwan. *J. Formos. Med. Assoc.* **2015**, *114*, 1170–1180. [CrossRef]
13. Liao, H.F.; Hwang, A.W.; Kang, L.J.; Liao, Y.T.; Granlund, M.; Simeonsson, R.J. Development of the FUNDES-Child and its implications for the education of Taiwanese children. In *An Emerging Approach for Education and Care: Implementing a World-Wide Classification of Functioning and Disability*; Castro, S., Palikara, O., Eds.; Routledge: London, UK, 2018; pp. 85–111.
14. Hwang, A.W.; Yen, C.F.; Liou, T.H.; Simeonsson, R.J.; Chi, W.C.; Lollar, D.J.; Liao, H.F.; Kang, L.J.; Wu, T.F.; Teng, S.W.; et al. Participation of Children with Disabilities in Taiwan: The Gap between Independence and Frequency. *PLoS ONE* **2015**, *10*, e0126693. [CrossRef]

15. Bedell, G. *The Child and Family Follow-Up Survey (CFFS)-Administration and Scoring Guidelines*, 2011; Unpublished Manual. Available online: http://sites.tufts.edu/garybedell/measurement-tools/ (accessed on 24 August 2020).
16. Chen, W.C.; Bedell, G.M.; Yen, C.F.; Liou, T.H.; Kang, L.J.; Liao, H.F.; Hwang, A.W. Psychometric properties of the Chinese version of the child and adolescent factors inventory (CAFI-C). *Res. Dev. Disabil.* **2017**, *68*, 111–121. [CrossRef] [PubMed]
17. Chiu, T.Y.; Yen, C.F.; Escorpizo, R.; Chi, W.C.; Liou, T.H.; Liao, H.F.; Chou, C.H.; Fang, W.H. What is the gap in activity and participation between people with disability and the general population in Taiwan? *Int. J. Equity Health* **2017**, *16*, 136. [CrossRef] [PubMed]
18. Kang, L.J.; Yen, C.F.; Bedell, G.; Simeonsson, R.J.; Liou, T.H.; Chi, W.C.; Liu, S.W.; Liao, H.F.; Hwang, A.W. The Chinese version of the Child and Adolescent Scale of Environment (CASE-C): Validity and reliability for children with disabilities in Taiwan. *Res. Dev. Disabil.* **2015**, *38*, 64–74. [CrossRef] [PubMed]
19. Mokkink, L.B.; Terwee, C.B.; Patrick, D.L.; Alonso, J.; Stratford, P.W.; Knol, D.L.; Bouter, L.M.; de Vet, H.C. The COSMIN checklist for assessing the methodological quality of studies on measurement properties of health status measurement instruments: An international Delphi study. *Qual. Life Res.* **2010**, *19*, 539–549. [CrossRef] [PubMed]
20. Chi, W.C.; Chang, K.H.; Escorpizo, R.; Yen, C.F.; Liao, H.F.; Chang, F.H.; Chiou, H.Y.; Teng, S.W.; Chiu, W.T.; Liou, T.H. Measuring disability and its predicting factors in a large database in Taiwan using the World Health Organization Disability Assessment Schedule 2.0. *Int. J. Environ. Res. Public Health* **2014**, *11*, 12148–12161. [CrossRef] [PubMed]
21. Ministry of Health and Welfare. *Regulations for the Classification, Categories, Grades of Disability and Standards in Disability Evaluation System*; Ministry of Health and Welfare: Taipei, Taiwan, 2014.
22. Costello, A.B.; Osborne, J. Best practices in exploratory factor analysis: Four recommendations for getting the most from your analysis. *Pract. Assess. Res. Eval.* **2005**, *10*. [CrossRef]
23. Sharma, S. *Applied Multivariate Techniques*; John Wiley and Sons, Inc.: New York, NY, USA, 1996; pp. 90–143.
24. Prinsen, C.A.C.; Vohra, S.; Rose, M.R.; Boers, M.; Tugwell, P.; Clarke, M.; Williamson, P.R.; Terwee, C.B. How to select outcome measurement instruments for outcomes included in a "Core Outcome Set"—A practical guideline. *Trials* **2016**, *17*, 449. [CrossRef]
25. Byrne, B.M. *Structural Equation Modeling with LISREL, PRELIS, and SIMPLIS: Basic Concepts, Applications, and Programming*; Psychology Press: Stanford, CA, USA, 2013.
26. Beauducel, A.; Wittmann, W.W. Simulation Study on Fit Indexes in CFA Based on Data with Slightly Distorted Simple Structure. *Struct. Equ. Modeling A Multidiscip. J.* **2005**, *12*, 41–75. [CrossRef]
27. Marsh, H.W.; Hocevar, D. Application of confirmatory factor analysis to the study of self-concept: First- and higher order factor models and their invariance across groups. *Psychol. Bull.* **1985**, *97*, 562–582. [CrossRef]
28. Dijkers, M.P. Issues in the conceptualization and measurement of participation: An overview. *Arch. Phys. Med. Rehabil.* **2010**, *91*, S5–S16. [CrossRef]
29. McDougall, J.; Bedell, G.; Wright, V. The youth report version of the Child and Adolescent Scale of Participation (CASP): Assessment of psychometric properties and comparison with parent report. *Child Care Health Dev.* **2013**, *39*, 512–522. [CrossRef] [PubMed]
30. Golos, A.; Bedell, G. Psychometric properties of the Child and Adolescent Scale of Participation (CASP) across a 3-year period for children and youth with traumatic brain injury. *NeuroRehabilitation* **2016**, *38*, 311–319. [CrossRef] [PubMed]
31. De Bock, F.; Bosle, C.; Graef, C.; Oepen, J.; Philippi, H.; Urschitz, M.S. Measuring social participation in children with chronic health conditions: Validation and reference values of the child and adolescent scale of participation (CASP) in the German context. *BMC Pediatr.* **2019**, *19*, 125. [CrossRef] [PubMed]
32. De Kloet, A.J.; Berger, M.A.; Bedell, G.M.; Catsman-Berrevoets, C.E.; van Markus-Doornbosch, F.; Vlieland, T.P.V. Psychometric evaluation of the Dutch language version of the Child and Family Follow-up Survey. *Dev. Neurorehabil.* **2015**, *18*, 357–364. [CrossRef] [PubMed]
33. Bedell, G.; Coster, W. Measuring participation of school-aged children with traumatic brain injuries: Considerations and approaches. *J. Head Trauma. Rehabil.* **2008**, *23*, 220–229. [CrossRef]
34. Liao, Y.T.; Hwang, A.W.; Liao, H.F.; Kang, L.J. Do we hear the child's voice? Supporting participation engagement in goal-setting for elementary school students with special needs: A case report. *FJPT* **2017**, *42*, 228–233. [CrossRef]

35. Liao, Y.T.; Hwang, A.W.; Liao, H.F.; Granlund, M.; Kang, L.J. Understanding the participation in home, school, and community activities reported by children with disabilities and their parents: A pilot study. *Int. J. Environ. Res. Public Health* **2019**, *16*, 2217. [CrossRef]
36. Liao, H.F.; Wu, P.F. Early childhood inclusion in Taiwan. *Infants Young Child* **2017**, *30*, 320–327. [CrossRef]
37. Hwang, A.W.; Lin, P.J.; Kang, L.J.; Chen, L.J.; Chen, H.J.; Liao, H.F. To envision professional development —The planning of school-based physical therapy in Taiwan. *FJPT* **2017**, *42*, 195–210. [CrossRef]
38. Imms, C.; Granlund, M.; Wilson, P.H.; Steenbergen, B.; Rosenbaum, P.L.; Gordon, A.M. Participation, both a means and an end: A conceptual analysis of processes and outcomes in childhood disability. *Dev. Med. Child Neurol.* **2017**, *59*, 16–25. [CrossRef]

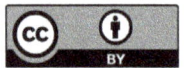

© 2020 by the authors. Licensee MDPI, Basel, Switzerland. This article is an open access article distributed under the terms and conditions of the Creative Commons Attribution (CC BY) license (http://creativecommons.org/licenses/by/4.0/).

MDPI
St. Alban-Anlage 66
4052 Basel
Switzerland
Tel. +41 61 683 77 34
Fax +41 61 302 89 18
www.mdpi.com

International Journal of Environmental Research and Public Health Editorial Office
E-mail: ijerph@mdpi.com
www.mdpi.com/journal/ijerph

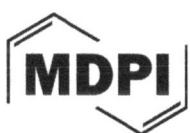

www.ingramcontent.com/pod-product-compliance
Lightning Source LLC
LaVergne TN
LVHW070439100526
838202LV00014B/1629